Survival Guide for
Anatomy & Physiology

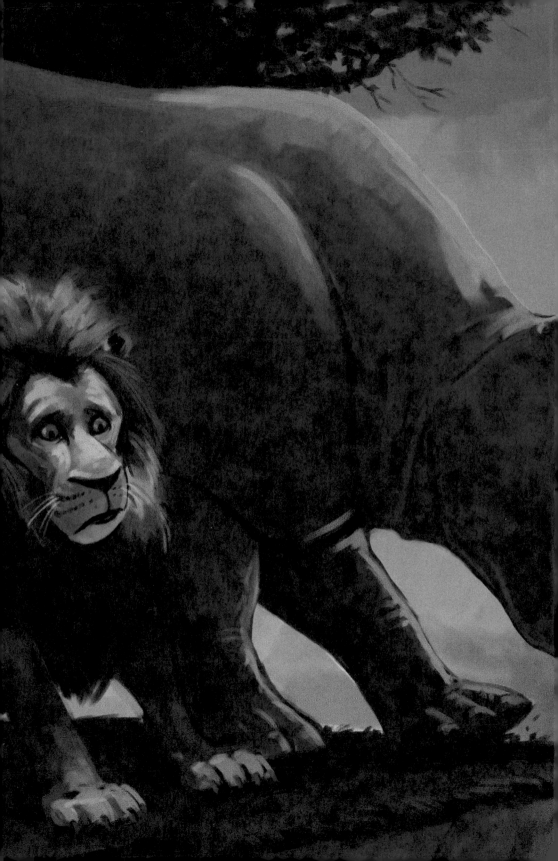

Survival Guide for
Anatomy & Physiology

2nd Edition

Tips, Techniques, and Shortcuts for Learning
about the Structure and Function of the
Human Body with Style, Ease, and Good Humor

Kevin T. Patton

Cartoons by Kevin Patton, Bill Colrus, and Joe Kulka

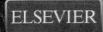

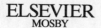

3251 Riverport Lane
St. Louis, Missouri 63043

Notices

Knowledge and best practice in this field are constantly changing. As new research and experience broaden our understanding, changes in research methods, professional practices, or medical treatment may become necessary.

Practitioners and researchers must always rely on their own experience and knowledge in evaluating and using any information, methods, compounds, or experiments described herein. In using such information or methods they should be mindful of their own safety and the safety of others, including parties for whom they have a professional responsibility.

With respect to any drug or pharmaceutical products identified, readers are advised to check the most current information provided (i) on procedures featured or (ii) by the manufacturer of each product to be administered, to verify the recommended dose or formula, the method and duration of administration, and contraindications. It is the responsibility of practitioners, relying on their own experience and knowledge of their patients, to make diagnoses, to determine dosages and the best treatment for each individual patient, and to take all appropriate safety precautions.

To the fullest extent of the law, neither the Publisher nor the authors, contributors, or editors, assume any liability for any injury and/or damage to persons or property as a matter of products liability, negligence or otherwise, or from any use or operation of any methods, products, instructions, or ideas contained in the material herein.

ISBN: 978-0-323-11280-2

Vice President and Content Strategy Director: Linda Duncan
Executive Content Strategist: Kellie White
Content Development Specialist: Joe Gramlich
Content Coordinator: Nathan Wurm-Cutter
Publishing Services Manager: Catherine Jackson
Senior Project Manager: Carol O'Connell
Design Direction: Brian Salisbury
Cover Illustration: Joe Kulka

Printed in the United States of America

Last digit is the print number: 9 8 7 6 5 4 3 2 1

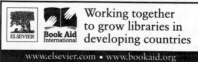

Working together
to grow libraries in
developing countries

www.elsevier.com • www.bookaid.org

Hi! I'm Kevin Patton, the author of this survival guide. I've enjoyed several decades of studying human anatomy and physiology—and also studying how to study this subject. Besides taking anatomy and physiology courses at the high school, college, and graduate levels, I have also taught it at all three levels. I still study A&P informally as I author A&P textbooks and as I prepare for the classes I teach at a community college and university. I study A&P several times each year at formal workshops and seminars. During this time, I've come to appreciate that the major keys to success in any A&P course are style and attitude. This book will help you with both by giving you some simple and clear tips on how A&P can be easily and quickly mastered.

This survival guide can be used easily in any A&P course with any textbook. In fact, you can use some of it in your other courses, too!

This survival guide for anatomy and physiology students begins with a quick and easy overview of some of the strategies my students and I have used to make our studies more productive—and therefore more fun and less time-consuming.

Scattered throughout the first section of this guide, I've included boxes conspicuously titled "Survival Tips" and other special boxed sidebars that cover topics of interest to many students. For example, a sidebar for returning or nontraditional students is offered, a sidebar for learners with special needs, a sidebar about learning in the laboratory, and a sidebar about using digital devices to help study A&P. You'll also find sidebars that highlight some of the more important points in this guide.

If you find that a thoughtful look at how you study has a positive effect on the efficiency of your studying—and I'm sure that it will—then I encourage you to talk to your professor, college librarian, or a learning center specialist to find out more ways to help yourself learn A&P and other subjects.

The second part of this guide is a handy compilation of diagrams, charts, and tables that serve as quick "field guides." This collection of resources will help you as you study in class, at home, in the lab, and even later in clinical or applied situations because they contain much of the essential information needed to understand the human body's structure and function. The diagrams are like pocket maps to the body, quickly getting you on the right road when you're lost. The charts and tables summarize facts in a way that will help you organize your own thinking about important concepts—and they will help you remember the details when they slip your mind.

The second part of this guide also includes a scattering of analogies and models that you will find helpful in learning some of the trickier concepts of A&P.

I suggest that you READ the first part of this survival guide right away. That'll get you on the right track. Then as you progress through your A&P studies, RAID the second part for maps, charts, and shortcuts to help you with specific concepts.

I'm using the analogy of survival in a wilderness throughout this book for at least two reasons. First, beginning students often do feel overwhelmed in an unfamiliar territory. Secondly, it is a good analogy—many of the skills you might use to survive in the wilderness have their counterparts in coping with your A&P course. And, as we shall learn, *analogies make learning easier.*

I'd love to get any feedback on this guide that you'd like to share with me—good or bad. Or perhaps you'd like to share some learning secrets you've discovered. Contact me at kevin@theAPstudent.org and follow me on my blog for A&P students at theAPstudent.org.

Kevin Patton
Weldon Spring, Missouri

Dedication

This book is dedicated (in no particular order) to Andrew, Aileen, Luke Baraka, Jenny-tamu, Tom, Pat, Rick, Will, Mallory, Jeanńe, Max, Sammee, David and Sue, Gary and Emogene, Sally, Kellie, Joe, Cathy, Dan, Heather, Corkey and Cooper the Wonder Dogs, members and staff of HAPS, Jules Jacot, Tom, Jeff, Gordon and Rosie, Carol, the Campolongos, Pat (a different Pat than the one mentioned previously), Michael, several Mikes, Audrey, fellow members of the Irish Diaspora, Laura, Ron Giedinghagen, Clyde, the SCC crowd, Jacqueline, Karen, Monica, Ellen, Virginia, Timba and Dante (I miss your hugs), Thomas Jefferson, Jessica, Kim, The Flying Wallendas, Ivor (David), TC Westfall, Monty Python, Roger Tory Peterson, Ann, Zoe, Mary Ann, Gene, Vicki, Stacey, John, Tracy, Katrita, Suzanne, Bob and the gang at NYCC, Robert H., Nurse Kelly, Yvonne, Gracie Allen, Alfred Court, NABT, Hal, Rev. Krista, The Royal Liechtenstein Circus, Takeshi, United Republic of Tanzania, Marlin and Carol Perkins, Sister Virginia, Alpha Calhoun, Miss Mudd, Jack and Mike, Flora, Dr. Mulligan, Professor Keller, Paris (the city), Big Al and Little Al, Jerry, Loretta, Leonardo Da Vinci, Gunther, Sarah and Michael, Flora, Wayne Franzen, Stormy, St. Louis Zoo and WBS alumni, Mary Ellen Whitehead, Ana Mary, Gregor Mendel, Jim, Miss Jones, C.V. Mosby and Catherine Anthony, DB, Ira, Peter, the Grimaldi family and the Monte Carlo Circus Festival, Marjorie, Andreas Vesalius, Caoimh'n, Steve, Mr. Bean, Michelle, SLU Pharm/Phys, Fr. John, CFA, Mysté, Greenway Network, Mahatma Gandhi, the Chieftains, Saitoti, Rhonda, Dora, Pam, Bill-Jim, Lucia, Margaret, Joe and Elaine, Dr. Greene, Ned Devine, W.B. Yeats, Mary Alice, and Julie Bowen.

Credits

Portions of this book are adapted from the following publications and are used here by permission.

Anatomy & Physiology by Kevin T. Patton and Gary A. Thibodeau
Essentials of Anatomy & Physiology by Kevin T. Patton, Gary A. Thibodeau, and Matthew M. Douglas
Lion Den (lionden.com)
Lion Tamers Guide to Teaching (LionTamersGuide.blogspot.com)
Structure and Function of the Body by Gary A. Thibodeau and Kevin T. Patton
The A&P Professor (theAPprofessor.org)
The A&P Student (theAPstudent.org)
The Electronic Professor (TheElectronicProfessor.org)
The Human Body in Health and Disease by Kevin T. Patton and Gary A. Thibodeau
Figure 1-2: *Barbara Cousins.*
Figure 1-7B: *Courtesy A. Arlan Hinchee.*
Figure 3-17: *Adapted from Guyton A, Hall J: Textbook of medical physiology, 11e, Philadelphia, 2006, Saunders.*
Figure 4-3: *Inset from Belcher AE: Blood disorders, St Louis, 1993, Mosby.*
Figure 4-25: *Abbas A, Lichtman A: Cellular and molecular immunology, 5e, Philadelphia, 2005, Saunders.*
Figure 5-17: *Barbara Cousins.*
Figure 5-19: *Adapted from Brundage DJ: Renal disorders. Mosby's clinical nursing series, St Louis, 1992, Mosby.*
Figure 6-1: *Barbara Cousins.*

CONTENTS

PART 2   Maps, Charts, & Shortcuts, 63

PART 1

Introduction to the Survival Skills

A s you begin a new course, you may feel as though you're wandering in a wilderness where the ideas are strange, the language unique, and the terrain unfamiliar. In other words, you feel a little lost. At times, you may even feel like you are being chased by wild animals. *Have no fear!* This guide provides a set of survival skills to help you in your trek through the strange and wondrous world of human anatomy and physiology (A&P).

Take the time to have a good look at the skills outlined in the following pages. Some you will find useful; others may not suit your style. The important thing is to give some thought to *your style* of learning and *your attitude* toward this great adventure that you're starting. I guarantee that any time given to working on your approach to studying will be returned to you at least tenfold!

> ■ **Choose the strategies that work for you—
> then use them!**

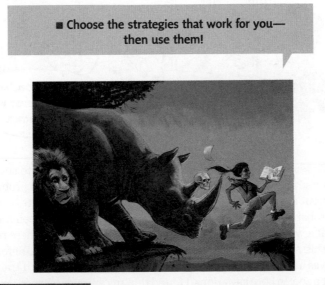

✧ SURVIVAL TIP

☑ The inside front cover lists the twelve Survival Tips. *Each time you start a new topic,* briefly check the list of Survival Tips to make sure you're not forgetting something.

1

Have a Winning Attitude

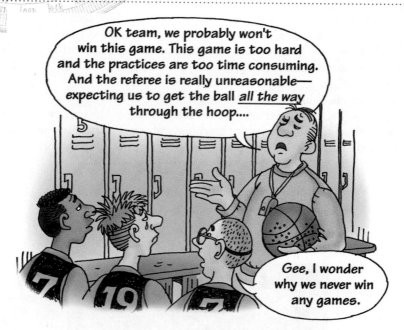

In the introduction to this guide, I stated that the major keys to success in any A&P course are *style* and *attitude*. I'll tell you more than you probably care to know about style in Survival Skill 2. For now, let's concentrate on attitude.

You've probably have heard a hundred times—or maybe it seems more like a million—that a winning attitude is an important key to success. There really is a lot of truth to this statement, especially when it comes to learning. Before I started teaching, I was a lion tamer in the circus (no kidding!); before that, I trained marine mammals at a zoo. In both situations, I found that my animals learned new behaviors really fast and really well *if they were having fun* or if they were *highly motivated*. If they were *both* having fun *and* highly motivated, the results were incredible!

With both my African lions and my sea lions, I was the one setting the learning goals—so it was up to me to set the attitude. I only asked my animals to do things that they found to be fun (by watching them play on their own), and I gave them food rewards and praise (lions, by the way, will do almost anything for a hug and a kind word). In your situation, however, setting the attitude is *up to you*. It's as simple as deciding to have a positive, winning attitude.

As goofy as it might sound, just telling yourself that you're successful in your A&P course is enough to dramatically improve your chances of success. It's just like the cases of patients who refuse to give in to their injuries or illnesses and who jump into their therapy with gusto—they're always the ones who exceed all normal expectations of recovery.

But what if you have a hard time resisting negative thinking? Do you tell yourself, "I'll never be able to understand this concept!"? That's OK. Researchers have found that a *little* bit of negativity actually helps you! If you have about one negative thought for every three positive thoughts about your studying, that's just about right. The trick is to put your negative thoughts to good use. For example, if you're thinking "I can't seem to focus after the first hour of studying," then that can be a useful thing. You can try breaking up your study time into smaller sessions, which may turn out to be a breakthrough for you.

Research also shows us that you'll have an even better chance at shining success in A&P if your "self-talk" takes the form of a question rather than a direct statement. In other words, it works far better if you ask yourself, "Can I pass the muscle test?" rather than simply telling yourself "I can pass the muscle test!" with no further thought. By answering the question "Can I pass the muscle test?" with thoughts about what you've already learned about muscles and what you can do to further prepare for the test, you'll be in a much better position to succeed.

One place you can always count on to find someone to help you maintain a winning attitude is your professor's office. Like a good animal trainer—or a winning coach—your professor will always take the time to talk to you about your studies and help you to keep the proper attitude. Even professors that might seem a little intimidating that first day of class will *always* turn out to be caring, willing helpers in your struggles with A&P. As President Emeritus of the Human Anatomy and Physiology Society (HAPS), and as a teacher of A&P instructors, I've gotten to know literally thousands of A&P teachers across North America and beyond. All of those people *love* A&P, and they *love* teaching it. They really enjoy helping people like you find success in a subject that is very exciting for them. When that enthusiasm rubs off—and it will—you'll be that much closer to reaching your goal.

> ■ Your professor will always take the time to talk to you about your studies and help you to maintain the proper attitude.

So what about the *fun* and the *motivation*? Let's start with the fun (a motto to live by). Your instructor's enthusiasm, if you open yourself up to it, will get you started on the road to having fun. Then, try to get into a study group. I'll talk more about the learning value of this strategy later in Survival Skill 8, but right now let's concentrate on the fun. Getting together with other A&P students for study sessions can be fun. Take turns hosting sessions by rotating who chooses times and places. Perhaps bring snacks or go out for snacks as a group. Make it as much a social gathering as an academic endeavor.

I'm not suggesting that you go out and party on the pretext that you're studying. I'm saying instead that studying as a group can be fun if you decide to make it fun. Laugh, joke around, gossip, whatever—but stay at least loosely focused on learning your topic. Set specific learning goals for session, and don't end the "party" until you've reached your objective or at least until you've made specific plans to meet your goals. As you and your classmates get to know one another better, you may want to try a social outing or two. Getting to know people outside the classroom or study session often makes your academic partnerships more effective.

Another way to make A&P fun is to involve people who aren't even in your A&P class. If you have friends or family members who might like to share some of the time you're spending with your A&P studies, perhaps you can involve them. I've known students who have had their partners or friends help them drill with flash cards (see Survival Skill 8). Some students have their children or younger siblings work along with them in drawing and coloring diagrams and sketches. Because you don't want to spend much more than 30 minutes at a time studying anyway (I'll discuss this later), most friends and family members won't object to cooperating with you for a few minutes. And if you are studying with someone you like sharing time with anyway, you're more likely to have fun.

Another way to have fun is to approach your studies with a sense of humor. Draw silly cartoons that illustrate key concepts. Make funny remarks in the margins of your notebook. Set your memorized lists to your favorite melodies. Try thinking of wild and crazy analogies or models for concepts that you are learning. Just have fun with it!

Now let's look at motivation. Sea lions are motivated by fish. Lions are motivated by fresh meat and hugs. My kids are motivated by hugs, smiles, candy, and Disney World (not in that order). What motivates you? Like most of us, you are probably motivated by a number of different things. How can you tie them into your success in A&P?

More than likely, you are taking this course because it's required for a physical education or health-related career that you are pursuing. Please don't look at this course as simply a hoop you need to jump through (with a C+ or better) to get a piece of paper that you want. Human A&P is the foundation for *ALL* of the clinical, therapeutic, and physical professional courses. A good understanding of A&P will almost always ensure success in your profession. What better motivation is there than this?

You may be thinking, "OK, I'm planning a career in physical therapy. Why do I need to understand the structure and function of the skin? My motivation for this topic is simply to get the grade." I've been there myself a few times. But you'd be surprised at how much *everything relates to everything else*. You are right; as a physical therapist, you'll probably be focused more on nerves, muscles, and joints than on the skin. However, you'd be surprised how much your understanding of nerves, muscles, and joints deepens when you have a solid understanding of the concepts behind the structure and function of skin. The trick is that you really can't fully appreciate this link until *you have learned all of it*. In other words, you need to know it before you can begin to understand *why* you need to know it!

> ■ Everything relates to everything else.

I hope that you can trust the professionals who designed and required you to take your A&P course and accept the fact that the topics presented in this course really will be important to you—and use that as your motivation to really understand it.

The bottom line to Survival Skill 1 is *know* that you can succeed—and you *will!*

◇ SURVIVAL TIPS

- ☑ My friend Bill Stark at St. Louis University taught me this trick for making A&P more fun: For each new topic that you learn, try to find a song that contains lyrics that are related to the topic, especially if it's a really silly connection or some really outrageous lyrics. For example, *Heartbeat* by Enrique Iglesias (amzn.to/Y7mX2b) would be appropriate for studying the cardiac pumping cycle. Rod Stewart's classic *You're in My Heart* (amzn.to/14n2uK7) can cover not only the study of the heart but also kidney function ("urine" my heart).
- ☑ Dr. Stark plays his favorites for the whole class before his lectures. Why not challenge the people in your study group to come up with the best—or goofiest—song? Search your music device . . . you probably already have a lot of A&P material there!

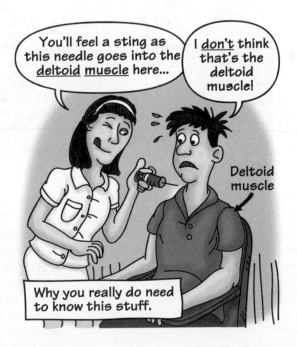

2

Know Your Learning Style

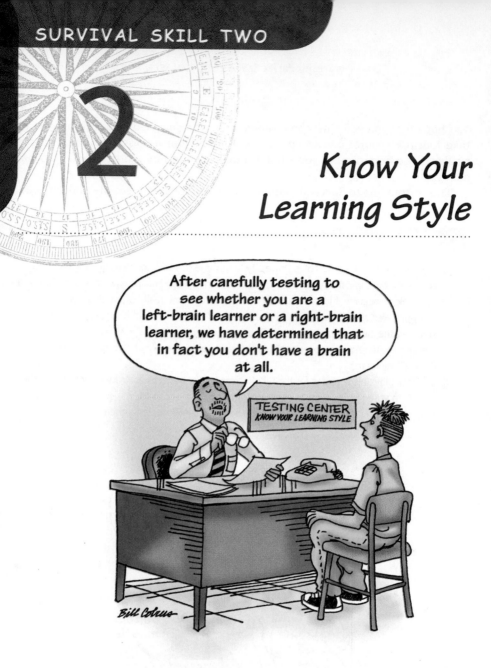

After carefully testing to see whether you are a left-brain learner or a right-brain learner, we have determined that in fact you don't have a brain at all.

TESTING CENTER
KNOW YOUR LEARNING STYLE

Bill Colrus

In the previous Survival Skill, we discussed attitude. Now let's think about style. Learning researchers have found that each of us has a certain style of learning. When we use the word *style* here, it doesn't refer to what kind of clothes we wear to school. Our learning style is the way we approach new information, process that information, and then use it. Being familiar with your own learning style can be a *major* key to successful learning. Knowing your style, you can approach new information in a way that will help you to learn it more efficiently.

Learning styles can be described in many different ways. For example, some learning specialists like to categorize people as being either left-brain learners or right-brain learners. This system is based on the notion that the part of the brain most involved with complex learning—the cerebrum—is divided into right and left halves.

Experiments with patients who have had the connections between these two halves cut by a surgeon show that the right side, when acting alone, seems better able to grasp spatial relationships, to interpret non-speech sounds such as music and animal sounds, and to interpret the sense of touch. The left side seems better able to govern functions of language, such as speaking and writing. Left-brain learners are said to be more logical and mathematical in their approach to learning, whereas right-brain learners tend to be more creative and nonlinear in their approach.

Although differences between learners are not solely related to the locations of different brain functions, it's certain that different people learn best in different ways. Using the metaphors of left-brain learning and right-brain learning, as well as many other learning metaphors, works.

Other approaches to learning style have been proposed, and you should be aware of some of them so that you can better understand the concept of learning style. One approach that I think is very useful is based on *how you use your senses* when you are learning.

People that learn best by *seeing* a demonstration are called *visual learners.* If you learn better by *hearing* an explanation, then you're probably an *aural* or *auditory learner.* If you need to put your hands on something and *feel* it or work with it, then you're a *kinesthetic* or *tactual learner.* If you learn best by *reading* about something, then you're a *reading learner.* Of course, some of these categories may overlap. For example, I think that I learn best visually (which explains why I have included so many illustrations in my textbooks and teaching presentations), but I am also strong in the tactual area (which explains why I enjoy the laboratory setting).

So why is it important to know your learning style? It's important because, if you know your strengths or preferences as a learner, you can arrange your learning activities to build on your strengths. For example, if you're a strong visual learner but are weak in auditory (aural) learning, then you will want to study primarily by drawing diagrams and charting concepts rather than spending most of your time listening to tapes of lectures. On the other hand, a strong auditory (aural) learner will do much better by listening to lecture tapes and spending a little less time with diagrams.

The first step that you must take is to determine *your own style* of learning. You can do this in several ways.

✧ **SURVIVAL TIP**

☑ For free online self-quizzes that help you to determine your learning style— and for learning advice after you've figured out your style—visit *Learning Styles* (my-ap.us/1oRcpE2).

One way to determine your own learning style is to ask a learning specialist to test you. Although formal tests are available, such testing could be as informal as a chat with a staff member at your college's learning center. Another way to discover your own learning style is to ask yourself questions with the use of a self-quiz method.

Here are a few self-quiz questions that will help you to determine your personal approach to learning—that is, your style:

☑ **Do I prefer a verbal explanation of a process or a written explanation?** If you prefer verbal explanations, then concentrate your studies on lectures and verbal dialog with your professor, tutors, members of your study group, and your lab partners. If you prefer written explanations, spend more time with your notes, class handouts, your textbook (yes, please do), and other written materials suggested by your professor or college librarian. You may also want to check out the many digital resources available on the Internet. (See the special box on computer use in Survival Skill 10).

☑ **Do I need to see, hear, or touch a model or specimen as I learn about a process?** If you need visuals or something else to hold in your hand, you'll find this course to be just your ticket! A&P involves models, specimens, and other gizmos that you can look at and play with as much as you want. Check with your professor for hints about what kinds of lab models and specimens are available for your studies. In addition, your school library will certainly have many visual and auditory resources, including animations and computer simulations, which might be useful to you.

☑ **Do I learn better at a particular time of the day?** Of course you want to schedule your classes, lab sessions, and study sessions for the times when you're at your peak performance level. If you can't do that, then at least take this into consideration and try to break up your study times so that you don't tax your concentration.

☑ **Do I learn better if I am physically active or eating or drinking while I study?** It's always a good idea to take breaks every 15 to 20 minutes while you're studying. When you take a break, move around as much as possible. Considering the benefits of exercise on general physical and mental health (including learning ability and memory), you may want to consider taking a short walk, briefly lifting weights, doing some isometric exercises, or perhaps performing some floor exercises during your break.

If you like to eat or drink while studying, consider the health consequences. I like to drink while I study, but beer destroys my concentration. Plain old water is absolutely the best thing you can drink while studying! You should be drinking several glasses of water throughout the day for good health anyway. Water prevents dehydration, which can affect your concentration, and it helps your body to maintain its proper function.

Watch what you eat, too. You don't want to succeed in A&P at the expense of becoming obese! The best snacks are small and frequent rather than part of one long eating binge. Depending on your own metabolic system, it's usually best to avoid foods that are very high in refined carbohydrates, such as sweets, breads, pasta, potato chips, corn chips, and pretzels. Instead, try nuts, vegetables, and fruits. A high ratio of refined carbohydrates—or too many carbohydrates during a short period of time—will cause your insulin levels to skyrocket and make you feel too sluggish to study effectively.

☑ **Do I prefer starting with the "big picture" and working toward the detail, or do I prefer starting with the detail and then assembling the big picture?** At the end of each chapter in nearly every A&P textbook, a section summarizes the important points of the chapter—a sort of "big picture" section. These short, easy-to-read outlines or lists help you to put the pieces presented in the text together to see how they fit with one another and allow the body to work as an integrated ("put together") whole. If you like starting with the big picture (which is my style), look at the end of the chapter and read the last part *first*. Then, after you have the big picture in your head, go back to the beginning of the chapter and read the material. If you instead prefer to start with smaller pieces and details, then read each chapter just as it's laid out in the book.

These and other questions will help you to identify your approach to learning. After you've done this, you can plan a learning strategy that will allow you to process new information in a way that will work best with your learning style.

✧ SPECIAL SURVIVAL SKILLS

Learners with Special Needs

Unless and until someone with special needs recognizes and names these special needs, learning can be difficult or impossible. I can't think of *any* disability or problem that could prevent someone from learning at least a little about how the body is put together and how it functions.

When dealing with any problem that might affect learning, it's always wise to form a network of support. First, your professor and your college's learning specialists will be able to help you identify your needs if you haven't already pinpointed them; then use these individuals to help you design a strategy to achieve success.

I once had a student tell me at the end of two semesters of A&P that she had a hearing impairment and that she would have probably gotten an A instead of a B if I hadn't occasionally faced away from her during my lectures and demonstrations, because she was then unable to read my lips. If only I had known at the beginning of the course—if she had *involved me* in her situation—I would have made a conscious effort to make sure that I always faced her and spoke clearly.

> ■ **It's always wise to form a network of support.**

I fully realize that it's often difficult (and perhaps even embarrassing) to talk to your professor about your problems, but *that's what we're here for!* Professors have experience and often some special training in dealing with a variety of difficulties. When we can't help you, we often know where you can get help, and we are *always* willing to work with you to help you succeed.

Continued

✦ SPECIAL SURVIVAL SKILLS—cont'd

Quite a few students have subtle learning problems that they don't recognize; they may only be aware that they're having some sort of difficulty. I remember one very bright student who really seemed to understand the concepts but just couldn't seem to get more than a D on her tests. After helping her all that I could, with little success, I referred her to our campus learning specialists. Right away, those specialists spotted a reading comprehension problem that affected this student's test-taking ability. When she developed a new test-taking strategy that was based on her work with a learning specialist, she raised her final grade to a B! That learner is now a successful health professional who still uses what she learned that semester to help her stay up to date in her field. The important thing is that she took the step of involving others in her situation.

The main thing to remember is that *your special need is part of your learning style.* If you can identify your special needs, you can almost always find a strategy that will help you succeed in learning about human anatomy and physiology (A&P).

✦ SURVIVAL TIPS

☑ If you're having *any kind* of difficulty that affects your learning, see your professor or your campus learning specialists. Usually these people can help you to identify the problem and find a strategy to deal with it.

☑ If you already know of a special need that affects your learning, talk to your professor or campus learning specialists *immediately.* The sooner you can form a team to help you with your learning, the better your chances are for great success.

Know the Language

3

When you travel to a new place, you may encounter people who speak a language different from your own. If you try to learn their language as quickly as possible, you'll enjoy your safari a lot more—and you'll understand a lot more about what is happening around you. The world of human anatomy and physiology has its own language. The best approach is to try and learn this new, strange language right away so that you don't miss anything important.

If you are unfamiliar with it, the scientific and medical terminology used in A&P can seem overwhelming. The length and apparent complexity of many terms often scare people who have not had training in or practice with scientific terminology. Although it requires knowledge of some basic word parts and a few rules for using them, scientific terminology is not as difficult as it seems. This handy introduction provides you with what you need to get started.

Following are a handful of survival tips to help you learn and use the terms that are related to A&P. At the end of this book, there are several tables that contain many of the most commonly used word parts as well as examples of how they are used. This handy summary does not attempt to teach you the entire field of scientific and medical terminology. However, with the information that is given here and a little practice, you will soon become comfortable with the basics that are required as you travel through your A&P course.

- ☑ **Most terms come from Latin and Greek.** Many scientific terms are derived from the Latin and Greek languages. This is because many of the anatomists, physiologists, and physicians who discovered the basic principles of the modern life sciences used these languages themselves so that they could communicate with each other without having to learn dozens of individual local languages. Thus, Latin and Greek have become the universal languages of scientific terminology. Many of the words used are derived from these classical languages, and so are some of their rules of use. The most useful rules are given in a later section.
- ☑ **Terms are made by combining word parts.** One set of rules for using Latin and Greek is essential to the understanding of scientific terminology. Both languages rely on the ability to combine word parts to make new words. Thus, almost all scientific terms are constructed by combining smaller word elements to make a specific term. Because of this combining technique, many

11

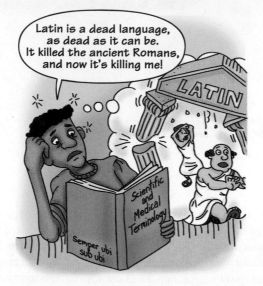

scientific terms appear at first glance to be long and complex. However, if you read a new term as a series of word elements rather than a single word, determining the meaning will be less imposing. One of the easiest ways to learn scientific terminology is to develop the ability to analyze new terms instantly to discover the word parts that comprise them. Different kinds of word parts are used, depending on exactly how they fit with other word parts to form a complete term.

■ Almost all scientific terms are constructed by combining smaller word elements.

A **prefix** is a word part that is added to the beginning of an existing word to alter its meaning. We use prefixes in English as well. For example, the meaning of *sense* changes when the prefix *non-* is added to make the word *nonsense*.

A **suffix** is a word part that is added to the end of an existing word to alter its meaning. Once again, suffixes are also sometimes used in English. For example, the meaning of *sense* changes when the suffix *-less* is added to create the word *senseless*. A complex term can have a series of suffixes, a series of prefixes, or both. For example, the word *senselessness* has two suffixes: *-less* and *-ness*.

A **root** is a word part that serves as the starting point for the forming of a new term. In the previous examples in English, the word *sense* was the root to which a prefix or a suffix was added. Word parts that are commonly used as roots can also be used as suffixes or prefixes to form a new term. In addition, several roots may be combined to form a larger root to which suffixes or prefixes can be added.

Combining vowels are vowels *(a, e, i, o, u, y)* used to link word parts, often to make pronunciation easier. For example, to link the suffix *-tion* to the root *sense,* we must use the combining vowel *-a-* to form the new term *sensation.* Using the *-e* that is already at the end of the word would make the term difficult to pronounce. A root and a combining vowel together—in this case, *sensa-*—is often called the *combining form* of the word part.

As in English, Latin and Greek word parts have *homonyms*—words with identical spellings and pronunciations that have different meanings. For example, the prefix *de-* could mean "down" as in *descending,* or it could mean "remove" as in *deoxygenate.* Thus, a word part may have different meanings in different contexts. With *synonyms,* however, different word parts may all have similar meanings. For example, *com-* in *compartment* and *con-* in *contract* both mean "together." This adds to the richness of scientific terminology, as it does in any language. However, it can be confusing.

✧ SURVIVAL TIPS

- ☑ If you pay attention to word parts as you pick up new terms, you will begin to learn them *quickly* and *easily.* Then, you'll find yourself recognizing the construction of terms that are completely new to you. And you'll be able to recall the meaning of terms you have learned much more easily.
- ☑ At the back of this book, there are some handy lists of commonly used word parts to help you get started with your "new language."
- ☑ Your A&P textbook may include translations of word parts in the chapter word lists, in the glossary, or in both places. If so, *pay attention to them.* By doing so, you'll eventually pick up the language easily.
- ☑ If your textbook doesn't include word parts, try keeping a print or digital scientific and medical dictionary handy. I recommend *Mosby's Dictionary of Medicine, Nursing & Health Professions* (amzn.to/X2a7zm).

☑ **Some terms use Latin plural forms.** Another set of rules for using Latin- and Greek-based terms that you will find useful relates to using nouns in their singular and plural forms. To form a plural in English, we often simply add *-s* or *-es* to a word. For example, the plural of the word *sense* is *senses.* Because we have adopted scientific terms into English to form sentences, we often simply use the pluralization rules of English and add the *-s* or *-es.* At times, however, you will run across an English term that has been pluralized according to Latin or Greek rules. As in ordinary English, some Latin-based forms are the same whether they are used as singular or plural. For example, the term *meatus* (a tube-like opening) is both singular and plural. This brief list will help you to distinguish between many plural and singular forms:

Singular	Plural	Examples
-a	-ae	ampulla → ampullae
-ax	-aces	thorax → thoraces
-en	-ina	foramen → foramina
-ex	-ices	cortex → cortices
-is	-es	neurosis → neuroses
-ix	-ices	appendix → appendices
-ma	-mata	lymphoma → lymphomata
-on	-a	mitochondrion → mitochondria
-um	-a	datum → data
-ur	-ora	femur → femora
-us	-i	villus → villi
-yx	-yces	calyx → calyces

☑ **Avoid confusing adjectives with nouns.** As in any communication in English, we sometimes convert nouns to adjectives to describe anatomical parts or physiological processes. This is usually done by adding the word parts *-ic* or *-al* to the end of a noun to make it an adjective. For example, if we want to describe something that pertains to the base of a structure, we could use *basal* or *basic*, as in *basal layer* or *basic solution*. Sometimes we even go crazy and add both endings, as in *anatomical,* which is the adjective form of the noun *anatomy*.

It would be accurate to state that the *femur* is a bone in the *femoral* region of the lower extremity or that the *facial* nerve has connections in the *face*.

When using these terms, the noun form can stand alone, but the adjective form needs a noun to modify or describe. For example, it is not proper to say "carpal" when you mean "carpal bones" or "carpus." Although saying "My carpals hurt" is often used in casual conversation, saying "My carpal bones hurt" is more accurate and less likely to be misinterpreted. If you really mean that your whole wrist hurts, it would be best to state "My carpal region hurts" or "My carpus hurts."

Likewise, referring to your "occipital" is not as clear as referring to your "occipital bone" or your "occiput."

☑ **Correct spelling is important.** Correct spelling of scientific terms is essential to their meanings. I know, I know! All this *AND* I have to learn the correct spelling of all these crazy words?! I'm afraid so, because it can literally spell the difference between the life and death of your future clients! In fact, mistakes in spelling terms or in acronyms and abbreviations are a major cause of death and injury. In some settings, spelling mistakes are grounds for discipline or dismissal from your job.

Correct spelling is especially important for terms that are very close in spelling but very different in meaning. For example, the *perineum* is the region of the trunk around the genitals and the anus, whereas the *peritoneum* is a membrane that lines the abdominal cavity and covers abdominal organs. Even a mistake in one letter can change the meaning of a word, as in the case of *ilium* (part of the bony pelvis) versus *ileum* (part of the small intestine).

American spellings of terms occasionally differ from those found in other forms of English, such as the English dialects used in Canada, Australia, and the United Kingdom. For example, *centimeter* (the American form) and *centimetre* are both correct. The American word *esophagus* is often spelled *oesophagus* in other parts of the world. Always use the spelling that is appropriate for your location and your intended audience.

☑ **Be aware of alternate terminology.** An important reference called the *Terminologia Anatomica* (*TA* or *Ta*) is an international list of gross anatomy terms, and the *Terminologia Histologica* (*TH* or *Th*) is an international list of microscopic anatomy terms. The *Terminologia Embryologica* (*TE* or *Te*) is for developmental anatomy terms. These lists are important because they contain the terms that have been agreed upon by working anatomists from around the world, to avoid confusion caused by having too many alternate names.

✦ SURVIVAL TIP

☑ Free digital versions of these anatomical terminology lists can be found online at *International Lists* (my-ap.us/Uv5lxp).

Although such lists are helpful, alternate terminology is still frequently encountered. Even the standard lists themselves often show alternate forms of the same term. Good reasons sometimes exist for using a newer term or a term that is more easily understood by your colleagues or in your region of the world. Do not forget that new terminology is slow to be adopted worldwide, so you may need to know newer and older terms to communicate easily with many different people.

Also remember that eponyms (terms based on the name of a person) are also frequently used in science and medicine. However, most eponyms are currently being phased out in favor of more descriptive terms. A brief list of some important eponyms and their alternatives is given later in this section.

When using eponyms, it is an increasingly common practice to drop the apostrophe and "s" at the end of an eponym. In other words, we do not use the possessive form of the name. For example, we use *Bowman capsule* instead of *Bowman's capsule* or *Parkinson disease* rather than *Parkinson's disease*. Likewise, *organ of Corti* is increasingly replaced by *Corti organ*. Be aware that not everyone follows this practice—you may sometimes encounter the possessive form.

✧ SPECIAL SURVIVAL SKILLS

Pronunciation

Correct pronunciation is important! Because many scientific terms are spoken, correct pronunciation is as important as correct spelling. Scientific terms can usually be pronounced phonetically—by sounding out each letter sound of each syllable. Check the pronunciation keys given in your textbook or dictionary if you are uncertain about how to pronounce any word that you encounter in A&P. Audio pronunciations are also provided with the electronic resources that accompany this textbook.

Regional differences in pronunciation and differences among different branches of science and medicine do exist. For example, the American pronunciation of vitamin is *VYE-tah-min*, but in many other parts of the world the pronunciation is *VIH-tah-min*. The term *centimeter* is correctly pronounced *SEN-tah-mee-ter*, but some health professionals have learned the pronunciation *SAWN-tah-mee-ter*.

Your A&P textbook may have audio pronunciation guides available as a digital resource. If so, it's worth using these guides to learn your language without forming bad habits and mispronouncing terms.

There are free digital pronunciation guides available online, too. I really like these two:

☑ *Talking Dictionary of English Pronunciation* (my-ap.us/SVQmx8)
☑ *Forvo: All the words in the world. Pronounced.* (my-ap.us/Y9BWIM)

Ask your A&P teacher about different pronunciations. He or she may be able to clarify which pronunciations are common in your region—or which are used in clinical versus basic science settings.

☑ **Practice new terminology.** As you know, practice makes perfect. Practice using the scientific terms in this or another book until you become comfortable with scientific terminology. It won't take long, and you will probably have fun doing it.

The easiest way to practice new terms is by using *flash cards*. I will walk you through this active learning strategy in Survival Skill 8 on page 37.

Plan a Learning Strategy

he intention to learn something is a step in the right direction, but intent alone is not in itself a learning plan. Rather, you must carefully plan a set of activities that will move you toward your goal of learning the essentials of human A&P. Consider two important aspects of a good learning strategy: 1) time management; and 2) a logical sequence of activities.

Time Management

For any plan to work, it must account for timing. A learning strategy must have its foundation in the careful planning of study time for your work in human A&P. To get started, here are a few tips that might help:

☑ **Put your time plan down on paper.** One good way to organize your plan involves three simple steps. First, make a monthly calendar. Make or buy a large sheet calendar that shows the whole month at a glance, or use one of the many handy monthly planners that you can find at your college bookstore. Those that are marked "Academic" or "Fiscal" usually run from July to July and thus work best for traditional semester or quarter systems. (If your computer or cell phone has a calendar, you can certainly use that as well.) Mark your test dates as soon as you know them, and add the days that assignments are due. If your professor has given you dates for particular lecture topics or lab activities, you may want to include these as well. Be sure to also mark this information for your other classes and to include other big events and occasions that are taking place in your life. Do this for the entire semester.

Second, make a weekly schedule. This is an ideal model of a typical week. Include time for your job, your classes, household or personal duties and chores; other commitments such as sports, clubs, or church; time for routine activities such as eating and sleeping; and of course, include plenty of time for studying—marking *specific* times for study each day.

Third, every day, make a *to-do list*. This should be a simple list of things that you must get done that day. Make your list the evening before or the first thing in the morning. Show which items are high priority and which are low priority, and be sure to cross items off of your list as you complete them. To do this, you need to *carry your list with you all the time.* The easiest way I've found is to use a 3- × 5-inch card. These cards fit almost anywhere, and they don't tear apart or get lost easily.

✧ SPECIAL SURVIVAL SKILLS

Time-Management Tools

You need to take time management seriously for success in your A&P course and beyond. Now is a good time to experiment with different tools to help keep your time organized and thus to keep your studies on track. Here are a few tools that I've found to be useful for time management.

- ☑ Your mobile device can be a great tool for managing your time. Get to know what built-in time-management features your device already has, and then look around for additional apps that may be helpful for you.
- ☑ For to-do lists, I recommend the free Evernote app (my-ap.us/14097f4). You can also use this app to clip notes, tips, and references from other online sources. For example, you could clip relevant anatomical charts from *Gray's Anatomy Online* (my-ap.us/Ya9uqj).
- ☑ Consider setting "study alerts" on your mobile device or electronic watch to remind you of your planned study times. This may sound goofy, but it really works! You may have a calendar app that is already built into your device, but I recommend the free Google Calendar app (my-ap.us/Uv8LAc), which can send you text messages at certain times to remind you to study.

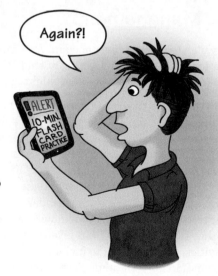

- ☑ For more ideas about time management tools for your mobile device check out *Top 50 Apps for Time Management* (my-ap.us/WGLfPs).
- ☑ Some folks like the low-tech route. That's OK, there are some great tools that are low tech. I recommend any of the great pocket or notebook calendars from the AT-A-GLANCE line (my-ap.us/111i2VW). The key, however, is to actually *write in* several daily study sessions before each new week starts. That will not only remind you, but also block the time off from other uses.

☑ **Don't short yourself on study time.** I recommend a combined total of about an hour and a half *every day* for a typical three- or four-credit A&P course. This covers both lecture and lab sections. Some students will need more time, and some (especially those who are using the study skills and shortcuts outlined in this book) can make do with a little less time. If you don't spend enough time working on your studies outside of the classroom, don't expect to be successful, no matter how smart you are. Maybe you didn't need this much time for other courses in high school or college, but *A&P is different.* You really will need all that time!

> ■ If you don't spend enough time working on your studies outside of the classroom, don't expect to be successful, no matter how smart you are.

A common error that is often seen by A&P professors occurs when students spend all of their study time on one or two long sessions just before a test or exam. Instead of spreading their study time out and including a little bit each day, these students wait until the last possible moment and then *cram* for hours and hours. Then, they wonder why they didn't do as well as they thought they would. Even if this has worked in the past for you, it will *NOT* work very well for your A&P course or for any course that follows it, so please don't even try this type of approach.

◆ **SURVIVAL TIPS**

☑ Use a three-step method for time planning:
1. Monthly calendar
2. Weekly schedule
3. Daily to-do list

☑ Once you have a plan, *FOLLOW IT!*

☑ **Break up your study sessions.** Divide your study time into 20- to 30-minute blocks if you can. This is the most efficient use of your study time. *Never* go over 90 minutes with study time—the extra time you spend will not do you any good and will probably increase your frustration level.

Use unconventional times to do some of your studying. For example, many of my auditory learners listen to taped lectures or study sessions while driving to work or school or doing their household chores. I've had several students listen to my taped lectures while working on an assembly line! Others carry their flash cards with them (see Survival Skill 8) and review them during unexpected breaks in their day, such as when waiting in line, just before class starts, and during television commercials.

> ◆ **SURVIVAL TIP**
>
> ☑ Most people can read or concentrate on a topic to be studied for only *20 to 30 minutes at a time!* For this reason, frequent breaks and short study sessions always work best.

☑ **Turn wasted time into study time.** There are so many minutes throughout the day that we can put to better use. Think of all the minutes that we spend standing in lines, riding the bus or carpooling, waiting for class to start, and so on. Even if it's just a minute or two, a quick look at a few flash cards or a brief review of your notes is a great way to keep up with your studies. As already noted, many brief study spurts throughout the day are much more effective for learning than one long study session.

☑ **Watch yourself.** Once a week—preferably at the same time each week so that you make a habit of it—briefly review what you did with your A&P studies during the previous week. Perhaps you can keep a list in your notebook or calendar. Write down an estimate of how many hours you spent on various study and learning activities, and specify exactly what you did and when. Alternatively, you could keep a detailed study journal in which you jot down what you did and then simply review that weekly. Doing this may seem like a waste of time, but it is a really effective way to develop time-management skills. Some people pay a lot of money to business coaches and life coaches to learn this simple trick—and you're hearing about it for next to nothing!

☑ **Learn when to say "no."** This is the hardest one for me, so I saved it for last. Teachers, like coaches and health professionals, get a kick out of helping people. This is normally a character strength, but if we don't limit ourselves to reasonable schedules, it can become a weakness. While you're studying A&P, you're going to have to put some things off or cancel them entirely if you want to succeed. Be selective: say "yes" to important requests and "no" to those that aren't so important.

Hanging with your friends is a great thing, and it certainly helps keep stress levels low, but if you say "yes" too often, when will you have time to study?

Perhaps the most difficult situations occur when your obligations outside of school are simply too demanding to allow for your academic success. The wisest decision for some students may be to quit or change a job or to temporarily rely on more childcare services than they're usually comfortable with. For others, the best thing to do may be to cut back on the course load and increase the number of semesters needed to complete the desired program. Often trying to do too much in too little time will guarantee that goals will not be met.

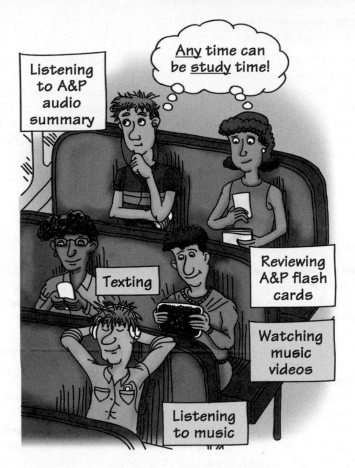

Logical Sequence of Activities

The sequence of learning activities within your budgeted study time should be determined by your learning style, any limitations that you may have to live with, and a look at what has worked for others. However, you will need to devise a plan. If you just perform your study and reading activities in a random manner, you'll be wasting a lot of time. Your overall efficiency is greatly enhanced by using a plan that suits you.

> ■ It will take you less time to study if you use an organized plan.

◆ SURVIVAL TIPS

☑ If you have trouble budgeting your time, perhaps you should seek the advice of your instructor or a learning specialist.

☑ Ask your librarian to help you find books about time management. Many good titles are available, but you may need your librarian's advice to choose one that is right for you.

☑ Many colleges and local communities offer seminars and workshops that address time management. Even information that is designed primarily for business executives can be extremely helpful to college students.

Here is a plan that has worked for many A&P students:

1. **Read the appropriate chapter in the textbook.** Use a reading strategy that suits your learning style (see Survival Skill 6). Don't even try to master all of the material with this first read through. Just get a rough idea of what's going on; a fuller understanding will come later. Whatever you do, don't read more than one chapter at a time!

2. **Attend the lecture or discussion class, and take careful notes.** Use a note-taking strategy that works for you (see Survival Skill 7).

3. **Review and organize your notes.** Do this as soon after class as possible—not more than 24 hours. Don't rewrite or copy your notes. That method often does more harm than good.

4. **Participate in related laboratory and demonstration activities.** Try to relate both the lecture and lab sections of the course to the topic—they're complementary courses. If you have the opportunity to do extra lab work or attend extra demonstrations, take advantage of it!

5. **Reread the textbook chapter.** This time through, you'll have a much better understanding of what's going on. Now is the time to highlight, underline, and take notes from the text.

6. **Work through some learning activities.** This is discussed in much greater detail in Survival Skill 8.

7. **Review the material with other students, perhaps in a study group.** This is the most overlooked—but often the most important—tip for success in A&P!

8. **Make a quick review of your notes just before the test.** Don't overdo it, though. A lengthy cramming session usually does more harm than good.

✦ SPECIAL SURVIVAL SKILLS

Returning Learners

Today more and more people are returning to college and university studies. Traditionally, most college students were recent high school graduates. Returning students who have been out of school for a few (or perhaps many) years are considered "nontraditional" by this standard. Nontraditional students often face challenges that are quite different from those experienced by traditional students.

I've been both a traditional and nontraditional college student myself, and I've faced many of the challenges that you might face while pursuing my college studies: I've worked full-time. I've had the responsibilities of having a spouse and children, and I've also been a single parent. I've worked in a volunteer organization. I've started my own business. I've dealt with divorce, family illnesses, and deaths. I've had personal setbacks and illnesses. I write this to let you know that I do understand what some of your challenges are, and I'm here to tell you this: As overwhelming as it might seem at times, you CAN succeed!

> ■ As overwhelming as it may seem at times, know that *you CAN succeed.*

Through the years, I've gathered a number of ideas that have helped me or my students face the challenges of being a nontraditional student. Perhaps some of them will be valuable to you.

- ☑ **Make an informal, *written* contract with your family or life partner.** This simple exercise will help you all to understand the seriousness of your commitment to pursue your studies—as well as each loved one's role in helping you to succeed. It will also avoid the conflicts that invariably result from misunderstandings and unspoken expectations.
- ☑ **Learn to live with dust under the bed, dirty dishes in the sink, and weeds in the garden.** For a time, your priorities will be elsewhere. Don't worry about it. If someone else has a problem with it, well, *it's his or her problem*, isn't it?
- ☑ **Work with your professor and the learning specialists at your school to learn about strategies for returning learners.** Quite a bit of wisdom is just waiting to be shared with you, but *you have to ask.*
- ☑ **Find other returning learners with whom you can network.** Many other returning learners would love to share the mutual support that you all can provide to each other. Sometimes frustrations can turn into joys when you have friends with whom to share them. If you can include other returning learners in your study group, you might find a special friend there. Often your learning center can refer you to others in your situation. In fact, many schools now have active programs for returning learners. My community college even has a special lounge on campus for returning learners as well as lunchtime seminars that cover topics of interest to returning learners!
- ☑ **If possible, postpone big events or life changes until after you've finished your studies.** If at all possible, don't plan to move, change jobs, change your marital status, have children, undergo a facelift, or try out for the Olympics while you're in school. Life-changing experiences and events can be exciting, but trying to do too many things at the same time while in school can be disastrous!

✧ SPECIAL SURVIVAL SKILLS—cont'd

☑ **Don't hold back.** Some returning learners are somewhat intimidated when they first reenter the classroom, and they don't jump into discussions or speak up with questions. The sooner that you realize that the years you've been away from the classroom give you an *advantage* over the younger traditional students, the easier it will be to *jump in* and get the most out of school.

☑ **Rely on your strengths.** I saved the best for last. Studies—including one that I conducted myself with our A&P students—show that returning learners usually do better in A&P than their classmates. Really! Just think about it. Returning learners have more life experience, more practice juggling the many competing pressures of life, and a more realistic view of the importance of succeeding in school. Bring the wisdom and "street smarts" that you've gained to A&P, and you'll do great!

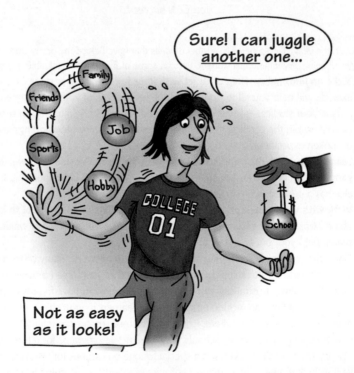

Arrange a Suitable Study Area

5

J ust as the timing of study activities is important, the location in which you work can be critical to learning A&P effectively. Because none of us lives in an ideal world, you may have to settle for less than the best. However, extra effort put into securing a prime study site could pay big dividends come test time.

There are three keys to learning that you should keep in mind when arranging a suitable study area:

1. *Focus.*
2. *Focus.*
3. *Focus.*

The following tips for promoting good, steady focus should be considered when selecting a study location:

☑ **Make sure that you have good access to the site.** Don't plan to study in an area that is closed during your planned study time or that is often being used by others before you get there. In addition, if you're hosting a study group, make sure that you choose a convenient location. If you live way out in the boonies and all your study partners live in town, then find somewhere midway to meet them.

☑ **Be sure that you have comfortable lighting.** Some learners do best in bright lighting, whereas others prefer moderately dim lighting. Despite all the stories that you've heard about Abe Lincoln studying by the light of the fireplace in his cabin, very dim light is not good for studying. Likewise, you may find reading easier in incandescent rather than fluorescent lighting, especially if you have a reading disability. If you have any difficulty with your vision while studying or if you experience headaches as a result, talk to a physician or an eye-care professional.

☑ **Ensure that the surroundings complement your learning style.** In other words, make sure that your site is comfortable. However, make sure it's not so comfortable that you'll tend to doze!

☑ **Analyze the background noise.** Few study locations are perfectly noiseless. Ask yourself whether your selected site has noise that will be tolerable (loud or soft; people sounds, music sounds, or machine sounds).

✓ **Eliminate distractions.** I've heard some students say that they study better with distractions such as being around playing children, watching videos, helping customers, and so on. Bunk. *NOBODY* studies more effectively with distractions. Studies show that even the best multitaskers are not nearly as productive as people who can stay focused. Sure, sometimes distractions are unavoidable. I'm just saying that you should *try* to avoid them.

✓ **Make sure that you have what you need to study.** If you need pens, pencils, paper, a computer, disks, a video player, a live band, books, tapes, a basketball, or whatever, make sure that you have them with you *before you begin to study.*

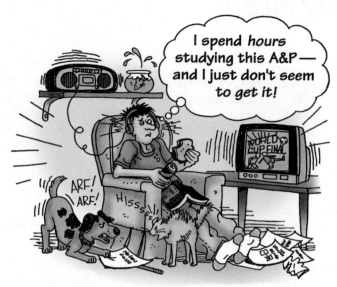

✧ SURVIVAL TIP

✓ Can't think of a good place to study? Try the following 12 places:
 1. College library
 2. Public library
 3. Student lounge
 4. Campus quad
 5. Local park
 6. Campus study room
 7. Bedroom
 8. Café
 9. Work (if your boss permits it)
 10. Parent room at a play spot
 11. Yard near your home
 12. Front, back, or side porch, balcony, or deck

Plan a Reading Strategy

6

lthough reading the right chapter is one element of the overall learning strategy, reading requires a strategy of its own. In the case of A&P textbooks especially, the "jump right into it" approach used for novels or magazine articles does not work very well. Instead, you must do some *pre*-reading and *post*-reading of a new chapter if you're going to understand it well.

Learning specialists have invented several reading strategies. A popular method that works well with most A&P textbooks is called the *SQ4R Reading Method*. The six steps of this method (Survey, Question, Read, Recite, Record, Review) are described below:

1. **SURVEY the chapter before you read it.** That is, glance over the start-of-chapter materials (such as word lists or brief outlines); then glance over the body of the chapter (paying more attention to the topic headlines, tables, and illustrations than the actual narrative), and the end-of-chapter materials (summary information). Leave the end-of-chapter questions or problems for a later step.

✧ SURVIVAL TIPS

- ☑ You may have heard about famous successful people, such as U.S. presidents, taking special training in reading to improve their speed and comprehension. Check out the many reading programs that may be available at your school, in your area, or on the Internet.
- ☑ Check out my video entitled *Reading & Raiding: Shortcuts to Using Your Textbook* (youtu.be/BR7NVHrFFpQ), which briefly summarizes specific advice for getting the most out of any A&P textbook.

2. **Ask yourself QUESTIONS.** Ask WHAT, WHY, and HOW as you survey the chapter, as you read the chapter, and after you're finished reading. Asking such questions will help you find answers as you read—thereby helping you focus on the important ideas. Always be willing to challenge what the textbook authors present to you in the text (just don't challenge us to a duel!). Doing this will help you to develop your critical thinking skills. Take your challenges to your study group or professor—this may spark a discussion that will really help you to understand the material more deeply.

3. **READ the chapter.** As you read, look for the main ideas, and look at how they're organized. Textbook authors put a lot of thought into how our chapters are organized, always building in a progression that we think will help you see the big picture. Try to get a feel for the rhythm and pace of the writing style. In addition, don't forget the tables, illustrations, and boxed sections. Much to our editors' dismay, textbook authors often leave certain things out of the narrative but instead put them into tables or illustrations where we think they make more sense. You'll miss these important ideas if you read only the narrative. (Remember, don't expect to "get it" all on your first read through. This is very technical stuff; it takes a few tries to really get it.)

✧ SURVIVAL TIPS

- ☑ Concentrate on what you're reading. If you can't concentrate, *put the book down and come back to it later.* Don't waste your time!
- ☑ Do *NOT* highlight or mark the text yet! That comes later.
- ☑ Some readers do well in understanding the connection between text and illustration by using the two-finger approach: using one finger to follow the text and the other to trace elements of the figure.

Unlike a novel, which you just read through, a textbook should be bitten off in pieces. Don't move to the next section until you've taken the time to stop and consider each **boldface term.** Textbook authors take the trouble to highlight them because THEY'RE IMPORTANT! In addition, take the time to make sure you answer any end-of-section review items before moving to the next section.

4. **RECITE aloud what you have just read.** When my daughter Aileen was first learning to read, she often used to recap aloud what she had just finished reading. No wonder her comprehension was so remarkable (do I sound like a proud Dad or what?). When I first tried this method, I felt pretty silly—like a little kid. However, you don't have to speak loudly, and it really does help. Recap aloud what you've read after each page or section; don't wait until the end of the chapter, or this tip won't help you.

5. **RECORD the main ideas.** Some people prefer to use a highlighting pen to highlight important terms and phrases as a method of recording the main

ideas for future use. You can go back later and review the portions you've highlighted. If you choose the highlighting method, make sure that you don't highlight everything—or it won't be very useful to you. You might also try writing yourself notes in the margins. I don't like this method much myself; I find it more effective to write down the main ideas in a special reading notebook that I keep. If you're an auditory (aural) learner, you might want to record your thoughts verbally into smartphone or digital recorder for later review. Whatever you do, *use your own words* as you write; don't simply parrot the text.

6. **REVIEW your textbook and reading notes often.** Review what you've read *every day*. As you review your own notes, compare them against the summary material at the end of the chapter. If you do this, an understanding of the material will seem to come to you rather effortlessly. When you review, don't try to focus on a complete understanding at first—such an understanding will grow with continued reviewing. If you're not progressing, see your professor for help with getting on the right track.

   After you've reviewed the chapter and your notes a few times, you're ready to tackle the end-of-chapter material in earnest. It's best to write out the answers to the questions or problems or to recite them aloud. If you just think them through without *actively* responding, you won't learn as quickly or efficiently.

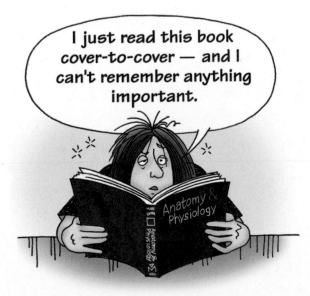

✦ SURVIVAL TIPS

☑ If you choose the highlighting method of recording, try using different colors of highlighting pens for different topics, different kinds of information, or different levels of importance.

☑ Some learners use Post-It notes in the margins or as page tabs as they record. These notes come in different styles and colors. Play around with them and see if you can develop your own customized system!

☑ Highlighting and adding in-text notes is easy with digital textbooks, too. In fact, on many e-book platforms, you can even share your highlights and notes with each other.

☑ Many similar methods of textbook reading exist, one of which might serve you better. Here are two:

1. *PQRST:* Preview, Question, Read, Summarize, and Test
2. *OK5R:* Overview, Key ideas, Read, Record, Recite, Review, and Reflect

☑ You can find details about these and other reading strategies at your college learning center or library, or review the many tips at *Reading Strategies* (my-ap.us/TlyIP3).

Analyze Your Note-Taking Skills

7

A s you may know, taking notes during a lecture or discussion improves both the comprehension (understanding) and retention (recall) of information. Because note taking requires the on-the-spot organization of information that is seen and heard during the class period, it improves *comprehension*. Because note taking reinforces information as it's recorded, it improves *retention*. Here are a few points to consider when planning a note-taking strategy:

> ■ Note taking is the key to comprehension, retention, and recall.

☑ **Know the professor's style.** Some professors present A&P in a well-organized manner, whereas others tend to ramble. Some speak very softly—or perhaps too loudly. Some may choose to follow the organization of the textbook very closely; others may decide to take a completely different approach. Being conscious of a professor's style will help you determine how you want to organize your notes, whether you'll need an audio recording to back up your notes, and where you want to sit in the classroom.

✦ SURVIVAL TIPS

☑ If your professor rambles during lectures, leave wide spaces between entries in your notebook. That way, if the professor returns to a previous point, you will have room to fill in more information.

☑ If your professor follows the textbook closely (bless his or her heart!), have the textbook handy, and highlight key points in it as you take notes. However, don't substitute highlighting for writing notes—you'll be sorry if you do!

☑ **Plan for note taking.** Know what style of note taking you will rely on, what materials you need to have with you, and how much lap or desktop space you require. Make sure that you're ready to start writing *before the professor begins class.*

☑ **Listen well.** Before you can take effective notes, you must hear what is being presented. This means making sure not only that you can perceive the sound but also that you understand the meaning. Try to clue in on the speaker's personal style to determine the main points and relationships between concepts.

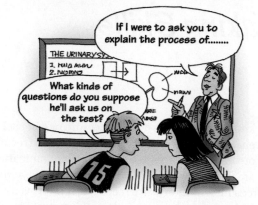

Most professors give a lot of clues that will help you. For example, if the professor says, "If I asked you to describe the function of a lysosome, what would you tell me?" then I bet he is thinking of asking something like that on a test or quiz. At the very least, the professor has raised an important question for you to think about. It amazes me how often in class I come right out and say "I often ask this on a test" and then watch as most of my students make no notation of this in their notebooks! It's no surprise that those who do take note of these comments always get those particular test items correct.

☑ **Structure your notes.** Because note taking helps you to organize the contents of a lecture, make sure that you're conscious of structure as you proceed.

1. *Know ahead of time whether you will use a formal outline style or your own personal modified outline style.* Here are some possible styles for note taking. You can use any of the outline formats shown here—or you can be creative and invent your own personal style of outlining!

Formal Outline:	*Modified Formal Outline:*
I. Heading	1. Heading
A. Subtopic	a. Subtopic
B. Subtopic	b. Subtopic
1. More about the subtopic	i. More about the subtopic
2. More about the subtopic	ii. More about the subtopic
a. Greater detail	(1) Greater detail
b. Greater detail	(2) Greater detail
(1) Even more detail	(a) Even more detail
(2) Even more detail	(b) Even more detail

Legal-Style Outline:

I. Heading
  I.1 Subtopic
  I.2 Subtopic
    1.2.1 More about the subtopic
    1.2.2 More about the subtopic
      1.2.2.1 Greater detail
      1.2.2.2 Greater detail
        1.2.2.2.1 Even more detail
        1.2.2.2.2 Even more detail

Bulleted Outline:

- Heading
  - Subtopic
  - Subtopic
    - More about the subtopic
    - More about the subtopic
      - Greater detail
      - Greater detail
        - Even more detail
        - Even more detail

2. *Be concise.* Don't try to take down every word; instead, use phrases, abbreviations, symbols, and diagrams to summarize the points made by the lecturer. For example, use symbols like *Ca* or *Ca^{++}* for calcium, *w/* for with, *w/o* for without, *#* for number, ☆ for something that is likely to be a test item, and *EZ* for enzyme—just to name a few. However, make sure that you know what your symbol or shorthand means later on, when it's not so fresh in your memory!

3. *Leave room between entries.* This way you can fill in more information if the professor returns to a point. Another method is to use only the right or left half of your notepaper. Some students fold each page of notes in half lengthwise to form a margin down the middle to leave a lot of room for adding things later.

4. *Try using highlighting pens or colored pencils to organize notes with color.* Use Post-It notes or tabs in a similar way; a variety of colors, shapes, and sizes of these exist.

✧ SURVIVAL TIP

☑ Leo Malone, one of my chemistry professors, required us to put a star in our notes next to any concept or fact that he introduced with a statement such as, "When you see something like this on the test. . . ." He even stopped class occassionally when he made such a statement to see if we'd put a star in our notes! This habit has stuck with me for decades. I still put a star on notes that I take during workshops, courses, meetings, or for any other work. In the classes that I teach, I put a star on the whiteboard when I want to emphasize that a point I'm making really is *worth remembering*. It works for me and my students—and I'm sure it will work for you!

☑ **Process your notes.** As soon after a lecture as possible—and certainly within 24 hours—work with your notes to clarify what you've written. Fill in any blank spots that you may have left, and write out abbreviated terms so that you'll know the meaning later. Don't completely rewrite or transcribe your notes, but be sure that everything is there and understandable. If you find a gap or a muddled section, check with a classmate or the lecturer for clarification.

> ■ Don't completely rewrite or transcribe your notes.

☑ **Write it out!** The most common error made when taking notes is being too brief. Write out complete thoughts rather than just key words or phrases, and draw diagrams or sketches if that helps you to understand the material. Write *as much as you can* during the class, and you'll thank yourself later. If you can't keep up with a fast-talking professor, then (with permission) record the presentation and go over your notes later with other students. In addition, write legibly; you want to be able to read it later!

☑ **Look for connections.** One of the great secrets to really understanding A&P is looking for how things are related to one another—and *making connections.* Your note-taking system can be used to recognize and keep track of connections in a number of ways.

The easiest way is to keep a section of your notebook (perhaps tabbed so that you can find it easily) for "connection pages." On the top of each connection page, write the name of a concept that keeps coming up during the course; then, as you process your regular notes, when you run across that concept again, add the new information to your connection page for that topic. For example, calcium has a variety of important roles in the body and will be discussed frequently. Every time calcium comes up in the discussion, add it to your "calcium page" in the "connections section" of your notebook. You'll probably end up with a lock-and-key page, a sodium page, a G protein page, a sodium cotransport page, a citric acid cycle page, a cytoskeleton page, a collagen page, and a receptor page. For more ideas about connection pages, visit *Concept Lists* (my-ap.us/XJW69G) for directions, tips, and even a video.

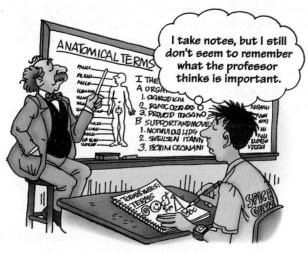

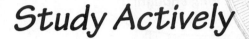

Study Actively

8

Many students feel that studying is the same as reading, so they spend study time only in reading and rereading the textbook and their class notes. Although reading is a part of a study plan, additional activities are required for your study time to be *effective*.

Some A&P students already have some skills in getting ideas into their short-term memories. Enough to pass the test. Then they relearn those ideas for the exam. But often, much of it is *gone* months or years down the road. *How can one get it all into long-term memory?*

The answer is easy ...

    Practice.

    Practice.

    Practice.

But what kinds of practice are helpful? Here a few aggressive methods for actively practicing your A&P concepts:

- ☑ **Answer the review questions found at the end of each chapter.** Write out the answers; don't just answer them in your head. The process of writing them out uses more parts of your brain and helps you to understand connections more clearly. It also helps you to remember concepts more easily later.

- ☑ **Do some or all of the activities in the study guide.** Often a study guide will accompany your A&P textbook and provide you with specific activities to work through the concepts of each chapter. Study guides help you to focus on what's important and promote active practice.

◇ SURVIVAL TIP

☑ The language of A&P really is a new, foreign language to most students. As I outlined in Study Skill 3, it really helps with vocabulary if you take a look at the word parts and their meanings, too. Many of my students have added this feature to their flash cards—and swear by it.

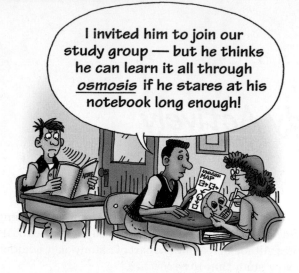

☑ **Keep up with the new vocabulary.** A number of years ago, a language professor published an article that stated that A&P students learn more new words than students in a freshman foreign language course! By far the easiest way to work on this new vocabulary is by making and using flash cards.

Write the term on one side of an index card and the meaning on the reverse side. Then simply review the deck of cards you'll have for each chapter. Don't try to cram with these cards; just look at the word, try to remember the meaning, and then check your answer by flipping the card over. Carry the deck with you, and review a few terms when you have a minute now and then. Some students tape their flash cards all over their homes so that they're constantly reviewing the material. If you tackle these new terms gradually but frequently, you'll know all the important words with hardly any effort!

Test your creativity by devising other vocabulary-strengthening activities. However, don't make the mistake of thinking that if you've mastered the vocabulary, you have a complete understanding of the topic. Vocabulary building is the *foundation,* not the whole thing.

☑ **Use computer-assisted tutorials, visualizations, and reviews.** Most A&P textbooks come with a link to a set of online study resources. Some of these are sort of like computer games, and they may make studying a little more fun. In addition, many stand-alone digital study resources for A&P are available on the Internet or in your college learning center or library. (For more hints, see the box about using digital devices to study A&P on page 45.)

☑ **Form a study group.** Get together with others in your course to discuss, review, and process A&P together. Ask each other test questions that you devise yourselves, and argue about the correct answers. Meet on a regular basis throughout the semester, not just before big tests or exams.

Using Flash Cards Effectively

Flash cards are commonly used to study the terms and basic facts in nearly *all* health science courses, not just A&P—so it's a good idea to develop advanced skills with flash cards now. There's a lot more to it than the flash cards you used in grade school to learn spelling and math facts!

Think about building your own *library* of flash cards over a lifetime. Because many terms, facts, and concepts come up later in the course and then in later courses, it's a good idea to keep them in a master set that is organized by subject or alphabetically. Steve Dina, one of my favorite professors, had a whole cabinet full of cards that he continued to use as he kept up with his specialty in biology.

A method of "adaptive" learning using flash cards is the Leitner System (LS). In this system, you arrange a set of boxes—let's say five in our example, marked A through E. After assembling the cards that you'll need to study, you put them all in the first box (box A). Then review the cards as described earlier. If you are successful with the first card, then put it into box B. If you didn't quite get it, then put it in the back of box A. That way, you'll see it again soon and can try the concept again.

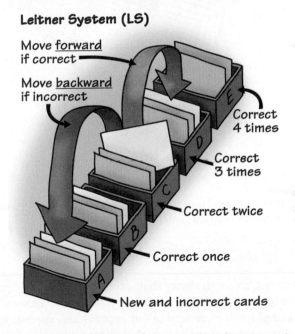

Leitner System (LS)

Move <u>forward</u> if correct

Move <u>backward</u> if incorrect

Correct 4 times

Correct 3 times

Correct twice

Correct once

New and incorrect cards

As you continue, successfully reviewed cards get pushed forward to the next box—but cards that give you trouble stay in the same box. Eventually, all of the cards from box A will have moved into box B. You then do the same thing again. This time, however, if you get a concept wrong, move the card back to box A (rather than keeping it in box B). Your review will probably go faster this time, because you've already had some success with all of these cards. Eventually, box B will be empty, and you can start over with box A, which should go even faster.

Keep going, moving the cards forward or back, until they've all made it through boxes B, C, and D into box E, which is the last box. You have now mastered this set of concepts! It's always a good idea to go back and review them all again later, but you're good to go for now.

Continued

✧ SPECIAL SURVIVAL SKILLS—cont'd

There are many variations of the Leitner System. The variation that I call *PALS*—Patton's Adapted Leitner System—works really well for A&P. Instead of using a bunch of boxes, you simply carry around a single deck of flash cards. As you work through them, correctly answered cards go all the way to the back of the deck, and incorrectly answered cards go somewhere in the middle. Those that you "almost" got can go further toward the back, and those that you really bombed should go closer to the front of the deck.

Patton's Adapted Leitner System (PALS)

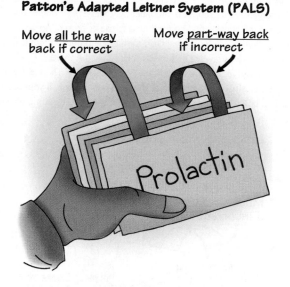

Move <u>all the way</u> back if correct

Move <u>part-way back</u> if incorrect

The PALS variation is not as precise the box-based system, but it works pretty much the same way, and it's more portable!

For more tips and turbo-charged methods of using flash cards to study A&P, check out the links, resources, and video *New Terms* (my-ap.us/TMTFZ1).

Believe it or not, research shows that attending a study group is one of the most effective learning strategies available! It helps if you have a group of people with mixed levels of natural talent or previous experience with the subject. The better students will learn more by teaching the weaker students; the weaker students will benefit from the peer tutoring by the better students. However, any mix of students should work.

> ■ Study groups are one of the most effective learning strategies.

How do you find study partners? I guess taking out an ad on Craigslist *might* work, but a safer bet is to just ask your lab partners or the people sitting near you in your A&P class if they would like to join a study group with you. If they're already in one, ask if you can join. If you're having trouble finding study partners, ask you professor or learning center to help.

For more advice on group study, please visit *Study Groups* (my-ap.us/116dblg).

☑ **Make a "concept map" of important concepts.** A *concept map* is a graphic representation of an idea that can take many forms. Here are a few examples of the different kinds of concept maps you might try:

1. ***Flow chart.*** A flow chart, such as the one shown on page 80 (Figure 1-6) in the second part of this book, shows the step-by-step process of building a protein. Figure 4-21 on page 313 shows yet another, simpler, style that pulls together many different concepts into one chart about blood flow. Many other examples of flow diagrams are provided in this book and in your textbook. How many can you find?

2. ***Circle diagram.*** A circle diagram is really just a flow chart in a circular arrangement. This is a favorite style among biologists, because so many biological processes are cycles (circles). Look at the examples on page 94 (Figure 1-10) of this book. Notice how the circle diagram is like a snake biting its tail: you always return to where you started.

3. ***Tree diagram.*** A tree diagram is really just an outline of topics and subtopics. To produce an outline such as the outline or summary found at the end of each textbook chapter, you have to know the organization and relationship of all of the ideas involved in a topic—making this is a great way to improve your understanding. If you incorporate sketches into your outline, you'll be even closer to a full understanding.

4. ***Full-color sketch.*** A sketch of a concept, especially if it involves colors, really kicks a lot of senses into gear to help you learn a concept. I know one student who draws out some concepts as a series of cartoon panels, as you might see in a comic book. I'm still pitching my editors with the idea that I'll someday produce a comic book version of our A&P text! Hey, if it works for *Classics Illustrated* and *Scientific American*—why not?

5. ***Tables.*** Create tables such as those found in Part 2 of this book. Such tables help you to draw information together in ways that show you *connections* between ideas. The simplest kind of table is called a *T-table* or a *T-chart.* Simply draw a huge letter "T" on a page, and then fill in your headings above the top bar and use the two regions below the bar as two columns to compare and contrast or to name and describe the concepts that you are studying. See *T-Charts* (my-ap.us/NPKtdd) for tips, examples, and links.

Be creative! Build concept maps out of clay, dough, or craft sticks. Paint a watercolor of the cell. Photograph or record your study partners acting out the citric acid cycle. Use your computer to animate the function of muscle cells. Have fun with it!

Your professor, learning center, or library will be able to help you learn how to do concept mapping. Visit *Concept Maps* (my-ap.us/YzQCEY) for examples, links, a video walk-through, and tips for making and using concept maps for A&P.

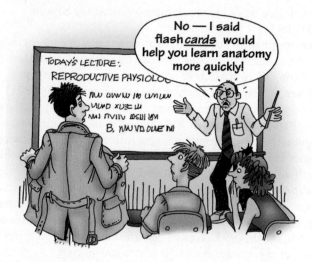

✧ SURVIVAL TIPS

☑ Tom Westfall, emeritus department chair at St. Louis University Medical School and a popular and award-winning teacher of pharmacology, suggests that his students learn drug names, their pharmacological classifications, and their actions by incorporating them into lyrics that can be sung to well-known melodies.

☑ When you have a particularly difficult concept or list of facts to deal with, try composing a poem or song that will help you learn it. The act of composing will help you organize your thoughts and understanding of the subject, and repeating the poem or song can help you remember the essential elements of the concept.

☑ Drawing diagrams and pictures of concepts is a great way to increase your understanding of those concepts. I've found that to be true as I sketch out the art concepts that I give to the illustrators of my A&P textbooks. My understanding is always clearer after drawing a picture or diagram because *I have to get the relationships right* before I can finish the picture.

☑ If you come up with a new idea for a diagram, table, or illustration that really helps you, send it to me. I may use your idea in the next edition of this book!

Use All Your Resources

9

Some learning resources are obvious: the textbook, the study guide, your notes, the professor, the course syllabus, and so on. Let's start with some of those:

☑ **Use your textbook resources.** Many students skip over the study aids that have been built into the chapters of their A&P textbooks. If you take the time to look them over and use them, you'll find that they actually help you to save time by quickly reinforcing your comprehension and learning of concepts. In addition, A&P textbooks also offer many online resources to help you learn A&P. Take the time at the beginning of your course to browse through these resources so that later you'll know what's available to help you.

☑ **Get to know your professors.** Getting to know your professors by chatting during office hours helps in a variety of ways. First, studies show that such contact improves your overall success in college. Second, it gives the opportunity for individualized mentoring. Mentoring helps you to grow as a student, the professor will often have specific advice to help you, and it opens a direct channel of communication for when you later need help quickly. An added bonus is that you are building your professional network, which can later help you obtain a scholarship, gain entry into an academic program, and perhaps even get a job.

☑ **Read the syllabus.** Many professors spend a lot of time and effort providing you with the information that you need to succeed right in the course syllabus. However, many students barely give the syllabus a glance, and even then it's usually only on the first day of the course. Refer to your syllabus often, and look for information and insights that can help you, including advice about how, where, and when to get help when you need it.

Other useful resources are often less obvious, so allow me to list some so that you don't miss any:

☑ **Teaching assistants, aides, and tutors.** Some colleges and universities provide tutors free of charge.

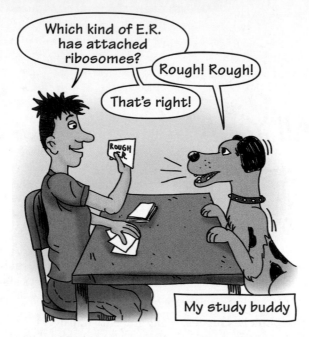

☑ **Study partners.** Classmates are the obvious choice, but other friends or family members can help you study. (Pets are unreliable study partners, in case you were wondering.)

☑ **Students who have recently taken the A&P course.** Consider organizing a group to find and recruit some former students who are willing to act as A&P coaches.

☑ **Campus learning center or library.** Besides providing study spaces, they may have books, media, and other resources (such as models, skeletons, or microscopes) specific to A&P. Perhaps even scheduled tutoring or study sessions.

☑ **Other A&P books.** Sometimes reading different wording and seeing different diagrams in an alternate A&P textbook can "shake things loose" for you when you are confused. Your library may have these books available. There are also many study guides available to help you to practice the concepts or offer insights into learning. For lab work, you may find anatomical atlases and medical references to be helpful.

☑ **Journals, newspapers, magazines, blogs, and related media.** Brief articles from *Science News, New Scientist, Discover,* and *Scientific American* are particularly useful for A&P students. Now would also be a good time to start reading professional journal articles to prepare you for your future career. Many of these have easy-to-read, brief articles of interest to A&P students at the beginning of each issue. To start, try subscribing to the free online articles from *Science* (my-ap.us/WyhAtP) and *Nature* (my-ap.us/ YiJxVE).

☑ **Video and related media.** Television series such as *Nova* and *Scientific American* as well as series and special programs from channels that are focused on science and learning are great resources. Check your college library or bookstore for videos in their collections that may help you. Check out my tips for getting the most out of YouTube video searches later in this chapter.

☑ **Study skills workshops.** Most colleges offer courses, seminars, and books that address study skills. No matter how good you already are, there is always something to learn from these courses. What surprises me is that many people—students and professionals alike—skip opportunities to learn how to learn more of what they need faster. Don't be one of those people!

◇ SURVIVAL TIP

☑ If you ever see the film *Fantastic Voyage* (amzn.to/Vse6aK) in your television listings or online video service, watch it! The special effects are really cheesy by today's standards, even though they won the film an Academy Award in 1966. However, the effects are good enough to show a neat concept for visualizing the inside of the human body. Use this imagery yourself, and take an imaginary fantastic voyage as you learn microscopic A&P. Other films that help you to visualize the inside of the body include *Innerspace* (amzn.to/YiSder), *Osmosis Jones* (amzn.to/UDAtuF), and *Antibody* (amzn.to/WyoHTb).

◇ SPECIAL SURVIVAL SKILLS

Using Your Digital Device to Study A&P

The widespread use of digital devices such as smartphones, tablets, advanced e-readers—in addition to personal and public computers—has revolutionized how we learn and study. You probably already use your digital device in some way in your own learning. You may have already taken my previous tips to heart and use it for time management, to signal study times, or to watch *Innerspace*.

But I'll bet there are still other ways to use these devices to improve your learning of A&P. Maybe these tips will spark some ideas:

☑ **Keeping and reviewing notes.**

Bring your device to class for note taking. But if you can't draw on your device, also have a paper notebook handy for drawing diagrams and sketches! Use a simple word processor to take your notes, and then store them on a cloud server so that you can access them anywhere.

Share your notes with classmates. Sharing your notes electronically by e-mail or by linking to files that are stored on a cloud server helps you and your classmates to catch things that each other may have missed. And it helps you catch up when you are sick and have to miss class or lab. You'll probably discover some note-taking methods that are used by other students that you'll want to adopt for yourself.

Continued

Highlight and mark up your notes. Most software lets you add highlights, hyperlinks, and embedded comments that help you to clarify or emphasize important concepts in your notes.

Illustrate your notes. Copy and paste illustrations from online sources of anatomical art, such as *Gray's Anatomy Online* (my-ap.us/Ya9uqj) or the *A&P Professor Image Library* (my-ap.us/a6RHQO).

Record written and audio notes. You're probably aware of the classic uses of your smartphone or digital recording device to record your teacher, yourself, or your study partners. Try using a recording pen such as Livescribe (my-ap.us/118AD2g) to record synchronized notes and audio that you can later review and share. You can even jump to a specific part of your notebook and hear the audio that is synched with that section! Check out my Livescribe Pencast example (my-ap.us/WRHLd1).

Clip notes from digital sources. Use a note database with a web-clipping function—such as the Evernote app (my-ap.us/14097f4)—to save useful written, video, and audio tidbits from your course website, from digital notes shared by others, and from virtually any other digital source.

☑ **Use a digital textbook.**

In addition to being a good value, digital textbooks—or e-textbooks—are amazing study tools. Most textbooks are available for a variety of platforms, thereby allowing you to continue using them as you move from one device to the next. They usually have built-in tools for highlighting, sharing your highlights, making and sharing comments and notes, clipping sections into a customized study guide, and more. My favorite feature is the ability to search the entire book quickly for every mention of a particular topic or specific concept—saving a lot of time looking here and there in a paper book.

☑ **Use programs and apps specifically designed for learning A&P.**

There are a great variety of tools available for a range of digital devices that allow you to visualize human A&P, to practice learning concepts, and more. Some are simple apps that focus on a specific concept or skill, whereas others are full-blown suites of powerful learning tools. Look around at what others in your class are using, or ask your professor for suggestions. Research your choice carefully—not all programs are as useful as they first appear to be! For example, some are geared for advanced students and professionals, whereas others are meant for little kids.

☑ **Use programs and apps that are not specifically for A&P.**

Use a flow-charting program to create concept maps. Many concept-mapping or mind-mapping tools are available. Flow-charting software for business is great for making concept maps. Software programs for illustration, drawing, and presentations often have built-in concept-mapping tools. For example, Microsoft Office's WordArt tools are great for concept mapping. Simple painting or drawing programs that are probably on your computer somewhere can also be very useful for making concept maps. Start online with Text 2 Mindmap (my-ap.us/WfWMYv), then try some of the others listed at *Concept Maps* (my-ap.us/YzQCEY).

Use software suites. Google Drive (my-ap.us/14sfiic) includes a free suite of word processing, presentation, and illustration tools that let you both store your work on a

✦ **SPECIAL SURVIVAL SKILLS—cont'd**

cloud drive and share your notes and concept maps with others. Other similar suites are also available.

Use digital flash-card systems. Flash-card apps and websites can make the adaptive learning described on page 37 fast, easy, and convenient. One example is Study Blue (my-ap.us/14wCexJ), an online flash card resource also available as a mobile app. Find more at *New Terms* (my-ap.us/TMTFZ1) and *Flash Cards* (my-ap.us/LzuowE).

Use digital references as well as scientific and medical software. Elsevier and other publishers have a variety of computer programs about related topics that may help you with A&P. For example, medical terminology and medical dictionary programs or databases will help to you learn the language of A&P. Medical, nursing, and allied health titles might help, as will certain health, physical education, and sports titles. For example, check out the anatomy resources at InteractElsevier (my-ap.us/UDWN7D).

☑ **Use your course digital resources.**

Use your textbook's digital resources. Nearly all A&P textbooks include digital resources such as audio summaries, audio pronunciation lists, practice questions, related articles and links, and a variety of useful learning tools that you'll miss out on if you skip them.

Use your course learning system. If your course uses a learning management system or has a course website, then don't skip any optional resources, such as discussion forums, wikis, chat rooms, and so on. You may be missing some helpful tips and advice.

☑ **Don't forget YouTube.**

YouTube (my-ap.us/TYKQLR) and similar video sharing services such as TeacherTube (my-ap.us/XT4Yul) have a huge collection of videos to help you study A&P. Check out The A&P Student Videos (my-ap.us/12anuoF) and Kevin Patton's YouTube channel (my-ap.us/VotXFA) to get started. Simply type your specific concept or study skill into the search bar to find a lot of help from other A&P teachers and students.

✦ **SURVIVAL TIP**

☑ You can save a lot of money on your trip through the A&P jungle by looking for free or low-cost options when hunting for resources. For example, your college may offer free tutoring and workshops—or discounted software deals. A lot of software for learning A&P on the Internet is free or very low cost. Save money on your textbook by opting for digital or binder-ready versions, which are great values. Do NOT *rent* your A&P textbook, though—you'll need it for many years to come as you progress through your next courses!

10 Prepare for Tests

preparing for a safari, *going* on the safari, and *coming back* from the safari are all part of a safe and successful adventure. Likewise, a safe and successful experience with A&P tests and exams requires three sets of strategies:

1. What you do *before* the test.
2. What you do *during* the test.
3. What you do *after* the test.

In this chapter, I'll give you a few tips on *preparing* for tests. Then, in the next chapter, we'll move on to what to do *during* and *after* a test.

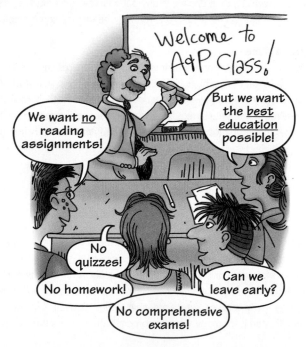

Obviously, you prepare for tests by studying the appropriate course material. We've already covered many strategies for doing that. However, a few special tricks may help you to deal with the testing situation itself. Following are some of tips that I have found to be the most useful.

☑ **Practice taking the test.** Sometimes professors provide sample questions or previous editions of an A&P test. Sample test questions may also appear in the study guide that accompanies your textbook. If you anticipate test questions in the style that your professor uses—which you can do after a test or two—then you can then make up your own questions and practice them with each other in your study group.

✧ SURVIVAL TIPS

☑ Practice taking essay (long-answer) tests by anticipating possible test questions (such as those at the back of each chapter in the textbook) and *writing out the answers*. As advised previously, writing out each answer exercises your brain in a whole different way than just answering review questions in your head. In addition, your written answers give you something to review later during your study process.

☑ My friend and former composition teacher Ron Giedinghagen always made us write all of our practice essays during a 50-minute class. This forced us to learn how to sketch out our ideas, organize our points, write the darn thing, and then proofread it in the shortest possible time. Practice writing essays under timed conditions, and you'll gain a very valuable skill. You'll also find yourself thinking more clearly when faced with test questions.

☑ **Stay healthy.** Don't overtax yourself by studying (especially doing any last-minute cramming) to a point that makes you sick, sleepy, or otherwise unable to operate at peak efficiency. Many students use extra caffeine or other stimulants to keep them awake as they study the night before an exam or even while taking the test. If you take caffeine (in coffee or soft drinks, for example) then use the normal amount and stay away from other stimulants.

☑ **Eat right.** As stated earlier in this book, consuming a lot of carbohydrates (especially sugars and starches) right before an exam will make you feel sleepy and make it hard to focus.

☑ **Be comfortable.** Within the limits of your particular situation, dress as comfortably as possible, and find a portion of the test room that suits you. Don't wear new shoes or a pair of pants that are too tight on test day!

✧ SURVIVAL TIP

☑ Prepare mnemonic devices (memory helpers) to help you learn lists of concepts. More information about this method is provided later in this book (see pages 60 and 160).

☑ **Make a final review of important concepts.** This review should be just a refresher right before the test; it should not be the first time that you look at the material in preparation for the test. Cramming is very seldom an effective strategy.

> ■ **Cramming is not an effective strategy.**

☑ **Get your head right.** Just before the test, clear your mind, and ask yourself, "Can I do this?" Try to find a positive answer by thinking about the practicing and other preparation that you've done. Try to get to a point where you are comfortable telling yourself, "I can do this!"

◆ SPECIAL SURVIVAL SKILLS

Test Anxiety

Nervousness during a test is something that we've all experienced. Generally, it's a *good* thing. Really! A bit of stress during a test of our knowledge or skills helps to keep our mind sharp and focused on the "threat" of a question—thereby helping us to answer it successfully. However, I think we've all had occasions when the stress was *too much*. We became so anxious during a test that it adversely affected our performance. Following are some proven tips for avoiding or managing such test anxiety.

☑ **Be prepared.** You will be much less likely to become overly anxious if you have the confidence that comes with good preparation for a test. If you've practiced possible test questions enough to be good at them and asked your teacher what to expect, then you won't be so nervous.

☑ **Write out your thoughts.** Studies show that, if you write out your thoughts on paper just before a test, you'll be less likely to become anxious and thus do better on the test. The action of writing along with sorting out your thoughts helps you to focus more on the positive than on the negative—an important skill we learned in the first chapter (see page 3). Learn more at *Trick to reduce test anxiety* (my-ap.us/XdoVes).

☑ **No last-minute cramming.** Before the test, don't sit with the crowd outside the classroom door frantically going over your notes. The anxiety that bubbles up in those groups—I can practically *feel* it as I walk by—does far more harm than good. Take a leisurely walk to gaze out the window or to watch the fish in the aquarium instead.

☑ **Don't forget to breathe.** If you find yourself getting anxious during a test, stop and close your eyes. Focus only on your breathing. Slow your rate of breathing gradually to about five breaths per minute, stretching out the exhalation as much as possible; pursing your lips slightly helps to slow exhalation. This will "reset" your stress response to the relaxation response. This technique works even better if you practice it daily. Learn more at *Don't forget to breathe!* (my-ap.us/dIdsS9).

☑ **Get help.** If your test anxiety is a real block to your performance and if it occurs frequently, then you can benefit by getting help from a professional who is trained to deal with test anxiety. Many colleges have such help available, or you can find a counselor on your own. It's worth it, isn't it, if it gives you a life skill that will help you to succeed?

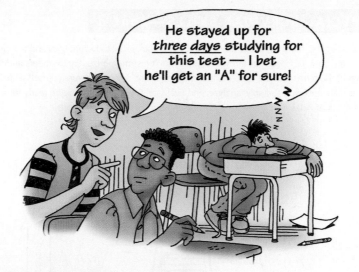

✧ SPECIAL SURVIVAL SKILLS

Climbing the Learning Pyramid

Imagine coming to a clearing in the jungle to find a huge, breathtaking pyramid. You notice steep steps that lead to a small platform at the top. You just know that taking in the view from the top of that pyramid will be an experience of a lifetime. You find the climb a bit tricky at first, and it's difficult to get your footing right on the narrow, steep steps. A few of the stones are loose or oddly shaped, and you have to regain your footing. As you climb higher, you find that it's not as easy as it was at first. Some stones are missing, and you have to figure out how to move higher without falling. The air is getting thinner, so you feel more worn out than expected—and you are finding it harder to focus. Finally, you reach the top! The view is magnificent. You can see so much more than you were able to when you were on the ground. You appreciate the clarity of the view, seeing things you would never see nor know otherwise, even more because of the great effort and perseverance put into the tricky climb to the top.

The learning pyramid—also called *Bloom's Taxonomy of Learning*—is an often-used model of how we all learn. As we learn new concepts, we must all start at the bottom of the pyramid, learning the basic facts. These facts provide the necessary, broad foundation. However, such facts are basically useless until we climb higher, where we gain an understanding of the meaning of those facts, learn to apply them, use them to analyze and evaluate different situations, and eventually find creative solutions to problems. It's hard enough to learn a large number of basic facts, but climbing higher can be very tricky and force us to deal with unexpected twists and missing information. If we want to succeed, however, we must stick to it and climb higher by overcoming the tricky parts—gaining more skills for dealing with those tricky parts as we climb.

> ■ Memorizing facts is the *first* step to learning, not the *last* step.

Continued

If you keep this model in mind, it will help to you plan your study strategies and test preparation. Start with the basic facts, such as terminology, but don't just memorize. Try to understand the meanings of the terms and the concepts that they represent. Then challenge yourself with "trick questions" that force you to apply, analyze, and evaluate. Only then will you be ready for a test that contains a mix of fact-based questions and "higher-order" or "tricky" questions.

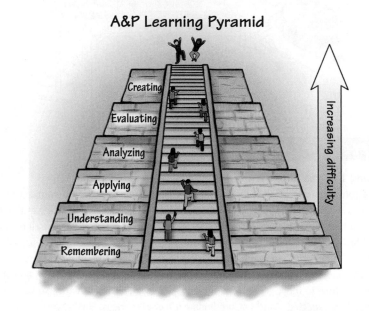

A&P Learning Pyramid

Creating

Evaluating

Analyzing

Applying

Understanding

Remembering

Increasing difficulty

11

Use Test-Taking Strategies During and After the Test

O nce you have begun the examination, you should still be implementing a strategy. Test taking is more than just passively spewing forth information. Rather, it's a process that requires thought, skill, and action. Many A&P students have found these *during-test strategies* to be useful:

☑ **Read the instructions.** Really, read them! So many students don't read the directions for a test because they're so anxious to get moving on the test itself. However, the instructions often include key items that will help you while you are taking the test and avoid the frustrations of not being able to figure out how to fill out your test forms.

☑ **Know the testing style.** Do what you can to find out specifics about the test's construction (for example, the format of the test, the number of items, the time given to complete the test, the wording of the test items, the level of complexity).

☑ **Skim over the test before you answer any questions.** Remember, read the directions for the entire test first. Next, briefly look at the style and content of all of the questions. It only takes a couple of minutes, and you'll know exactly what you're up against.

☑ **Skip questions that stump you.** If you come across a puzzling question, save it for later (when you know better how much time you can devote to it). It's not worth fretting over one question when it's eating up time that you could be spending on questions that you're able to answer well.

☑ **Know how to evaluate objective items logically.** Your college learning center should be able to provide you with some help learning how to apply principles of logic to objective tests. If you can't find help there, ask your librarian. Librarians *always* know where to find help!

☑ **Understand the nature of each item.** Is it a fill-in, matching, or multiple-choice section? Short answer or long answer (essay)? Are there any special

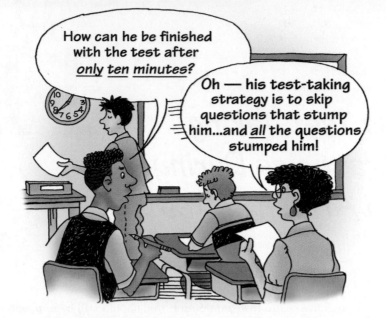

instructions? Is there more than one correct answer? Can the same answer appear more than once? Must the answer be written in complete sentences?

☑ **Analyze the wording.** Watch for key qualifying words, such as *all, every, always, never, sometimes, often,* and *usually.* Underline them. Absolute qualifiers such as *always* and *never* in a TRUE/FALSE item usually make the statement false. Determine whether the answer should be singular or plural, as well as the part of speech (noun, verb, adverb, adjective). If any part of a TRUE/FALSE item is false, *then the entire statement is false.* In essay questions or short-answer questions, look for key words such as *compare* (tell how things are alike), *contrast* (tell how things are different), *interpret* (give your explanation or meaning), and *discuss* (give a complete account). Your campus learning center may have a list of such words and their exact meanings.

☑ **Eliminate choices.** If several choices are offered (or occur to you) and all seem likely to be correct, try to eliminate those that are *least likely*. Such analysis may trigger a thought that leads you to the correct choice.

☑ **If you have to, guess.** If blank answers are scored the same as wrong guesses and you're really stumped, guess anyway. If you studied, your answer will be an *informed* guess, which is certainly better than a blank.

☑ **Plan your answers.** Essay and short-answer questions require a logical presentation if you want the maximum points from the grader. I find it easiest to jot down a brief outline of the answer first—just a list of phrases that summarize the main points. Take a quick look at your micro-outline. Do the points flow in a logical order that leads to your main point? If not, rearrange them. After you have a clear micro-outline, write out your answer.

☑ **Understand the directions.** This is especially important for this type of item, because it will determine the approach you take when planning your response. Amazingly, many students *don't even read the directions!* How much more strongly can I emphasize the importance of doing this? Don't assume that you know how the professor wants you to fill out the test just because you recognize the format.

There's the famous story of the incredibly difficult exam that one student finished, with a perfect score, in only 2 minutes. The directions on that test ended with the phrase, "and only answer one item, of your choosing, out of the 200 items given here." Only that one student bothered to read the directions thoroughly enough to see it. I think this is probably one of those mythical campus legends, but it makes a good point!

☑ **Understand the question.** Although key words are important, they're not the question itself. Take some time to mull over the question to be sure that you know what the question is really asking. If you don't understand the question or if you don't understand the directions, then ask your professor or the test proctor. Unless you've been instructed to not ask questions, any question that you ask is worth asking—it might make the difference in whether you answer the test question correctly.

☑ **Start with a thesis statement.** A thesis statement is simply a sentence that summarizes the core of your answer succinctly. Usually a rephrasing of the question makes a suitable thesis statement.

☑ **Arrange your points logically.** After stating your thesis, support it with a series of paragraphs (or sentences) that back it up. Organize these paragraphs in a manner that presents the material in the most convincing way possible.

☑ **If possible, make a concluding statement.** A restatement of the thesis (although not in exactly the same words) works best. A concluding remark is a good style point, and it allows you to emphasize your main point.

☑ **Don't dance around the central issue.** Many students feel that weaving circles around an issue that they don't understand completely will fool the grader into believing that they do understand it. It's likely that the grader will not only see that critical content is missing but also that he or she will become irritated with the student. Irritating the grader is not a good strategy for subjectively graded items!

✧ SURVIVAL TIP

☑ My friend Mary Ellen Whitehead gives her students this nifty RACES method for dealing with multiple-choice items:

R̲ead the question carefully.

A̲nalyze the question to see what's really being asked.

C̲ircle any words that might affect the meaning of the question (such as *except, not*).

E̲liminate as many choices as you can.

S̲elect the best choice from the remaining items.

As soon as you walk out of a test, you should then begin employing your *after-test strategies.* These are often ignored by most students, but they could be the *most critical thing you do for success* in the course. Here are some suggestions:

☑ **Dissect the test as soon as it's over.** Some students plan to meet up as they exit a test so that they can "debrief" each other about what happened. This is sort of an autopsy of the test. Which items were hardest? Which were easiest? Why? Write everything down, including all of the items and topics that you can remember—while it's all still fresh in your memory. Doing this as a group helps you to remember more, and it also gives you different perspectives. Discussing a test as soon as it's over will help you to better prepare for the next test.

☑ **Analyze each test.** When you get your graded test back, don't just glance at it. Thoroughly analyze what went wrong and what went right. Were there specific concepts that you messed up? Were there whole topics that were missing from your preparation? Are there specific types of questions that give you trouble? Some students make a grid that lists the items that they missed on each test. Such a grid helps you to visualize any patterns that you may not have noticed.

☑ **Fix what's broken.** If you thoughtfully evaluate your test analysis, you'll likely find some weak spots. The next step is to strengthen those areas. Do you need better test-taking skills? Do you need to work more on test anxiety? Are there concepts that you have yet to master? All of these issues can be fixed by going back and getting help with them. Sometimes, you may just need more practice with them. By the way, don't just blow off going back to re-learn concepts from a previous test because you think you won't need them again. In A&P, you *will* need them again. They'll probably pop up again later in A&P, and you'll certainly see them again in later courses.

☑ **Maintain what's not broken.** Don't ignore those concepts or test skills that you mastered for a particular test. Give some thought to what gave you that success. What preparation did you do? Were there new strategies you tried that seem to help you? Thinking this through and perhaps even jotting your ideas in a notebook will help you to refine your study strategies, improve your success, and trim the time that it takes you to study.

✧ SURVIVAL TIPS

☑ For more help with test-taking strategies and resources, visit *Taking Tests* (my-ap.us/VBLaAx).

☑ For strategies to use when taking online tests, visit *Online Tests* (my-ap.us/WlaWye).

☑ For test analysis tips, including a sample test analysis grid, visit *Test Item Analysis* (my-ap.us/WFR8io).

☑ For strategies to employ when taking lab tests, see Survival Skill 12.

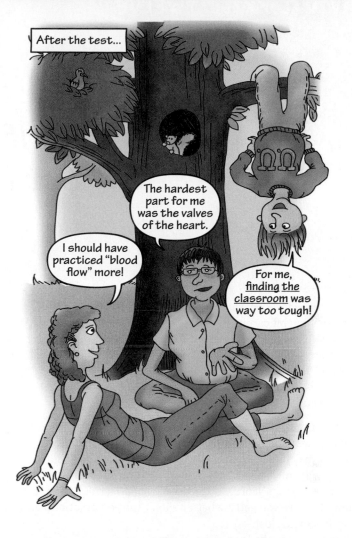

12

What To Do If You Get Lost

*E*xpect to get lost occasionally. Anyone who has traveled on a safari—or even on a daytrip off campus—can tell you that this happens. If you know what to do, you can get back on the right track—and perhaps even have an adventure along the way. If you don't know what to do, it could be dangerous, and you may never find your way back.

So, what *do* you do when you find yourself lost in your A&P course? Here are some possible strategies for getting back on track:

☑ **Try not to get lost in the first place.** Keep track of your progress—not on a map, but by keeping a record of your scores and other indicators of your progress. It may be as simple as regularly checking your course's online grade book, or it may involve keeping your own scorecard and continually updating your current average score. I suggest also keeping track of your progress with your practice. Are you getting better each time you practice a concept? If not, you may be getting lost.

☑ **Admit when you are lost.** A lot of people have trouble with this one. You've heard something like this before: "No, I'm not lost . . . it's got to be around here someplace!" Yeah, maybe, but probably not. If you get help *right away*, you'll get back on track before you get so lost it's hard to get back.

☑ **Check the map.** Your syllabus and your textbook are your primary maps. Go back and look at them again. Is there something that you missed? Do you need to review a section or two? Do you have supplemental maps, such as study guides, online resources, lab manuals, that you can check?

☑ **Ask your guide.** Guide? What guide? Your professor, of course. Some students have the idea that the professor's place is up at the front of the class and that's it. Nope. We A&P professors want you ask us for help when you get lost. You don't have to apologize for taking up our time—it's our job to help you when you need it. We're surprised and dismayed that more students don't ask us for help. Just ask. Really.

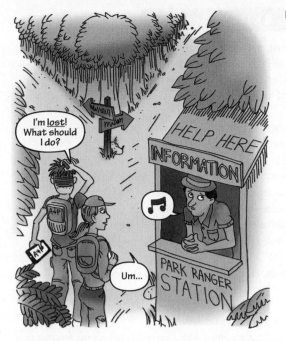

☑ **Join the auto club.** Not the *auto* club, but its academic equivalent. Your college probably has a learning center or library with staff and resources to help you when you get lost in any course, including A&P. They often have special programs to help students, including workshops and study skills courses that could get you back on the right track. These resources and programs are often free or very low cost. And often underused by the students that can use them.

☑ **Don't think you won't get lost.** My dad, who was a frequent traveler, always said, "You can't get lost if you are in a car, plane, or ship." However, he got lost a lot. Even the most experienced and talented traveler gets lost sometimes. If you get stubborn and think, "I can't be lost, I've never gotten lost!" then you are in big trouble. I can't tell you how many times we A&P professors hear, "But I'm getting an A in all my other courses!" A&P is a rigorous journey, and even the best students get off track occasionally. The trick—and you already know this—is to admit when you are lost and then ask your guide for help.

✦ SPECIAL SURVIVAL SKILLS

English as a Second Language

If English is not your primary language, A&P could prove especially difficult. In A&P, we tend to use the English vocabulary of science rather than the conversational English that may be more familiar to you. In other words, it's English, but it's not ordinary English—it's a Latin-based terminology system, as I described in Survival Skill 3.

For some of you who already speak a Latin-based language, the terminology of A&P may come quickly to you—and you may even be able to help coach some of the native English speakers in your class. However, you'll still have some extra work to do to manage the use of those terms in English conversation, in your textbook reading, and on your tests and exams.

Here are some tips that may make things go better for you:

☑ **Take advantage of ESL-friendly textbook features.** Many A&P textbooks provide lists of new words in each chapter and often pronunciation guides as well. Perhaps there are even audio pronunciations and audio chapter summaries available online with

Continued

✧ SPECIAL SURVIVAL SKILLS—cont'd

your textbook resources. If not, it may be worth investing in a second A&P book that is easier for you to use. Some ESL students have found that an A&P textbook in their primary language is a good option for a supplement to help them understand the course's textbook. Check first to see if there is an existing translation of your course's A&P text.

☑ **Take it slow.** Don't put off your reading or your review of your notes. The sooner you get started with that, the slower you can take it.

☑ **Ask questions.** As you read or review your notes, write down any questions that you have. Regularly take these questions to your professor during office hours to get help. You can also ask questions of other students in your class.

☑ **Join or organize a study group.** The very best way for those who are having difficulty with English to succeed in A&P is to join a study group that includes native English speakers. By helping you, they'll be gaining some improvement themselves, so *everybody* benefits!

☑ **Use your college ESL resources.** Even if you usually prefer to "do it on your own," now is not the time to be stubborn. Your college may already have an ESL program or counselors that can help you. There may also be some student support groups to help you find the resources or strategies you need.

☑ **Use the Internet to help you.** Occasionally, looking up a concept on the Internet in your primary language can help get you over a rough spot. You'll still need to learn it and think it in English. However, studying in your native language may help you when you need extra assistance. Likewise, you may want to use online translation services to get you through a rough spot.

✧ SURVIVAL TIP

☑ For more advice and links for non-native English speakers, visit *ESL* (my-ap.us/11zVq9y).

✧ SPECIAL SURVIVAL SKILLS

The Student Laboratory

The laboratory portion of the typical A&P course is in some ways a unique beast. I've collected a few ideas for how to make the student laboratory the best possible experience:

☑ **Safety is always first!** Do you remember me mentioning that I used to be a lion tamer? Lion tamers are sticklers for safety. Lion taming seems like a foolhardy and reckless occupation, but the reality is far different. Lion tamers never take a step into the cage without every possible safety precaution being in place. We are absolute tyrants about safety! Why? Because one little mistake often means death. My friends the Flying Wallendas of high-wire fame are the same way about safety precautions. The only people that I know of who are pickier about safety are scientists, for the same reason. A mistake in the lab—even a student lab—can make you as dead as

✧ SPECIAL SURVIVAL SKILLS—cont'd

my friend, Wayne Franzen, who was killed by one of his tigers when he wore an unfamiliar new costume that startled his cats, or as Karl Wallenda, who fell to his death from the high wire as a result of a badly rigged cable.

I've seen or heard of far too many preventable injuries in student labs, and they are awful. So *please* heed all of the safety precautions printed in your lab manuals, posted in your labs, and articulated or published by your school or your professor. In addition, use common sense.

☑ **Use the "field method" to identify anatomic structures.** Roger Tory Peterson, the famous naturalist and birder, developed a method for the field identification of birds that has since been used for everything from identifying sparrows to spotting enemy aircraft. The Peterson method focuses on "field marks": these are the one or two characteristics that distinguish particular birds or airplanes from similar birds or airplanes. I used this method to tell the difference between my lions: one had a scar on the nose, another had a notch in his ear, and yet another had an odd color to his mane. Simply approach tissues, bones, bone markings, muscles, and other structures that you need to identify in lab courses as you would animals in the field. Focus on the one or two characteristics that make a certain tissue different from all of the others.

Peterson's method also makes use of range maps that show where different birds are likely to be found. Do the same with lab specimens. Where are adductor muscles likely to be found? They are found on the insides of the limbs. So where would you start looking for the adductor longus?

Use a little tip from field geography, too. It could take you all day to find the Mississippi River on a map if you have no clue what a river is. When learning bone markings, how can you find the supraorbital foramen when you have no idea what a foramen is? Study types of things—like types of muscles, types of bones, and so on—before studying the specific examples assigned to you.

☑ **Remember that the laboratory is a playground.** Yes, the laboratory is a place to explore, but this doesn't mean that you should just goof around for no good reason. It does mean that labs are intended to be fun, hands-on opportunities to play with specimens, models, and experimental equipment. Therefore, approach it that way. Don't just try to get by with the minimum activity. If you linger and look a little deeper or turn the model around this way and then another way, you'll find a deeper understanding of what you were supposed to find and discover the connections that help you to draw concepts together into the *big picture*. Kinesthetic (tactual) learners will especially benefit from this aspect of the lab course, often in ways that bring home points from the lecture or discussion portions of the course.

☑ **Use flash cards.** Flash cards are especially useful for certain lab activities. My students like to draw pictures of lab specimens on one side of a card and then put the name or description on the other side. I even had one student who brought in a camera and took photos of her dissections so that she could make flash cards! Your cell phone may have a camera—feel free to use it as a learning tool in the lab.

Continued

✧ SPECIAL SURVIVAL SKILLS—cont'd

☑ **Use mnemonic devices.** Archeologists have recently uncovered evidence that mnemonic devices were used by the ancient Greeks thousands of years ago in their famous schools. You may have seen one of those famous memory experts that can spout off of all the names on a page in the phone book by using mnemonic devices. Mnemonic devices are little sayings or mental images that you use to help you remember a concept.

For example, the acronym *IPMAT* has been used by generations of students to help them learn the phases of the cell cycle: <u>i</u>nterphase, <u>p</u>rophase, <u>m</u>etaphase, <u>a</u>naphase, and <u>t</u>elophase. The mnemonic sentence *"On old Olympus's tiny tops, a friendly Viking grew vines and hops,"* is listed in this book as a mnemonic for learning the names (in order) of the 12 pairs of cranial nerves. Each word in the phrase begins with the same letter as the name of a cranial nerve. You can find it in the note following Table 3-8. A far raunchier version exists that I won't share here, but maybe you can figure one out.

The sillier the phrase or mental image you use—or perhaps the more ribald—the easier it is to remember and the more useful it is as a memory aid.

Although mnemonic devices are useful as you begin to learn new material, you want to continue practicing to the point that you don't need them anymore. A mnemonic aid is like a crutch that is used when you have a broken leg: you want to progress to the point where you can walk without it.

☑ **Dissect like an artist.** Some of the best anatomists have in fact also been great artists; I don't know of any anatomists who were also axe murderers. I don't think this is purely coincidental. Artistic finesse when pulling apart structures without destroying them or removing them from their relative position in the body is far more effective than the hacking style of an axe murderer. Your goal is to find structures so that you can understand how the body is constructed, not to make hamburger in the shortest possible time.

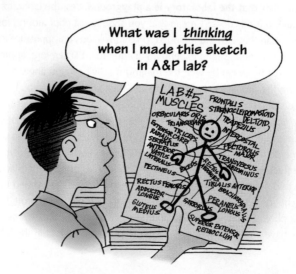

✦ SPECIAL SURVIVAL SKILLS—cont'd

☑ **You don't have to be a great sketch artist.** However, you should *sketch a lot*. Draw everything! Don't sweat and slave over creating a masterpiece—even if you're capable of creating a masterpiece (wait until after lab and work on your masterpiece over the weekend). However, do take enough time with it so that you can recognize key features later on when you use your sketches to study. In addition, label as much as you can. A sketch without any labels is pretty useless, except maybe as a coaster.

☑ **Come to the lab prepared.** Read what you will be doing in lab *before you do it*. If you don't come prepared, then half of the time spent in the lab will be spent just trying to figure out what to do. The other half of your time will be spent trying to rush through the activity without any appreciation of the concepts behind it. Preparation also means reading the portions of the textbook that relate to the lab activity. Preparation is probably the greatest key to using the student lab to its greatest potential.

☑ **Use many resources.** When you're trying to find anatomic specimens or interpret results from a physiology demonstration or experiment, don't rely solely on your textbook and lab manual. Often, your specimen will not look like the pictures in these books. No organ or tissue looks exactly like any other. Therefore, find out where you can purchase or borrow a lab atlas, an anatomy atlas, a histology book, and other useful resources. In addition, many useful resources for A&P lab can be found on the Internet (you can use a search engine to find them). Here's one to start with *Learning Anatomy in the Lab* (my-ap.us/YspQdQ).

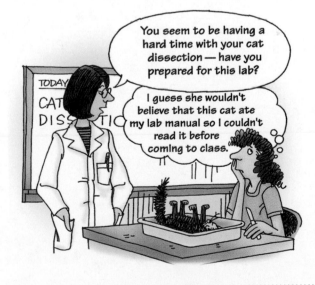

✧ SURVIVAL TIP

☑ My friend Mary Ellen Whitehead offers the FIRST strategy for developing mnemonic sentences:

        Form a word.
        Insert the letters.
        Rearrange the letters.
        Shape a sentence.
        Try combinations.

PART 2

Maps, Charts, and Shortcuts

When you're on safari, among your most valuable tools are your field guides. Field guides are handy pocket references that help you to quickly identify plants, animals, minerals, stars, and other natural features that you see on your safari. Each guide may include labeled illustrations or photographs, range maps of where a particular feature is likely to be found, and checklists to keep track of what you've seen.

This **Maps, Charts, and Shortcuts** section is a brief field guide to the human body that lays out the essential anatomic maps, functional diagrams, and summary tables needed for a basic understanding of human structure and function.

> ■ This Survival Guide is *not* a comprehensive review of A&P. Rather, it is a guide that will show you important landmarks and shortcuts that you can use alongside your textbook, lab manual, class notes, and other learning materials.

We begin in Chapter 1 with some the basic "lay of the land": the stuff the body is made of, the anatomic directions, the names of the body parts and systems, and a rough idea of how the body stays balanced. In later chapters, we'll find maps and lists that will help us explore each of the major territories of the body. These tools will bring topics into focus and clarify difficult concepts.

This section is organized into the major themes covered in a typical human A&P course. These may be presented in a slightly different order than they are in your textbook or course, but you will have no difficulty finding them. Where appropriate, analogies and other tips that illustrate complex topics or that help you to avoid hazards as you trek through the A&P jungle are briefly outlined in boxed sidebars called *Field Notes*.

✦ FIELD NOTES

Using Models and Analogies

Professional scientists use models and analogies all the time to explain complex concepts, so it's no wonder that models and analogies are used so often when teaching A&P—they work!

A **model** is a simplified version or description of something. For example, a model airplane is a simpler version of an airplane. It's a lot smaller than the real airplane, and it has far fewer parts and details than the real airplane. However, a model airplane can teach you a great deal about a real airplane, especially if you've never seen one before. Although in many respects the model is not at all like the real airplane, it's similar enough to teach you something about the real airplane. Likewise, when a scientist talks about the lock-and-key model of enzyme action, you can imagine that the enzyme molecule acts like a key in a lock when it interacts with a specific molecule to either break it apart from (unlock it) or put it together with another molecule (lock it up). An enzyme isn't really a key, but the model of a key in a lock works to demonstrate how enzymes really do work.

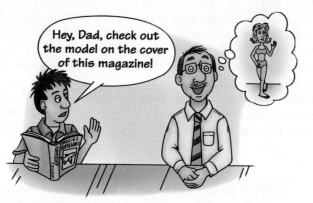

An **analogy** compares something with which you're familiar to something with which you're not familiar in order to explain it. It really is a way of using something as a model that probably doesn't seem to resemble the real thing at first glance. For example, going to school is like driving a car. As with driving, schoolwork requires that you "stay on the road" and don't stray from the path defined by your learning objectives. As with driving, if you go too fast or too slow (or become distracted), you will not be able to keep up with "traffic" (the pace of learning in your course). Thus, the idea of driving a car becomes a way for us to understand schoolwork in a different way.

In science, we often use analogies to help explain how something works. For example, parts of the immune system act like the military. There is nonspecific (innate) immunity that includes many general strategies that you would use against any invader. In the military, that could be bullets from your gun, defensive walls, and alarms that sound if there's an attack. In the body, it includes your defensive skin, the mucous membranes, the phagocytic cells that gobble up invading particles, and the chemicals that are released to sound an alarm in your body. Specific (acquired) immunity occurs when we develop specific mechanisms to combat specific invaders. In the military, we may develop special artillery to use against the armor of a specific enemy or use a unique plan of attack with an enemy that is not susceptible to more common forms of attack. Actually, this analogy has many elements of similarity; perhaps you can think of some yourself.

The great thing about analogies is that, because they are familiar and different from the new concept that we are trying to learn, they make it easy to remember the various elements of the new concept and to understand how it works in a simplified way.

This book uses the analogy of a safari—a voyage of discovery—to describe some successful ways to study A&P. We don't really come across any wild animals, swamps, or thick jungles in our course, but the analogy will be useful as we learn some "survival skills" that will really help us throughout our course.

1

The Body as a Whole

Navigation Guide

A. Science Methods

Anatomy and **physiology** are sciences. Science is a logical approach to studying nature. In **life science**, we study the nature of living organisms; in **physical science**, we study the nature of the nonliving physical universe. Thus, anatomy is a logical approach to studying structure and physiology is a logical approach to studying function.

This section outlines a few essential tools in understanding anatomy and physiology within the broader umbrella of life science.

The Scientific Method

Using detailed observations and vigorous tests, or *experiments*, scientists winnow out each element of an idea or **hypothesis** until a reasonable conclusion about its validity can be made. Rigorous experiments that eliminate any influences or biases that are not being directly tested are called *controlled experiments*. If the results of observations and experiments are repeatable, they may verify a hypothesis and eventually lead to enough confidence in the concept to call it a **theory**. Theories in which scientists have an unusually high level of confidence are sometimes called *laws*. Experiments may disprove a hypothesis, which often leads to the formation of new hypotheses to be tested.

Figure 1-1 summarizes some of the basic concepts of how new scientific principles are developed. As you can see, science is a dynamic process of getting closer and closer to the truth about nature, including the nature of the human body. Science is definitely not a set of unchanging facts, as many people in our culture often assume.

FIGURE 1-1
Scientific Method.

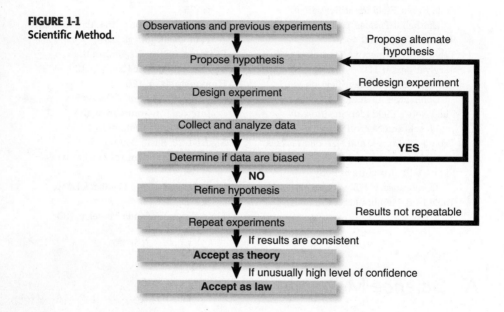

Levels of Organization

Knowledge of the different levels of organization—from the smallest parts of the body to the largest parts—will help you to understand the basic concepts of human A&P. The smallest parts of the body are the atoms that make up the chemicals or molecules of the body (Figure 1-2). Molecules, in turn, make up microscopic parts called *organelles* that fit together to form each cell of the body. Groups of similar cells are called *tissues,* which combine with other tissues to form individual organs. Groups of organs that work together are called *systems*. All of the systems of the body together make up an individual organism.

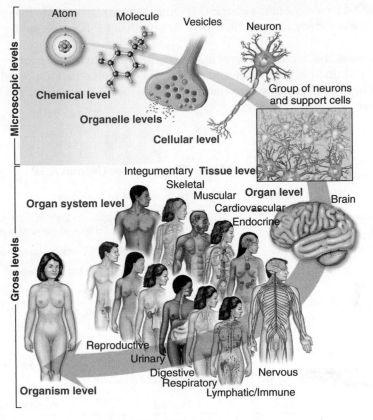

FIGURE 1-2 Levels of Organization.

Metric System

The **metric system**—also called the **International System of Units (SI)**—is the measuring system used in all of the sciences. Unlike the English system of measurement that many Americans are used to, the metric system is based on *decimal units*. Decimal units are units that are based on subdividing or multiplying each basic unit by multiples of 10. In the English system, on the other hand, many units may be divided or multiplied by 12 or by some other factor.

For example, to measure length, one could use the **meter** unit. A meter is a bit longer than the *yard* unit of the English system. If one wanted to measure a sports field, meters would be a handy unit to use. However, to measure the distance between cities, a unit a thousand times bigger would be better. The **kilometer** is equivalent to a thousand meters. The prefix *kilo-* shows the multiplying factor to be a thousand. But to measure a tiny blood cell, a meter is too large a unit to use easily. So we use the unit *micrometer* (μm)—one-millionth of a meter—to measure blood cells. The prefix *micro-* shows the dividing factor of a million.

Table 1-1 lists some of the metric (SI) units that are often used to measure size (length) when studying A&P. Start here to get a feel for how the metric system works.

The tables that follow will serve as a handy reference to use when you encounter other SI units in your studies, such as units of volume that are based on the **liter**. They will also help you to convert between metric units and English units, if needed.

✳ TABLE 1-1 — Common Metric Units of Size Used in A&P

Unit	Symbol	Equal to	Used to Measure
Centimeter	cm	1/100 m	Objects visible to the eye, such as the length of a limb or the entire body
Millimeter	mm	1/10 cm	Very large cells and groups of cells
Micrometer (micron)	µm	1/1000 mm	Most cells and large organelles
Nanometer	nm	1/1000 µm	Small organelles and large biomolecules
Angstrom	Å	1/10 nm	Molecules and atoms

✳ TABLE 1-2 — Basic Units of the Metric System

Basic Unit	Metric	English	English/Metric
Time	second	second	same
Length	meter (m)	yard	1.09 yards/1 meter
Volume	liter (l or L)	quart	1.06 quarts/1 liter
Mass	gram (g)	ounce	0.035 ounce/1 gram
Temperature	degree Celsius (° C)	degree Fahrenheit (° F)	1.8° F/1° C

✳ TABLE 1-3 — Prefixes Used in the Metric System*

Prefix	Written Description	Numeric Description
Less Than One Basic Unit		
nano-	one billionth	0.000000001
micro-	one millionth	0.000001
milli-	one thousandth	0.001
centi-	one hundredth	0.01
deci-	one tenth	0.1

✳ TABLE 1-3   Prefixes Used in the Metric System—cont'd

Prefix	Written Description	Numeric Description
More Than One Basic Unit		
deka-	ten	10.00
hecto-	one hundred	100.00
kilo-	one thousand	1000.00
mega-	one million	1,000,000.00

*An example may help illustrate the extremely small amount of material represented in a "parts per million" (ppm) or "parts per billion" (ppb) sample analysis. One part per million corresponds to a single penny in $10,000.00; one part per billion corresponds to 1 minute in 2000 years. Detecting even smaller quantities of certain materials (e.g., parts per trillion or less) in a body fluid or an environmental sample is now possible with the use of extremely sophisticated laboratory equipment. However, detecting such an extremely small amount of a particular material in a sample analysis may have no bearing on disease or environmental damage.

✳ TABLE 1-4   Common Unit Conversions

Multiply	By	To Get	Multiply	By	To Get
Time			**Volume**		
seconds	1000	milliseconds	liters	1.06	quarts
seconds	0.00167	minutes	liters	0.26	gallons
minutes	60	seconds	liters	1000	milliliters
milliseconds	0.001	seconds	liters	100	centiliters
Length			liters	10	deciliters
meters	1.09	yards	centiliters	0.01	liters
meters	3.28	feet	centiliters	10	milliliters
meters	100	centimeters	centiliters	0.1	deciliters
meters	1000	millimeters	deciliters	0.1	liters
centimeters	0.01	meters	deciliters	10	centiliters
centimeters	10	millimeters	**Mass**		
centimeters	100,000	micrometers	grams	0.035	ounces
millimeters	0.001	meters	grams	0.001	kilograms
millimeters	0.1	centimeters	grams	1000	milligrams
			milligrams	0.001	grams
			kilograms	1000	grams
			kilograms	2.21	pounds

✳ TABLE 1-5   Temperature Conversions

As you can see from Table 1-2: Basic Units of the Metric System, 1° C is a larger unit than 1° F. In fact, a Celsius degree is $\frac{9}{5}$ (1.8) times the size of a Fahrenheit degree. When you convert temperature readings from one form to another, this discrepancy in size must be taken into account. During the conversion from Celsius to Fahrenheit, 32° is added to account for the fact that, on the Fahrenheit scale, the freezing point of water is 32° (rather than 0°, as it is on the Celsius scale).

To convert ° C to ° F:
Multiply ° C by $\frac{9}{5}$ and add 32
_____ °C × $\frac{9}{5}$ + 32 = _____ ° F
For example, to convert 35° C to ° F:
35° C × $\frac{9}{5}$ + 32 = 95° F

To convert ° F to ° C:
Subtract 32 from ° F and multiply by $\frac{5}{9}$
(_____ ° F − 32) × $\frac{5}{9}$ = _____ °C
For example, to convert 101° F to ° C:
(101° F − 32) × $\frac{5}{9}$ = 38.3° C

✳ TABLE 1-6   Body Temperatures in Celsius and Fahrenheit

°C	°F	°C	°F	°C	°F	°C	°F
35.0	95.0	37.8	100.0	36.4	97.6	39.2	102.6
35.1	95.2	37.9	100.2	36.6	97.8	39.3	102.8
35.2	95.4	38.0	100.4	36.7	98.0	39.4	103.0
35.3	95.6	38.1	100.6	36.8	98.2	39.6	103.2
35.4	95.8	38.2	100.8	36.9	98.4	39.7	103.4
35.5	96.0	38.3	101.0	37.0	98.6	39.8	103.6
35.7	96.2	38.4	101.2	37.1	98.8	39.9	103.8
35.8	96.4	38.6	101.4	37.2	99.0	40.0	104.0
35.9	96.6	38.7	101.6	37.3	99.2	40.1	104.2
36.0	96.8	38.8	101.8	37.4	99.4	40.2	104.4
36.1	97.0	38.9	102.0	37.6	99.6	40.3	104.6
36.2	97.2	39.0	102.2	37.7	99.8	40.4	104.8
36.3	97.4	39.1	102.4				

B. Biochemistry

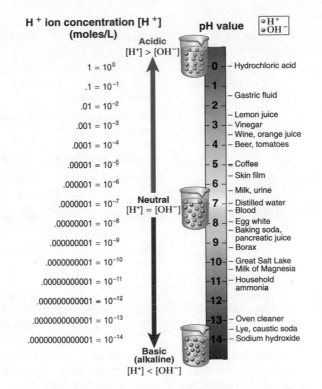

FIGURE 1-3 pH Scale. The term **pH** is literally an abbreviation for a phrase that means "the power of hydrogen" and is used to mean the relative H^+ ion concentration of a solution. As you can see on the left side of figure, the pH value is the negative of the base-10 logarithm of the H^+ ion concentration. The pH indicates the degree of *acidity* or *alkalinity* of a solution. As the concentration of H^+ ions increases, the pH goes down, and the solution becomes more acidic; a decrease in H^+ ion concentration makes the solution more alkaline, and the pH goes up:

- A pH of 7 indicates neutrality (equal amounts of H^+ and OH^-)
- A pH of less than 7 indicates acidity (more H^+ than OH^-)
- A pH greater than 7 indicates alkalinity (more OH^- than H^+)

The overall pH range is often expressed numerically on a logarithmic scale of 1 to 14. Keep in mind that a change of 1 pH unit on this type of scale represents a 10-fold difference in the actual concentration of H^+ ions. (The scale on the left side of the diagram shows the actual concentrations of H^+ in moles per liter or molar concentration as an ordinary number and then expressed as an exponent [logarithm] of 10. You can see that the pH scale is simply the negative of the exponent of 10.)

✳ TABLE 1-7   Examples of Important Biomolecules

Macromolecule	Subunit	Function	Example
Carbohydrates			
Glucose	Simple sugar (hexose: $C_6H_{12}O_6$)	Stores energy	Blood glucose
Ribose	Simple sugar (pentose: $C_5H_{10}O_5$)	Plays a role in the expression of hereditary information	Component of RNA
Deoxyribose	Simple sugar (pentose: $C_5H_{10}O_4$)	Plays a role in the storage and transmission of hereditary information	Component of DNA
Glycogen	Glucose	Stores energy	Liver glycogen
Lipids			
Triglycerides	Glycerol + three fatty acids	Store energy	Body fat
Phospholipids	Glycerol + phosphate + two fatty acids	Make up cell membranes	Plasma membrane of cell
Steroids	Steroid nucleus (four-carbon ring)	Make up cell membranes; needed to make some hormones	Cholesterol, various steroid hormones, estrogen
Prostaglandins	20-carbon unsaturated fatty acid that contains a five-carbon ring	Regulate hormone action; enhance the immune system; affect the inflammatory response	Prostaglandins E and A
Proteins			
Functional proteins	Amino acids	Regulate chemical reactions	Hemoglobin, antibodies, enzymes
Structural proteins	Amino acids	Component of body support tissues	Muscle filaments, tendons, ligaments
Nucleic Acids			
DNA	Nucleotides (sugar, phosphate, base)	Encodes hereditary information	Chromatin, chromosomes
RNA	Nucleotides (sugar, phosphate, base)	Helps decode hereditary information; acts as an RNA enzyme; may silence gene expression	Transfer RNA (tRNA), messenger RNA (mRNA), double-strand RNA (dsRNA)

✳ TABLE 1-7		Examples of Important Biomolecules—cont'd	
Macromolecule	**Subunit**	**Function**	**Example**
Nucleotides and Related Molecules			
Adenosine triphosphate (ATP)	Phosphorylated nucleotide (adenine + ribose + three phosphates)	Transfers energy from fuel molecules to working molecules	ATP present in every cell of the body
Creatine phosphate (CP)	Amino acid derivative + phosphate	Transfers energy from fuel to ATP	CP present in muscle fibers as backup to ATP
Nicotinic adenine dinucleotide (NAD)	Combination of two ribonucleotides	Acts as a coenzyme to transfer high-energy particles from one chemical process to another	NAD present in every cell of the body
Combined or Altered Forms			
Glycoproteins	Large proteins with small carbohydrate groups attached	Similar to functional proteins	Some hormones, antibodies, enzymes, cell membrane components
Proteoglycans	Large polysaccharides with small polypeptide chains attached	Lubrication; increases thickness of fluid	Component of mucous fluid and many tissue fluids in the body
Lipoproteins	Protein complex that contains lipid groups	Transport lipids in the blood	Low- and high-density lipoproteins
Glycolipids	Lipid molecule with attached carbohydrate group	Component of cell membranes	Component of membranes of nerve cells
Ribonucleoprotein	Combination of RNA nucleotide and protein	Enzyme-like actions such as splicing mRNA	Small nuclear ribonucleoproteins (snRNPs or "snurps") that make up the spliceosome structure in a cell

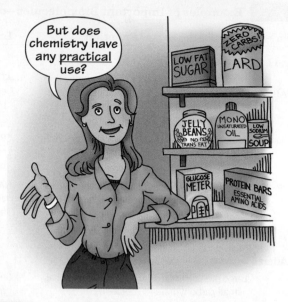

✳ TABLE 1-8 — Major Functions of Human Lipid Compounds

Function	Example
Energy	Lipids can be stored and broken down later for energy; they yield more energy per unit of weight than carbohydrates or proteins do
Structure	Phospholipids and cholesterol are required components of cell membranes
Vitamins	Fat-soluble vitamins: vitamin A forms retinal (necessary for night vision); vitamin D increases calcium uptake; vitamin E promotes wound healing; and vitamin K is required for the synthesis of blood-clotting proteins
Protection	Fat surrounds and protects organs
Insulation	Fat under the skin minimizes heat loss; fatty tissue (myelin) covers nerve cells and electrically insulates them
Regulation	Steroid hormones regulate many physiological processes; for example, estrogen and testosterone are responsible for many of the differences between females and males; prostaglandins help to regulate inflammation and tissue repair

✳ TABLE 1-9 — Major Functions of Human Protein Compounds

Function	Example
Provide structure	Structural proteins include the keratin of the skin, hair, and nails; parts of cell membranes; tendons
Catalyze chemical reactions	Lactase (enzyme in the intestinal digestive juice) catalyzes chemical reactions that change lactose into glucose and galactose
Transport substances in the blood	Proteins classified as albumins combine with fatty acids to transport them in the form of lipoproteins
Communicate information to the cells	Insulin (a protein hormone) serves as chemical message from the islet cells of the pancreas to cells all over the body

✳ **TABLE 1-9** **Major Functions of Human Protein Compounds—cont'd**

Function	Example
Act as receptors	Binding sites of certain proteins on the surfaces of cell membranes serve as receptors for insulin and various other hormones
Defend the body against many harmful agents	Proteins called *antibodies* or *immunoglobulins* combine with various harmful agents to render those agents harmless
Provide energy	Proteins can be metabolized for energy

✳ **TABLE 1-10** **Comparison of DNA and RNA Structure**

	DNA	RNA
Polynucleotide strands	Double; very long	Single or double; short
Sugar	Deoxyribose	Ribose
Base pairing	Adenine–thymine (A–T)	Adenine–uracil (A–U)
	Guanine–cytosine (G–C)	Guanine–cytosine (G–C)

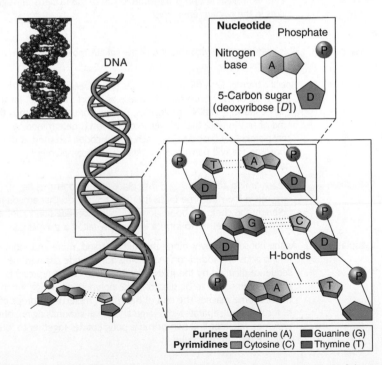

FIGURE 1-4 The Deoxyribonucleic Acid (DNA) Molecule. This representation of the DNA *double helix* shows the general structure of a nucleotide and the two kinds of *base pairs*: adenine (A) *(blue)* with thymine (T) *(yellow)* and guanine (G) *(purple)* with cytosine (C) *(red)*. Note that the G–C base pair has three hydrogen bonds, whereas the A–T base pair has two. *Hydrogen bonds (H-bonds)* are extremely important for maintaining the structure of this molecule.

✳ **TABLE 1-11**   **Summary of Protein Synthesis**

Step	Location in the Cell	Description
Transcription		
1	Nucleus	One region or gene of a DNA molecule "unzips" to expose its bases
2	Nucleus	According to the principles of complementary base pairing, RNA nucleotides already present in the nucleoplasm temporarily attach themselves to the exposed bases along one side of the DNA molecule
3	Nucleus	As RNA nucleotides align themselves along the DNA strand, they bind to each other and thus form a chain-like strand called *messenger RNA* (mRNA); this binding of RNA nucleotides is controlled by the enzyme RNA polymerase
Preparation of mRNA		
4	Nucleus	As the preliminary mRNA strand is formed, it peels away from the DNA strand; this mRNA strand is a copy or *transcript* of a gene
5	Nucleus	The spliceosome edits the mRNA molecule by removing noncoding portions of the strand (introns) and splicing the remaining pieces (exons)
6	Nuclear pores	The edited mRNA strand is transported out of the nucleus through pores in the nuclear envelope
Translation		
7	Cytoplasm	Two subunits sandwich the end of the mRNA molecule to form a ribosome
8	Cytoplasm	Specific transfer RNA (tRNA) molecules bring specific amino acids into place at the ribosome, which acts as a sort of "holder" for the mRNA strand and tRNA molecules; the kind of tRNA (and thus the kind of amino acid) that moves into position is determined by complementary base pairing: each mRNA codon exposed at the ribosome site will permit only a tRNA with a complementary *anticodon* to attach
9	Cytoplasm	As each amino acid is brought into place at the ribosome, an enzyme in the ribosome binds it to the amino acid that arrived just before it; the chemical bonds formed, called *peptide bonds,* link the amino acids together to form a long chain called a *polypeptide*
10	Cytoplasm	As the ribosome moves along the mRNA strand, more and more amino acids are added to the growing polypeptide chain in the sequence dictated by the mRNA codons (each codon represents a specific amino acid to be placed in the polypeptide chain); when the ribosome reaches the end of the mRNA molecule, it drops off of the end and separates into large and small subunits again; often enzymes will later link two or more polypeptides together to form a whole protein molecule

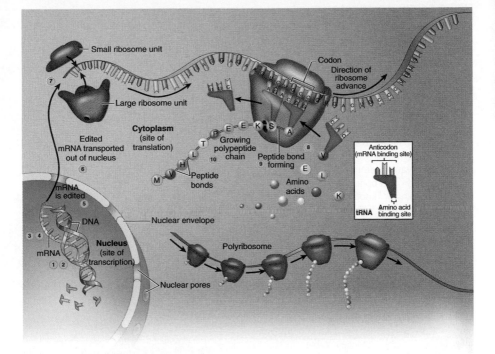

FIGURE 1-5 Protein Synthesis. Each of the numbered steps in the figure is further outlined in Table 1-11. Protein synthesis begins with transcription, a process in which an mRNA molecule forms along one gene sequence of a DNA molecule within the cell's nucleus **(1, 2,** and **3)**. As it is formed, the mRNA molecule separates from the DNA molecule **(4)**; the mRNA is edited **(5)**, and it leaves the nucleus through the large nuclear pores **(6)**. Outside of the nucleus, ribosome subunits attach to the beginning of the mRNA molecule and begin the process of translation **(7)**. During translation, transfer RNA (tRNA) molecules bring specific amino acids, which are encoded by each mRNA codon, into place at the ribosome site **(8)**. As the amino acids are brought into the proper sequence, they are joined together by peptide bonds **(9)** to form long strands called *polypeptides* **(10)**. Several polypeptide chains may be needed to make a complete protein molecule. Amino acids are identified by color codes and abbreviations.

FIGURE 1-6 Structural Levels of Protein.
Primary structure: This is determined by the number, kind, and sequence of amino acids in the chain, which is ultimately determined by a gene.
Secondary structure: Hydrogen bonds stabilize folds or helical spirals. A *motif* is a commonly occurring pattern with a specific function.
Tertiary structure: Globular shapes are maintained by strong (covalent) intramolecular bonding between side groups (R groups) of various amino acids and by stabilizing hydrogen bonds. These may include *domains* or "knots" with specific functions.
Quaternary structure: This results from bonding between more than one polypeptide unit. Various enzymes, including chaperonins, help to fold and combine polypeptides.
Native state: The final, functioning shape of a protein is often called its *native state*. The native states of the strong *structural proteins* found in tendons and ligaments are fibrous or thread-like, insoluble, and very stable. In contrast, *functional proteins* such as enzymes, certain protein hormones, antibodies, albumin, and hemoglobin have native states that are globular (ball-shaped) and often soluble and that have chemically reactive regions that are often flexible and dynamic.

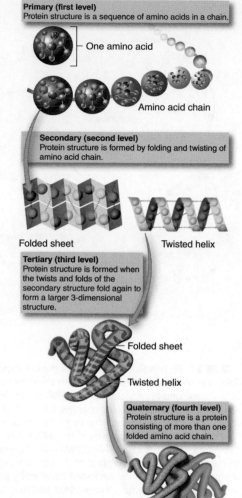

Primary (first level)
Protein structure is a sequence of amino acids in a chain.

One amino acid

Amino acid chain

Secondary (second level)
Protein structure is formed by folding and twisting of amino acid chain.

Folded sheet   Twisted helix

Tertiary (third level)
Protein structure is formed when the twists and folds of the secondary structure fold again to form a larger 3-dimensional structure.

Folded sheet

Twisted helix

Quaternary (fourth level)
Protein structure is a protein consisting of more than one folded amino acid chain.

Cooking Up Some Proteins

An often-used analogy to help us understand how proteins are synthesized in the cell is that of cooking. Of course, making proteins is not really the same as cooking up Grandma's carrot cake, but there are some useful similarities that help us to better understand the cellular processes. Use the accompanying table to follow this story of cooking that is really about making protein molecules.

You want to make carrot cake, so you go to your bookshelf (nucleus), where you keep your collection (genome) of cookbooks (DNAs). You find the recipe (gene) that you want and make a photocopy of it (transcribe mRNA) so that you don't mess up the cookbook. Before leaving the bookcase (nucleus), you notice that Grandma wrote a bunch of stuff in the margins of the recipe that you don't really need. So you black out (edit) the stuff you don't need (introns) and leave the essential parts (exons) of the recipe (mRNA) intact.

You leave the bookcase (nucleus), go through the door (nuclear pore), and go to the kitchen (cytoplasm), where you put the recipe (edited mRNA) near the mixing bowl (rRNA). Next, you read (translate) the first word (codon) of the recipe (gene) and recognize the ingredient (specific amino acid), so you get it in its proper measuring cup (tRNA) and put it in the mixing bowl (rRNA). You read (translate) the next ingredient (amino acid) and get the appropriate kind of measuring cup or scoop (tRNA) to get that ingredient (specific amino acid) and put it into the mixing bowl (rRNA). Pretty soon you have a whole bunch of ingredients in the bowl (rRNA). These ingredients, after some mixing and baking (protein folding), will become a yummy carrot cake (polypeptide/protein).

However, you like your carrot cake with cream cheese icing, so you go back to the cookbook collection (genome) and start the process again, this time using a different recipe (different gene) to make a different part of the dish (different polypeptide). When that's done (translated), you can put the icing on the cake to finish your favorite dessert (complete protein).

For a brief rundown of the protein synthesis process, check out *DNA* (my-ap.us/12BUmXF).

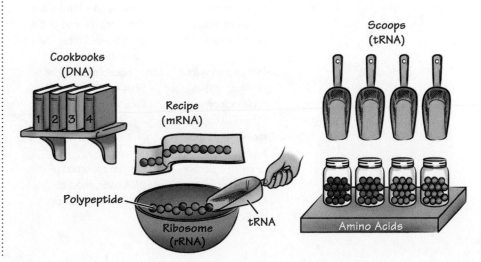

Continued

✧ FIELD NOTES—cont'd

Acronym	Name	Cooking Analogy	Role in Cell Function
	Amino acid	Individual ingredient used to make a dish	A chemical group that links with other amino acids to form a polypeptide chain and eventually a whole protein
	Codon	Word (in a recipe) that represents an individual ingredient; made up of any combination of 26 letters	Word (in a gene) that represents an individual amino acid; made up of any combination of four nucleotide bases
	Cytoplasm	The kitchen, where the making of the dish takes place	Area outside of the nucleus where the translation of proteins takes place
DNA	Deoxyribonucleic acid	The cookbook	The cell's "master copy" of the genetic code; a chromosome
	Editing	The process of blacking out unneeded parts of a copy of an individual recipe	The process of removing some segments of a gene (introns) in the mRNA that are not needed for translation
	Exon	A part of the recipe copied from a cookbook that you need to make the dish	The part of the gene that remains after introns are removed; the part of the gene needed for translation
	Gene	Individual recipe (one of many recipes in a cookbook or an individual copy of a recipe used when cooking)	The sequence of codons in DNA or RNA that codes for a specific amino acid
	Genome	Your entire collection of cookbooks, most of which are in a bookcase	The entire collection of DNA code, most of which is in the nucleus

✧ FIELD NOTES—cont'd

Acronym	Name	Cooking Analogy	Role in Cell Function
	Intron	A part of the recipe copied from a cookbook that you don't really need to make the dish	The part of the gene that is removed from the mRNA before it's translated into a protein
mRNA	Messenger RNA	Individual recipe (copied from a cookbook) that lists the ingredients and the order in which they are added	Serves as working copy of one protein-coding gene
	Nucleus	Bookcase where you keep all of your cookbooks	Cell structure that contains most of the cell's genome
	Polypeptide strand	The batter, yet to be processed (cut, folded, and so on)	Product of protein synthesis that is yet to be trimmed, folded, and possibly combined with other polypeptides to form a whole protein
	Folding	Baking the batter	Folding the polypeptide strand into primary, secondary, and tertiary structures
	Assembling	Stacking layers of a cake, icing a cake, or otherwise combining products of separate cooking events	Tertiary proteins, which are assembled using the same or different genes, can be combined to form larger quaternary proteins
	Various enzymes (e.g., chaperonins, ubiquitins)	Various cooking implements (e.g., tongs, spoons, mixers)	Enzymes function at many different stages of protein synthesis to help assemble, cut, and fold the polypeptide/protein molecule

Continued

✦ FIELD NOTES—cont'd

Acronym	Name	Cooking Analogy	Role in Cell Function
	Protein	The final, ready-to-serve form of a dish	The complete folded protein, ready to be used for any of many cell functions
rRNA	Ribosomal RNA	The mixing bowl into which the ingredients specified by a recipe are poured in the correct order	A component of the ribosome (along with proteins); attaches to RNA and participates in translation
snRNP	Small nuclear ribonucleoprotein	Black marking pen used to black out unneeded parts of an individual copy of a recipe	A component of the spliceosome; attaches to mRNA transcript to facilitate editing (the removal of introns and the splicing of exons) into the final version of mRNA
	Transcription	The process of copying an individual recipe from a cookbook	The process of copying a gene from DNA to a strand of mRNA
tRNA	Transfer RNA	A measuring cup that carries only one unit of an ingredient at a time and that can only be used for one type of ingredient	Carries a specific amino acid to a specific codon of mRNA at the ribosome during translation
	Translation	The process of reading a recipe, translating the instructions, and then making the dish	The process of using genes on mRNA to construct a polypeptide chain on a ribosome

C. Cell Biology

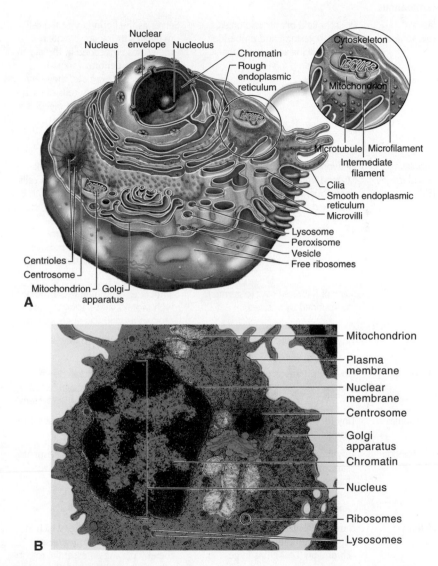

FIGURE 1-7 Typical Cell.
A, An artist's interpretation of human cell structure.
B, A color-enhanced electron micrograph of a cell.
Both of these images show the many mitochondria, which are known as the *power plants of the cell*. Note, too, the innumerable dots that border the endoplasmic reticulum. These are ribosomes, which are the cell's *protein factories*. Other cell structures are described in Table 1-12.

※ **TABLE 1-12**   **Some Major Cell Structures and Their Functions***

Cell Structure	Description	Functions
Membranous		
Plasma membrane	Phospholipid bilayer reinforced with cholesterol and embedded with proteins and other organic molecules	Serves as the boundary of the cell, maintains its integrity; protein molecules embedded in the plasma membrane perform various functions: for example, they serve as markers that identify cells of each individual, as receptor molecules for certain hormones and other molecules, and as transport mechanisms
Endoplasmic reticulum (ER)	Network of canals and sacs that extend from the nuclear envelope; may have ribosomes attached	Ribosomes attached to rough ER synthesize proteins that leave cells via the Golgi apparatus; smooth ER synthesizes membrane lipids, steroid hormones, and certain carbohydrates used to form glycoproteins as well as removes and stores Ca^{++} from the cell's interior
Golgi apparatus	Stack of flattened sacs (cisternae) surrounded by vesicles	Synthesizes carbohydrate, combines it with protein, and packages the product as globules of glycoprotein
Vesicles	Tiny membranous bags	Temporarily contain molecules for transport or later use
Lysosomes	Tiny membranous bags that contain enzymes	Digestive enzymes break down defective cell parts and ingested particles; a cell's "digestive system"
Peroxisomes	Tiny membranous bags that contain enzymes	Enzymes detoxify harmful substances in the cell
Mitochondria	Tiny membranous capsule that surrounds an inner, highly folded membrane embedded with enzymes; has small, ring-like chromosome (DNA)	Catabolism; adenosine triphosphate (ATP) synthesis; a cell's "power plants"
Nucleus	A usually central, spherical, double-membrane container of chromatin (DNA); has large pores	Houses the genetic code, which in turn dictates protein synthesis, thereby playing an essential role in other cell activities, namely cell transport, metabolism, and growth

✴ TABLE 1-12 Some Major Cell Structures and Their Functions—cont'd

Cell Structure	Description	Functions
Rafts	Stiff groupings of membrane molecules that travel together within the fluid mosaic of the plasma membrane (like a raft)	Many different functions, including organizing membrane regions, forming caveolae, cytokinesis, and cell transport
Caveolae	Tiny indentations of plasma membrane formed from membrane rafts	Capture extracellular material and move it into or across the cell
Nonmembranous		
Ribosomes	Small particles assembled from two tiny subunits of rRNA and protein	Site of protein synthesis; a cell's "protein factories"
Proteasomes	Hollow protein cylinders with embedded enzymes	Destroy misfolded or otherwise abnormal proteins manufactured by the cell; "quality control" mechanism for protein synthesis
Cytoskeleton	Network of interconnecting flexible filaments, stiff tubules, and molecular motors within the cell	Supporting framework of the cell and its organelles; functions in cell movement (using molecular motors); forms cell extensions (microvilli, cilia, flagella)
Centrosome	Region of cytoskeleton that includes two cylindrical groupings of microtubules called *centrioles*	Acts as the microtubule-organizing center (MTOC) of the cell; centrioles assist with the formation and organization of microtubules
Microvilli	Short, finger-like extensions of plasma membrane; supported internally by microfilaments	Increase a cell's absorptive surface area
Cilia and flagella	Moderate (cilia) to long (flagella) hair-like extensions of plasma membrane; supported internally by the cylindrical formation of microtubules, sometimes with attached molecular motors	Cilia move substances over the cell surface or detect changes outside of the cell; flagella propel sperm cells
Nucleolus	Dense area of chromatin and related molecules within the nucleus	Site of formation of ribosome subunits
Vault	Tiny capsule formed from tapered pieces that fit together into a barrel shape	Docks with nuclear pore complex and shuttle molecules to and from the nucleus; perhaps plays other transport roles

*Some (but not all) of these structures are visible in Figure 1-7.

⟡   FIELD NOTES

Drive a Cell Around the Block

When I visit my favorite car dealer, Al over at Subaru, he always wants me to take one of the new cars around the block to see how great it is. Well, it always is great, because Al puts me in a car loaded with all kinds of cool options.

If I do decide to buy a car from Al, I probably won't get all those options. Some, like the fax machine, I really don't need. Others, like the racing wheels, are nice, but I can't afford them. In addition, I'll probably ask for an extra option that wasn't on the car I test-drove—like all-weather floor mats, because I'm a slob.

So why did Al put me in the car with all the options he knew I couldn't afford? Well, how would I know if I did want them if I'd never experienced them?

It's the same with the "generalized" or "typical" cell that you see in most textbooks. First, remember that it's a cartoon cell anyway and not a realistic image of a cell. Second, it's like the car that Al gave me to test drive: it has a lot of options that you're not likely to see very often all on one cell. However, when it comes time to study a type of cell with a particular option, you'll have already test-driven a cell with that option. In addition, every once in a while, you'll run across a cell that has a feature that wasn't in the typical cell that you first studied. However, by then, you'll be an expert on cell parts, and it won't faze you at all.

✳ **TABLE 1-13**   **Functional Anatomy of Cell Membranes**

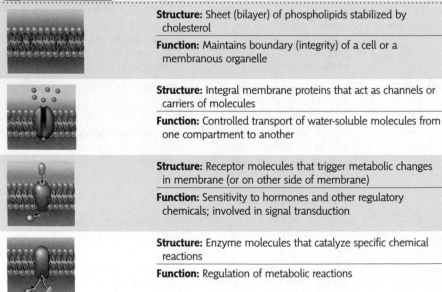

	Structure: Sheet (bilayer) of phospholipids stabilized by cholesterol
	Function: Maintains boundary (integrity) of a cell or a membranous organelle
	Structure: Integral membrane proteins that act as channels or carriers of molecules
	Function: Controlled transport of water-soluble molecules from one compartment to another
	Structure: Receptor molecules that trigger metabolic changes in membrane (or on other side of membrane)
	Function: Sensitivity to hormones and other regulatory chemicals; involved in signal transduction
	Structure: Enzyme molecules that catalyze specific chemical reactions
	Function: Regulation of metabolic reactions

✳ TABLE 1-13   Functional Anatomy of Cell Membranes—cont'd

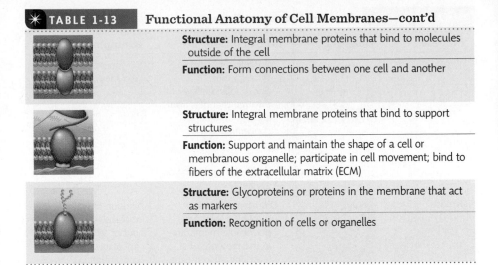

Structure: Integral membrane proteins that bind to molecules outside of the cell

Function: Form connections between one cell and another

Structure: Integral membrane proteins that bind to support structures

Function: Support and maintain the shape of a cell or membranous organelle; participate in cell movement; bind to fibers of the extracellular matrix (ECM)

Structure: Glycoproteins or proteins in the membrane that act as markers

Function: Recognition of cells or organelles

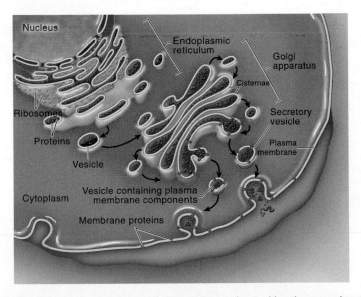

FIGURE 1-8 The Cell as a Protein Factory. Polypeptides synthesized by ribosomes (see Figure 1-5) are delivered to the **endoplasmic reticulum (ER)**, where they are trimmed and folded. Small **vesicles** then transport these proteins from the ER to the **Golgi apparatus,** which then processes and packages them. After entering the first *cisterna* of the Golgi apparatus, a protein molecule undergoes a series of chemical modifications and then is sent (by means of a vesicle) to the next cisterna for further modification, and so on, until it is ready to exit the last cisterna. When it is ready to exit, a molecule is packaged in a membranous **secretory vesicle** that migrates to the surface of the cell and "pops open" to release its contents into the space outside of the cell. The vesicle membrane, including any **integral membrane proteins (IMPs)**, then becomes part of the plasma membrane. Some vesicles remain inside the cell for some time and serve as storage vessels for the substance to be secreted.

✳ **TABLE 1-14** **Passive Transport Processes**

Process	Diagram	Description	Examples
Simple diffusion		Movement of particles through the phospholipid bilayer or through channels from an area of high concentration to an area of low concentration (i.e., down the concentration gradient)	Movement of carbon dioxide out of all cells
Osmosis		Diffusion of water through a selectively permeable membrane in the presence of at least one impermeant solute (this often involves both simple and channel-mediated diffusion)	Diffusion of water molecules into and out of cells to correct imbalances in water concentration
Channel-mediated passive transport (facilitated diffusion)		Diffusion of particles through a membrane by means of channel structures in the membrane (i.e., particles move down their concentration gradient)	Diffusion of sodium ions into nerve cells during a nerve impulse
Carrier-mediated passive transport (facilitated diffusion)		Diffusion of particles through a membrane by means of carrier structures in the membrane (i.e., particles move down their concentration gradient)	Diffusion of glucose molecules into most cells

◇ FIELD NOTES

What's a Gradient?

Understanding passive transport—and many other processes in the body—requires the understanding of what **gradients** are and how they work.

Put simply, a gradient is a *graded* difference as you move between one point and another. For example, as you move from the cold outdoors in the winter to the warm indoors, you'll notice a *gradual* change in air temperature. That's a temperature gradient. In the figure below, you can see that, when you put sugar into a cup of tea, there is a concentration gradient of sugar particles. There are sugar particles per drop where the sugar crystals are dumped in. The concentration *gradually* changes as one gets farther from that point.

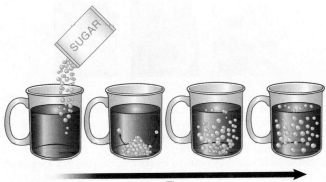

Time

In nature, particles are always moving. As they collide, they tend to spread out. The closer the particles are to one another, the more collisions there are, and the faster they tend to move apart. We can describe this overall outward spread as "moving down the concentration gradient" or moving from an area of high particle concentration to an area of low particle concentration. Such diffusion (spreading) is visible with the sugar in the hot tea pictured.

But there are many gradients encountered in A&P in addition to concentration gradients. There are also temperature gradients. For example, there's a temperature gradient between the skin and your internal organs—it gets warmer the deeper you go. There are also pressure gradients. For example, the blood pressure (fluid pressure) in your heart and large arteries (the vessels that drain the heart chambers) is higher than the blood pressure in your smaller arteries.

Generally, things tend to move *down* a gradient. That is, they move from high toward low. Dissolved particles move from high concentration toward low concentration. Heat moves from high temperature (warm) areas toward lower temperature (cooler) areas. So heat flows from your body's core toward the skin. Fluids flow from areas of high pressure toward areas of low pressure. So blood flows from the heart into the arteries.

As things move down their gradients, they are moving toward an **equilibrium**—a balanced state in which there is no distinct gradient. As a system becomes "equal" along what was once a gradient, we say that *equilibration* occurs.

Knowing what a gradient is and how it works will be useful many times as you travel through the jungle of A&P.

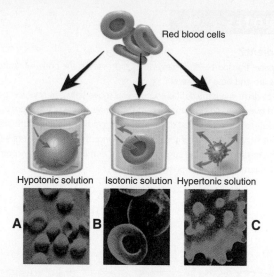

FIGURE 1-9 Osmosis. Osmosis is the diffusion of water through a selectively permeable membrane when impermeant solutes are present. Water moves down its concentration gradient toward equilibrium, but the impermeant solutes cannot move across the membrane. This causes a change in water volume and water pressure (**osmotic pressure**). The *potential osmotic pressure* of a solution is a prediction of whether it is likely to gain or lose water by osmosis. **Hypotonic** (literally "low pressure") solutions lose water by osmosis to the cells that are placed in it. **Isotonic** ("equal pressure") solutions are at equilibrium, and there is no net osmosis into or out of cells. **Hypertonic** ("high pressure") solutions gain water by drawing it out of cells.
A, Normal red blood cells placed in a *hypotonic* solution may swell (as the scanning electron micrograph shows) or even burst (as the drawing shows). This change results from the inward diffusion of water (osmosis).
B, Cells placed in an *isotonic* solution maintain a constant volume and pressure because the potential osmotic pressure of the intracellular fluid matches that of the extracellular fluid.
C, Cells placed in a solution that is *hypertonic* to the intracellular fluid lose volume and pressure as water osmoses out of the cell and into the hypertonic solution. The "spikes" seen in the scanning electron micrograph are rigid microtubules of the cytoskeleton. These supports become visible as the cell "deflates." Because their edges look "scalloped" under a light microscope, these are called *crenated* cells.

✳ TABLE 1-15   Active Transport Processes

Process	Diagram	Description	Examples
Pumping		Movement of solute particles from an area of low concentration to an area of high concentration (i.e., up the concentration gradient) by means of an energy-consuming pump structure in the membrane	In muscle cells, pumping of nearly all calcium ions into special compartments or out of the cell
Phagocytosis (endocytosis)		Movement of cells or other large particles into the cell by trapping them in a section of plasma membrane that pinches off to form an intracellular vesicle; a type of vesicle-mediated transport	Trapping of bacterial cells by phagocytic white blood cells
Pinocytosis (endocytosis)		Movement of fluid and dissolved molecules into a cell by trapping them in a section of plasma membrane that pinches off to form an intracellular vesicle; a type of vesicle-mediated transport	Trapping of large protein molecules by some body cells
Exocytosis		Movement of proteins or other cell products out of the cell by fusing a secretory vesicle with the plasma membrane; a type of vesicle-mediated transport	Secretion of the hormone prolactin by pituitary cells

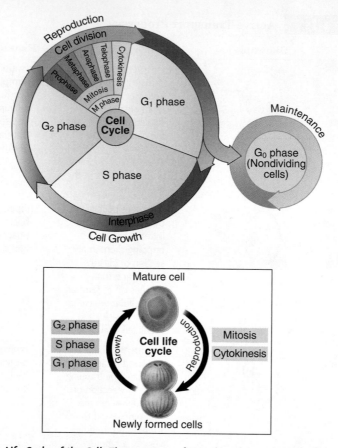

FIGURE 1-10 Life Cycle of the Cell. The processes of growth and reproduction of successive generations of cells exhibit a circular (cyclic) pattern. Newly formed cells grow to maturity by synthesizing new molecules and organelles (G_1 and G_2 phases), including the replication of an extra set of DNA molecules (*S phase*) in anticipation of reproduction. Mature cells reproduce (*M phase*) by first distributing the two identical sets of DNA (produced during the S phase) via the orderly process of mitosis and then by splitting the plasma membrane, cytoplasm, and organelles of the parent cell into two distinct daughter cells (cytokinesis). Daughter cells that do not go on to reproduce are in a maintenance phase (G_o).

✳ TABLE 1-16	Summary of the Cell Life Cycle

Phase of Cell Life Cycle	Description
Cell Growth	**Interphase**
Protein synthesis	Proteins are manufactured according to the cell's genetic code; functional proteins (enzymes) direct the synthesis of other molecules in the cells and thus the production of more and larger organelles and the plasma membrane; sometimes called the *first growth phase* or the G_1 *phase* of interphase; see Table 1-11 (p. 78)
DNA replication	Nucleotides, which are influenced by newly synthesized enzymes, arrange themselves along the open sides of an "unzipped" DNA molecule, thereby creating two identical daughter DNA molecules; this produces two identical sets of the cell's genetic code, which enables the cell to later split into two different cells, each with its own complete set of DNA; sometimes called the *(DNA) synthesis stage* or *S phase* of interphase: see Table 1-17 (p. 97)
Protein synthesis	After DNA is replicated, the cell continues to grow by means of protein synthesis and the resulting synthesis of other molecules and various organelles; this *second growth phase* is also called the G_2 *phase*
Cell Reproduction	**M Phase**
Mitosis or meiosis	The parent cell's replicated set of DNA is divided into two sets and separated by an orderly process into distinct cell nuclei; mitosis is subdivided into at least four phases: prophase, metaphase, anaphase, and telophase
Cytokinesis	The plasma membrane of the parent cell "pinches in" and eventually separates the cytoplasm and the two daughter nuclei into two genetically identical daughter cells

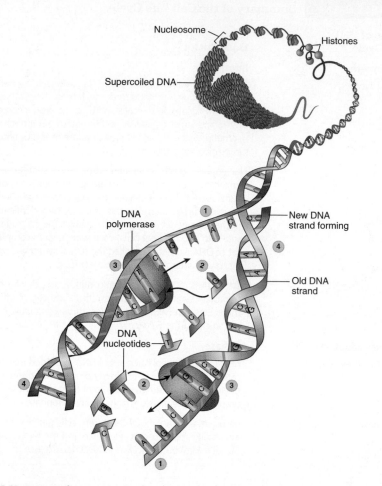

FIGURE 1-11 DNA Replication. Replication of the entire set (genome) of DNA molecules prepares the cell for reproduction, when one set will go to one daughter cell and the other set to the other daughter cell.

1, The tightly coiled DNA molecules uncoil, except for small segments. (Because these remaining tight little coils are denser than the thin, elongated sections, they absorb more stain and appear as *chromatin granules* under the microscope. By contrast, the thin, uncoiled sections are invisible because they absorb so little stain.) As the DNA molecule uncoils, its two strands come apart.

2 and 3, Along each of the two separated strands of nucleotides, a complementary strand forms. Intracellular fluid contains many DNA nucleotides. By the mechanism of *obligatory base pairing* and with the work of specific enzymes, nucleotides become attached at their correct places along each DNA strand. This means that "new" thymine from the intracellular fluid attaches to the "old" adenine in the original DNA strand. Conversely, new adenine attaches to old thymine. In addition, new guanine joins old cytosine, and new cytosine joins old guanine.

4, DNA nucleotides are added in different directions in each of the two strands of the mother DNA molecule and connected to each other by the enzyme *DNA polymerase*. This results in the end of one mother strand not being copied. The loss of useful code is prevented by the presence of **telomeres** (literally, "end roots"), which are strands of "extra" nucleotides that can be lost without affecting the coding part of the chromosome. As telomeres shorten, they eventually disappear, unless they are rebuilt by the enzyme *telomerase*. Telomerase contains a bit of RNA that provides the code for rebuilding the telomere sequence.

FIGURE 1-11, cont'd By the end of this part of the growth phase, each of the two DNA strands of the original DNA molecule has a complete new complementary strand attached to it. Each half of the DNA molecule, or strand, in other words, has duplicated itself to create a whole new DNA molecule. Thus two new chromosomes now replace each original chromosome. However, at this stage (before cell reproduction has actually begun), they are called **chromatids** instead of chromosomes. The two chromatids that have been formed from each original chromosome contain duplicate copies of DNA and therefore contain the same genes as the chromosome from which they were formed. Chromatids are present as attached pairs; their point of attachment is called the **centromere.** The numbers refer to the steps described in Table 1-17.

✳ TABLE 1-17   Summary of DNA Replication

Step	Description
1	DNA molecules uncoil and "unzip" to expose their bases
2	Nucleotides already present in the intracellular fluid of the nucleus attach to the exposed bases according to the principle of obligatory base pairing
3	As nucleotides attach to complementary bases along each DNA strand, the enzyme DNA polymerase causes them to bind to each other
4	As new nucleotides fill in the spaces left open on each DNA strand, two identical daughter molecules are formed; as the parent DNA molecule completely unzips, the two daughter molecules coil to become distinct, but genetically identical, DNA double helices called *chromatids*

These steps are illustrated in Figure 1-11.

✳ TABLE 1-18   The Major Events of Mitosis

Prophase	Metaphase	Anaphase	Telophase
1. Chromosomes shorten and thicken (from coiling of the DNA molecules that compose them); each chromosome consists of two chromatids attached at the centromere	1. Chromosomes align across the equator of the spindle fiber at its centromere	1. Each centromere splits, thereby detaching two chromatids that compose each chromosome from each other and elongating in the process (DNA molecules start uncoiling)	1. Changes that occur during telophase essentially reverse those that took place during prophase; new chromosomes start elongating (DNA molecules start uncoiling)
2. Centrosomes move to opposite poles of the cell; spindle fibers appear and begin to orient between opposing poles		2. Sister chromatids (now called *chromosomes*) move to opposite poles; there are now twice as many chromosomes as there were before mitosis started	2. A nuclear envelope forms again to enclose each new set of chromosomes
3. Nucleoli and the nuclear membrane disappear			3. Spindle fibers disappear

Continued

✳ **TABLE 1-18**	**The Major Events of Mitosis—cont'd**

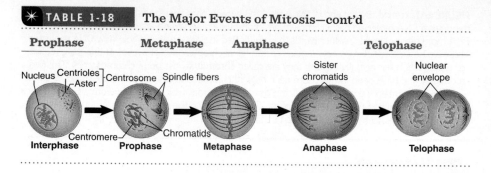

Prophase	**Metaphase**	**Anaphase**	**Telophase**

D. Tissues

A tissue is a group of similar cells that perform a common function. Tissues can be thought of as the fabric of the body, which is "sewn together" to form the organs of the body and to hold all of the organs together as a whole.

Each tissue specializes in performing at least one unique function that helps to maintain homeostasis, ensuring the survival of the whole body. The arrangement of cells in one tissue may form a thin sheet that is only one cell deep, whereas the cells of another tissue may form huge masses that contain millions of cells. Regardless of the size, shape, or arrangement of cells in a tissue, the cells are all surrounded by or embedded in a complex extracellular material that often is called simply a **matrix.**

A good understanding of the major tissue types will help you to understand the next highest levels of organization of the body: organs and organ systems.

Although a number of subtypes are present in the body, all tissues can be classified by their structure and function into four principal types:

1. **Epithelial tissue** covers and protects the body surface, lines the body cavities, specializes in moving substances into and out of the body or particular organs (via secretion, excretion, and absorption), and forms many glands. The cells in epithelial tissue are usually very close together, with very little extracellular matrix.
2. **Connective tissue** functions to support the body and its parts, to connect and hold them together, to transport substances through the body, and to protect the body from foreign invaders. The cells in connective tissue are often relatively far apart and separated by large quantities of matrix.
3. **Muscle tissue** produces movement; it moves the body and its parts. Muscle cells are adapted for contractility and produce movement by shortening or lengthening the contractile units that are found in cytoplasm. Muscle tissue also produces most of the heat of the body.
4. **Nervous tissue** may be the most complex tissue in the body. It specializes in communication between the various parts of the body and in the integration of their activities. This tissue's major function is the generation of complex messages that coordinate the body's functions.

◇ FIELD NOTES

Fabric of the Body

I usually wear a sport coat in class when I'm teaching. I do it partly because I want to look suave and sophisticated, but mostly I wear a jacket because that room is always cold, no matter what time of year.

The jacket is sort of like an organ of the body. It has its own distinct function, but it also works with my other clothes to keep me warm and stylish (just like an organ is part of a system and of the whole organism).

However, when you look at the jacket, you see that it's made up of several different fabrics. Each fabric has its own structure and function. The wool in the outer shell looks great and keeps me warm. The silky lining makes it easy to move around in. The thick padding in the shoulders makes me look even more macho than usual. The leather patches on the elbows resist wear and tear on the wool sleeves.

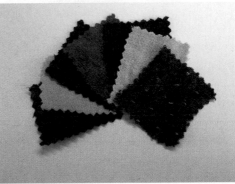

Likewise, organs of the body are each made up of different tissues. Tissues are the fabrics of the body. In fact, the English word *tissue* comes from the Old French word for "woven fabric," which underscores the proper way to think of tissues. Like different fabrics, each tissue has its own structural and functional characteristics that contribute to the structure and function of the whole organ and therefore of the whole body.

As you learn the tissues, keep this analogy in mind. If you think of each tissue as a different kind of fabric—paying attention to its structural characteristics and how that determines its function in the body—you'll find **histology** (tissue biology) to be fun and easy.

TABLE 1-19   Major Tissues of the Body

Tissue Type	Structure	Function	Examples in the Body
Epithelial tissue	One or more layers of densely arranged cells with very little extracellular matrix May form either sheets or glands	Covers and protects the body surface Lines body cavities Transports substances (absorption, secretion, excretion) Glandular activity	Outer layer of skin Lining of the respiratory, digestive, urinary, reproductive tracts Glands of the body
Connective tissue	Sparsely arranged cells surrounded by a large proportion of extracellular matrix that often contains structural fibers (and sometimes mineral crystals)	Supports body structures Transports substances throughout the body	Bones Joint cartilage Tendons and ligaments Blood Fat
Muscle tissue	Long fiber-like cells that are sometimes branched and that are capable of pulling loads; extracellular fibers sometimes hold muscle fibers together	Produces body movements Produces movements of organs such as the stomach and heart Produces heat	Heart muscle Muscles of the head, neck, arms, legs, and trunk Muscles in the walls of hollow organs such as the stomach and intestines
Nervous tissue	Mixture of many cell types, including several types of neurons (conducting cells) and neuroglia (support cells)	Communication between body parts Integration/regulation of body functions	Tissues of brain and spinal cord Nerves of the body Sensory organs of the body

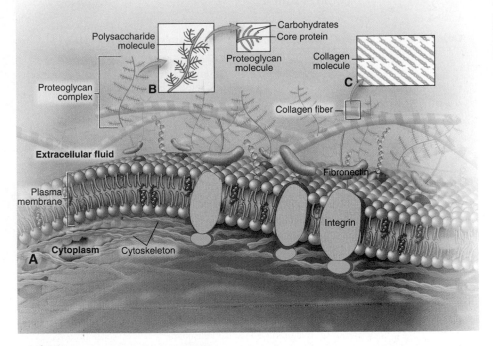

FIGURE 1-12 Extracellular Matrix (ECM).
A, The ECM is made up of water, proteins and glycoproteins, and proteoglycans that often form large bundles or complexes that bind together and to the cells of the tissue. Although the makeup of ECM varies from tissue to tissue, it usually includes some connections to **Integrins** in the plasma membranes, thereby allowing for structural integrity as well as communication and coordination within the tissue.
B, A detailed view of a **proteoglycan** complex shows many proteoglycans—each with a protein backbone and attached carbohydrate subunits—all held together by a polysaccharide chain.
C, Detailed view of a collagen bundle showing the individual **collagen** fibers within it.
See Table 1-20 for additional details.

✳ **TABLE 1-20**   **Components of the Extracellular Matrix (ECM)***

Component	Example	Description	Function	Example of Location
Water		Water molecules along with a small number of ions (mostly Na^+ and Cl^-)	Solvent for dissolved ECM components; provides fluidity of ECM	All tissues of the body
Proteins and glycoproteins	Collagen	Strong, flexible structural protein fiber	Provides flexible strength to tissues	Tendons, ligaments, bones, cartilage, many tissues
	Elastin	Flexible, elastic structural protein fiber	Allows flexibility and elastic recoil of tissues	Skin, cartilage of ear, walls of arteries

Continued

✳ **TABLE 1-20**   **Components of the Extracellular Matrix (ECM)—cont'd**

Component	Example	Description	Function	Example of Location
	Fibronectin	Rod-like glycoprotein	Binds ECM to cells; communicates with cells through integrins	Many tissues of the body, such as the connective tissues
	Laminin	Glycoproteins arranged as a three-pronged fork	Binds ECM components together and to cells; communicates with cells through integrins	Basal lamina (basement membrane) of the epithelial tissues
Proteoglycans	Various types	Protein backbone with attached chains of various polysaccharides:		
		Chondroitin sulfate	Shock absorber	Cartilage, bone, heart valves
		Heparin	Reduces blood clotting	Lining of some arteries
		Hyaluronate	Thickens fluid; lubricates	Loose fibrous connective tissue, joint fluids

*Not all components are present in all ECM; examples of only some of the many major ECM components are provided. Some components are illustrated in Figure 1-12.

◆ **SURVIVAL TIPS**

☑ The absolutely ONLY way to learn tissue identification is:
   Practice.
   Practice.
   Practice.
   It's only by looking at a lot of different samples, over and over, that you start to "get" what to look for. If you don't practice, no amount of shortcuts will help you.

☑ An easy way to practice is to use flash cards. Put the name of the tissue on one side of the card and a photo of a sample of that tissue on the other side. This works even better if you make several cards for each tissue type, each with a different photo (search online for samples). Use the PALS method (see page 38), and carry around a deck of flash cards with you to review many times throughout the day, every day.

☑ For more tips on learning tissues, see *Histology* (my-ap.us/KR4tvs) as well as *Tissues* (my-ap.us/VOjdpl).

☑ Don't skip the FIELD NOTES on the following pages. They contain many shortcuts and hints for handling easily confused tissue types.

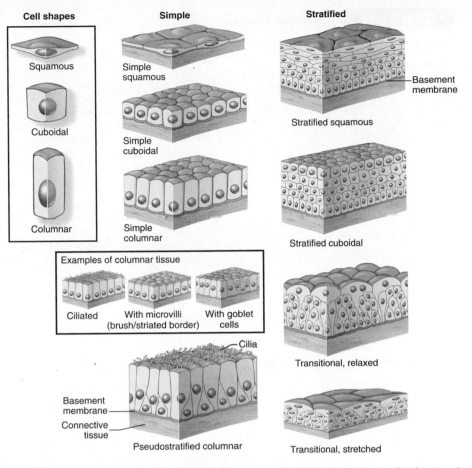

FIGURE 1-13 Classification of Epithelial Tissues. Tissues are classified according to the shape and arrangement of their cells. The color scheme of these drawings is based on a common staining technique used by histologists called *hematoxylin and eosin (H&E)* staining. H&E staining usually renders the cytoplasm pink and the chromatin inside the nucleus a purplish color. The cellular membranes, including the plasma membrane and the nuclear envelope, do not usually pick up any stain and thus may be transparent.

See Box 6-2 for information about cross sections of membranous tissues.

✳ **TABLE 1-21** **Classification Scheme for Membranous Epithelial Tissues**

Shape of Cells*	Tissue Types	Shape of Cells*	Tissue Types
One Layer		**Several Layers**	
Squamous	Simple squamous	Squamous	Stratified squamous
Cuboidal	Simple cuboidal	Cuboidal	Stratified cuboidal
Columnar	Simple columnar	Columnar	Stratified columnar
Pseudostratified columnar	Pseudostratified columnar	(Varies)	Transitional

*In the top layer (if more than one layer is present in the tissue).

✴ TABLE 1-22   Epithelial Tissues

Tissue	Location	Function
Membranous		
Simple squamous	Alveoli of lungs Lining of blood and lymphatic vessels (called *endothelium;* classified as connective tissue by some histologists) Surface layer of the pleura, pericardium, and peritoneum (called *mesothelium;* classified as connective tissue by some histologists)	Absorption by diffusion of respiratory gases between alveolar air and blood Absorption by diffusion, filtration, and osmosis Absorption by diffusion and osmosis Secretion
Stratified squamous Nonkeratinized Keratinized	Surface of the mucous membrane lining the mouth, the esophagus, and the vagina	Protection
	Surface of the skin (epidermis)	Protection
Transitional Relaxed Stretched	Surface of the mucous membrane lining the urinary bladder and the ureters	Permits stretching Protection
Simple columnar Without surface specialization With microvilli (brush/striated border) Ciliated With goblet cells	Surface layer of the mucous lining of the stomach, the intestines, and part of the respiratory tract	Protection Secretion Absorption Moving of mucus (by ciliated columnar epithelium)

✳ **TABLE 1-22**	**Epithelial Tissues—cont'd**	
Tissue	**Location**	**Function**
Pseudostratified columnar	Surface of the mucous membrane lining the trachea, the large bronchi, the nasal mucosa, and parts of the male reproductive tract (epididymis and vas deferens); also lines the large ducts of some glands (e.g., parotid)	Protection
Simple cuboidal	Ducts and tubules of many organs, including the exocrine glands and the kidneys	Secretion Absorption
Stratified cuboidal/columnar	Ducts of the sweat glands and mammary glands; lining of the pharynx; lining of part of the epiglottis; lining of part of the male urethra	Protection
Glandular	Glands	Secretion

Use Your Imagination for Cross Sections

When you look at photomicrographs of epithelial tissues or other structures that are tube-like, sac-like, or folded into complex shapes, it is sometimes hard to imagine what you are really looking at. As Diagram A shows, when you cut a tube on a cross section, the slice looks like a ring (if cut at a right angle) or an oval (if cut at an oblique or slanted angle). Diagram A also shows that, if the tube is bent where the cut is made, it can also look like an oval on the slide. Diagram B shows what happens when you have many tubes next to one another: your slice has many round or oval rings, depending on the angle of the cut. Diagram C shows what can happen when a membrane such as the intestinal lining is folded into complex shapes. The slice may look like a sort of zigzag line of cells. However, if it is shown at a high magnification, it may just look like a series of parallel rows. Try sketching out the "big picture" of the context of various tissue samples shown in the photomicrographs of your lab manual and textbook as well as those seen in your lab class—and then keep them in your notebook. By doing so, you'll be preparing yourself for later A&P course topics and later courses by learning to identify the context of a tissue on sight.

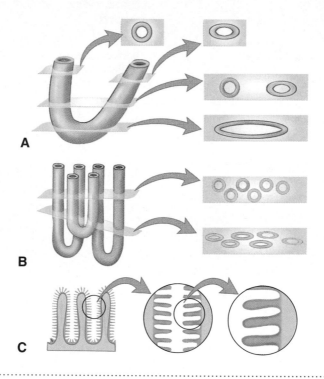

✳ **TABLE 1-23**   Structural Classification of Multicellular Exocrine Glands

Shape*	Complexity†	Type	Example
Tubular (single, straight)	Simple	Simple tubular	Intestinal glands
Tubular (coiled)	Simple	Simple coiled tubular	Sweat glands
Tubular (multiple)	Simple	Simple branched tubular	Gastric (stomach) glands
Alveolar (single)	Simple	Simple alveolar	Sebaceous (skin oil) glands
Alveolar (multiple)	Simple	Simple branched alveolar	Sebaceous glands
Tubular (multiple)	Compound	Compound tubular	Mammary glands
Alveolar (multiple)	Compound	Compound alveolar	Mammary glands
Some tubular; some alveolar	Compound	Compound tubuloalveolar	Salivary glands

*Shape of the distal secreting units of the gland.
†Number of ducts that reach the surface.

SURVIVAL TIPS

☑ As you look at tissue samples under a microscope or in your lab manual, textbook, or histology atlases, they are often labeled with the original location of the tissue in the sample. They may not be labeled with the general type. For example, your instructor may provide a slide labeled "kidney tubules" or "thyroid" so that you can find simple cuboidal epithelium. Why? Because tissues from those locations should provide a good sample of this tissue type.

☑ When you look at tissue samples provided by your instructor, don't expect a particular tissue type to be the only tissue present. For example, if your instructor gives you a sample of stratified squamous epithelium, it will also contain the underlying connective tissue. It's *up to you* to figure out which part is the tissue on which you want to focus.

☑ As you observe the prepared sectional slides of epithelial tissue, it is important that you first identify the "exposed" space. Since membranous epithelium covers the body or lines a cavity, there is always an exposed space. After you have identified the exposed space, classify the shape (squamous, cuboidal, or columnar) of the cells. Then determine the number of layers (simple or stratified).

FIELD NOTES

Field Identification of Epithelial Tissues

Look at the detailed descriptions and samples from your lab manual and textbook as you review these tips. That way, you can easily visualize the specific characteristics being described.

Simple Squamous Epithelium

Viewed from the side, as in a cross section, simple squamous epithelium looks like a thin line of cells, often with distinguishable nuclei. Viewed as a sheet from above, simple squamous epithelium looks like a two-dimensional layout of polygonal or rounded tiles, each with a central nucleus.

Stratified Squamous Epithelium

Nonkeratinized stratified squamous epithelium typically has a dense concentration of nuclei of the columnar and cuboidal cells near the basement membrane that becomes less dense toward the free surface. Most of the squamous cells near the free surface should have identifiable nuclei.

Keratinized stratified squamous samples will be from the epidermis (outer layer) of the skin. They will look similar to nonkeratinized specimens except that they have distinct additional layers overlying the top layers of squamous cells. This layer has no distinguishable nuclei.

Simple Cuboidal Epithelium

The cuboid shape of cells is easily seen in cross sections of kidney tubules. Because the sample is formed by many tubules cut at an angle, you will see many circles and loops made of simple cuboidal epithelium. Similar specimens are seen in thyroid tissue or tissues from other glands and glandular ducts.

Simple Columnar Epithelium

Simple columnar sheets often line cavities with deeply folded or grooved walls. The specimen, then, will appear to zigzag when viewed in a cross section. One surface of the sheet is always free, however, even though the free surfaces may fold back and touch one another. A goblet cell is easily recognizable by the very large bubble (vesicle) in the center or near the top. Because the vesicle contains clear, unstained mucus, it will appear more lightly colored than the surrounding material.

Pseudostratified Columnar Epithelium

On initial examination, pseudostratified epithelium resembles simple columnar epithelium. However, the telltale double row of nuclei gives it away. As in simple columnar epithelium, goblet cells may be present. Cilia look like distinct, tiny hairs along the free surface. Some specimens may have some areas of matted cilia or even "bald" spots. Under low magnification, the cilia look like "fuzz" on the free edge.

Transitional Epithelium

Transitional epithelium resembles nonkeratinized stratified squamous epithelium at first glance. Transitional epithelium, however, often has rounded cuboidal cells in the top layer (rather than only squamous cells). Depending on the individual specimen, you may see a great variety of shapes scattered throughout the tissue—some of them may have a sort of distorted teardrop shape. This variety gives transitional tissue a rather unorganized appearance as compared with the other epithelial types. Occasionally, transitional cells have two nuclei—an unusual characteristic that can help you to distinguish transitional epithelium from other epithelial types that have just one nucleus per cell.

⟡ SURVIVAL TIPS

☑ The terms *mucous* and *mucus* are often confused. *Mucus* is a noun that names a glycoprotein–water solution. *Mucous* is an adjective that describes something that is covered with mucus. Thus, mucous membranes are covered with mucus.

☑ To understand the shape of epithelial cells, you can use a soda can analogy. Imagine a soda can that has been completely smashed; this would represent a squamous-shaped cell. A soda can that has only been smashed halfway would represent a cuboidal-shaped cell. A soda can that has not been smashed would represent a columnar-shaped cell. Finally, soda cans arranged in all of these shapes would represent stratified transitional epilthelium.

✳ TABLE 1-24   Connective Tissues

Tissue	Location	Function
Fibrous		
Loose fibrous (areolar)	Between other tissues and organs Superficial fascia	Connection
Adipose (fat)	Under skin Padding at various points	Protection Insulation Support Reserve food Regulation of other tissues
Reticular	Inner framework of spleen, lymph nodes, and bone marrow	Support Filtration Blood production Immunity
Dense Fibrous		
Irregular	Deep fascia Dermis Scars Capsules of the kidneys, spleen, lymph nodes, and so on	Connection Support
Regular collagenous	Tendons Ligaments Aponeuroses	Flexible but strong connection
Elastic	Walls of some arteries	Flexible, elastic support
Bone		
Compact bone	Skeleton (outer shell of bones)	Support Protection Calcium reservoir

Tissue	Location	Function
Cancellous (spongy) bone	Skeleton (inside of bones)	Support Provides framework for blood production

Cartilage

Tissue	Location	Function
Hyaline	Part of nasal septum Covering articular surfaces of the bones Larynx Rings in the trachea and bronchi	Firm but flexible support Connection between structures
Fibrocartilage	Disks between the vertebrae Pubic symphysis	
Elastic	External ear Eustachian or auditory tube	

Blood

Tissue	Location	Function
	In the blood vessels	Transportation Protection

◆ **SURVIVAL TIPS**

☑ When classifying connective tissues, pay close attention to the matrix. Identify whether the matrix is protein (fibrous), protein (ground substance), or fluid. Use available resources (textbook, lab manual, atlas, or Internet sources) to familiarize yourself with the differences among these matrices.

☑ Many cells that are found in connective tissues are named according to their actions. Cells that produce matrix often have the suffix -blast ("make"). Cells that destroy matrix during remodeling have the suffix -clast ("break"). Cells that are in a relatively inactive mode have a -cyte ("cell") suffix. The first part of the name tells the specific kind of matrix involved: fibro- ("fiber"), chondro- ("cartilage"), or osteo- ("bone"). Thus, fibroblasts make fibers, chondroblasts manufacture cartilage matrix, and osteoblasts lay down bone matrix.

◆ FIELD NOTES

Field Identification of Connective Tissues

Look at the detailed descriptions and samples from your lab manual and textbook as you review these tips. That way, you can easily visualize the specific characteristics being described.

Loose Fibrous (Areolar) Connective Tissue

Areolar tissue's widely spaced fibers and variety of cell types make it an easy tissue to identify. The elastin fibers appear as dark, thick, jagged strands that may form branches. Collagen fibers form bundles that often appear as hazy pink or light purple crisscrossing lines.

Adipose Connective Tissue

Unlike other connective tissue cells, adipose cells are very close to one another. The large fat globule inside of each cell pushes the cytoplasm and organelles into a thin, dark ring around the inside of the cell membrane. The nucleus often appears as a bulge in the ring. The most obvious characteristic of this tissue is the presence of large fat vesicles, which generally look clear, yellowish, or light pink. The overall appearance is that of a host of large bubbles. Adipose tissue is often surrounded by areolar tissue, from which it develops.

Reticular Tissue

Reticular tissue is characterized by a network of extremely thin reticular fibers that are either stained darkly so that they can be seen easily or not stained, which makes them practically invisible under ordinary magnification. Reticular cells can be seen against the fibers, with cell shapes that seem to conform to the branches of the reticular meshwork.

Dense Fibrous Connective Tissue

Regular dense fibrous tissue usually has a roughly parallel arrangement of either collagen or elastic fibers. Collagen appears in wavy bundles stained pink or bluish. Elastin appears as thick fibers stained dark violet or blue. Darkly stained fibrocytes are scattered between fibers or fiber bundles, often in groups.

Irregular dense fibrous tissue is virtually the same as regular tissue in composition. Irregular tissue is different because the fibers appear as chaotic swirls rather than parallel lines.

Hyaline Cartilage Tissue

The collagen fibers of hyaline cartilage are not distinct in the matrix, which has a smooth, pinkish, or lavender appearance in many preparations. The chondrocytes are usually pink to violet and appear to have shriveled within their respective lacunae. Because of chondrocyte shrinkage, a clear ring appears around the inside of many lacunae.

Fibrocartilage Tissue

Fibrocartilage may appear alongside hyaline cartilage and sometimes looks very much like it. However, the distinct fibrous appearance of fibrocartilage's matrix is the determining factor.

Elastic Cartilage Tissue

In many preparations, elastin fibers stain very darkly. This makes their presence easy to detect and allows one to distinguish elastic cartilage without any problem.

Compact Bone Tissue

A cross section of compact bone has rings of lamellae that surround several adjacent central canals. The lamellae resemble rings in an onion slice. The central canals are either clear or nearly black, the lamellae are buff to orange, and the osteocytes are brown or black. The canaliculi often appear as wavy hairlines that radiate out from the lacunae.

✧ FIELD NOTES—cont'd

Trabecular Bone Tissue

Trabecular bone (cancellous or spongy bone) is distinguished by its rather disorganized array of trabecular beams of bone surrounded by myeloid tissue. The bone pieces may look like slivers of compact bone, with lamellae that often do not form complete circles. The myeloid tissue contains a scattering of blood cells, which appear as tiny, dark circles. Myeloid (hematopoietic) tissue may also have a net-like formation of very thin collagen fibers called *reticular fibers*. In some preparations, the bone tissue is pink and the myeloid cells are dark red.

Blood Tissue

A prepared blood smear is a drop of blood smeared on a slide and stained. The RBCs are the more numerous, smaller cells stained pink to orange-red. RBCs have no nuclei. The WBCs are much larger, with distinct, often distorted nuclei. Lab Exercise 34 has more complete details.

✧ FIELD NOTES

Field Identification of Muscle and Nerve Tissues

Look at the detailed descriptions and samples from your lab manual and textbook as you review these tips. That way, you can easily visualize the specific characteristics described.

Skeletal Muscle Tissue

Skeletal muscle preparations include very large cells with the characteristic striped pattern. The striping is very fine, so good focusing technique is critical with this specimen. The muscle fibers are generally parallel to one another in a longitudinal section, with the stripes at right angles across each fiber. Unlike the other types of muscle, skeletal muscle fibers have many nuclei per cell. The nuclei are often up against the cell membrane. Some fibrous connective tissue may be seen between the muscle cells.

Cardiac Muscle Tissue

Cardiac muscle striations are less distinct than those seen in skeletal muscle. Cardiac fibers have single nuclei, they usually have branches, and they do not taper at their ends. Many fibers attach end to end via intercalated disks, which appear as fine, dark (sometimes purple) lines at a right angle to a seemingly continuous fiber.

Smooth Muscle Tissue

Unlike other muscle cells, smooth muscle fibers are unstriated and have single nuclei. In some preparations, the cells are pink and the nuclei are purple or black. At first glance, you may confuse smooth muscle tissue with dense fibrous (regular) connective tissue. Smooth muscle is not wavy, like dense fibrous tissue sometimes is, and it has a more even distribution of nuclei than dense fibrous tissue.

Nerve Tissue

In a smear of spinal cord tissue, the neurons and glia are scattered randomly on the slide. The neurons are extremely large, each with a body that has a single nucleus. Neuron projections crisscross throughout. The glia appear as tiny, dark dots.

✳ TABLE 1-25   Muscle and Nervous Tissues

Tissue	Location	Function
Muscle		
Skeletal (striated voluntary)	Muscles that attach to bones	Movement of bones
		Generation of body heat
	Extrinsic eyeball muscles	Eye movements
	Upper third of the esophagus	First part of swallowing
Smooth (nonstriated, involuntary, or visceral)	In the walls of the tubular viscera of the digestive, respiratory, and genitourinary tracts	Movement of substances along the respective tracts
	In the walls of the blood vessels and the large lymphatic vessels	Changing the diameter of the blood vessels, thereby aiding in the regulation of blood pressure
	In the ducts of glands	Movement of substances along ducts
	Intrinsic eye muscles (iris and ciliary body)	Changing the diameter of the pupils and the shape of the lens
	Arrector muscles of hairs	Erection of hairs (gooseflesh)
Cardiac (striated involuntary)	Wall of the heart	Contraction of the heart
Nervous 	Brain	Excitability
	Spinal cord	Conduction
	Nerves	

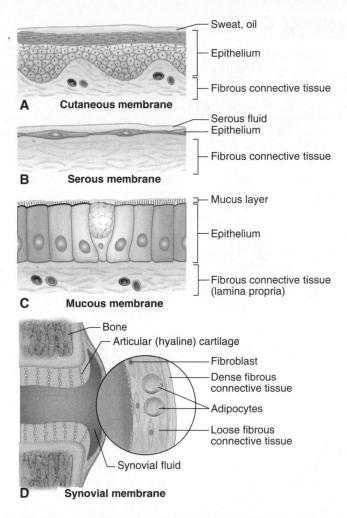

A   **Cutaneous membrane**
- Sweat, oil
- Epithelium
- Fibrous connective tissue

B   **Serous membrane**
- Serous fluid
- Epithelium
- Fibrous connective tissue

C   **Mucous membrane**
- Mucus layer
- Epithelium
- Fibrous connective tissue (lamina propria)

D   **Synovial membrane**
- Bone
- Articular (hyaline) cartilage
- Fibroblast
- Dense fibrous connective tissue
- Adipocytes
- Loose fibrous connective tissue
- Synovial fluid

FIGURE 1-14 Structure of Body Membranes. The term **membrane** refers to a thin, sheet-like structure that has many important functions in the body. Membranes cover and protect the body surface, line the body cavities, and cover the inner surfaces of hollow organs such as the digestive, reproductive, and respiratory passageways. Some membranes anchor organs to each other or to bones, whereas others cover the internal organs. In certain areas of the body, membranes secrete lubricating fluids that reduce friction during organ movements, such as the beating of the heart or lung expansion and contraction. Membrane lubricants also decrease friction between bones and joints. Two major categories or types of body membranes exist:
A, B, and **C, Epithelial membranes** are composed of epithelial tissue and an underlying layer of supportive connective tissue.
D, Connective tissue membranes are composed exclusively of various types of connective tissue; no epithelial cells are present in this type of membrane.
See Table 1-25 for more information about membranes.

✳ **TABLE 1-26**   **Membranes of the Body**

Type	Superficial Layer	Deep Layer	Location	Fluid Secretion	Function
Epithelial					
Cutaneous (skin)	Keratinized stratified squamous epithelium (epidermis)	Dense irregular fibrous connective tissue (dermis)	Directly exposed to the external environment	Sweat; sebum (skin oil)	Protection, sensation, thermoregulation
Serous	Simple squamous epithelium	Fibrous connective tissue	Lines body cavities that are not open to the external environment	Serous fluid	Lubrication
Mucous	Various types of epithelium	Fibrous connective tissue (lamina propria)	Lines tracts that open to the external environment	Mucus	Protection, lubrication
Connective					
Synovial	Dense fibrous connective tissue	Loose fibrous connective tissue	Lines joint cavities (in movable joints)	Synovial fluid	Helps hold joints together, lubricates, cushions

E. Body Plan

◇ **SURVIVAL TIPS**

☑ You can't explore a new territory without some idea of the general "lay of the land." Many students skim over this material or study it "just enough" to pass their first quiz. *They don't realize that it's a critical foundation on which rests nearly everything else in the course.* Take the extra time and effort to become *comfortable* with the plan of the human body.

☑ Be familiar with the *anatomical position*. This position involves a person standing straight with the toes forward, the arms to the side, and the palms forward. Imagine that the person is facing you. If you always imagine a person in this position as you look at individual body parts such as organs, you'll generally have the correct perspective. This works especially well when all you have is a verbal description of an organ or a location in the body.

☑ Try labeling yourself with sticky notes or mark up an old T-shirt with the names of the anatomical directions and regions of the body. It's goofy, I know, but it can really help you slow down and focus on the terminology. If you forget to take off some of the sticky notes? Great! When you find them later (or when someone else does), you'll have another chance to review.

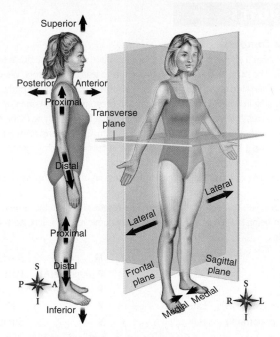

FIGURE 1-15 Directions and Planes of the Body. The transparent glass-like plates that divide the body into parts represent cuts or *sections* that can be made along a particular axis or line of orientation, which is called a *plane*. There are three major **body planes** that lie at right angles to each other. They are called the *sagittal* (SA-jih-tul), *coronal* (kuh-RO-nul), and *transverse* (or *horizontal*) planes. Literally hundreds of sections can be made in each plane, and each section made is named after the particular plane along which it occurs.

Sagittal plane: The lengthwise plane that runs from front to back is called the *sagittal plane*. This plane divides the body or any of its parts into right and left sides. If a sagittal section is made in the exact midline and results in equal and symmetrical right and left halves, then the plane is called a *midsagittal plane*.

Coronal plane: This is the lengthwise plane that runs from side to side and that divides the body or any of its parts into anterior and posterior portions; it is also called a *frontal plane*.

Transverse plane: This is the crosswise plane that divides the body or any of its parts into upper and lower parts; it is also called a *horizontal plane*.

The anatomic directions are listed in Table 1-17.

✧ FIELD NOTES

The Anatomic Compass

When I'm out on safari, I always have a map. I have to make sure that the guide knows where he or she is going, right? The main reason I have it, though, is to learn the territory. We use maps of the body all the time when studying anatomy, too, to learn the territories of the body.

When I'm traveling in a new territory and look at a geographic map, I often don't know which way to hold it. However, that's easily corrected by looking at the little thing in the corner that looks like a compass face with arrows marked *N* (north), *S* (south), *E* (east), and *W* (west). It's called a *rosette*, I guess because it looks kind of like a little rose. It tells me which way to look at the map and match the map features up with what I'm actually seeing.

To make the reading of anatomic figures a little easier, an *anatomic rosette* is used throughout this book (Figure 1-16).

On many figures, you will notice a small compass rosette similar to those seen on geographic maps. Rather than being labeled *N*, *S*, *E*, and *W*, the anatomic rosette is labeled with abbreviated anatomic directions:

A	Anterior	**M**	Medial
D	Distal	**P** *(opposite A)*	Posterior
I	Inferior	**P** *(opposite D)*	Proximal
L *(opposite M)*	Lateral	**R**	Right
L *(opposite R)*	Left	**S**	Superior

When I travel, it doesn't take long before I get somewhat familiar with the "lay of the land" and don't really need to check the rosette on the map anymore. It's the same with the anatomic rosette. At first, you may need to use it quite a bit to become oriented to a diagram, but after a while, you'll be so familiar with the body and its organs that you won't need it anymore.

FIGURE 1-16 Anatomic Rosette.

✧ **FIELD NOTES—cont'd**

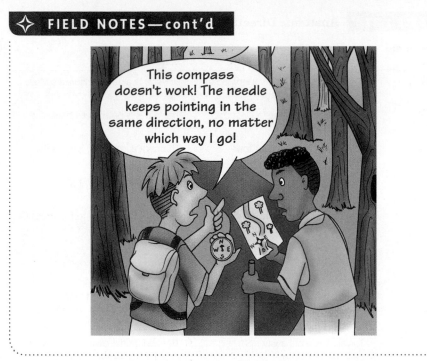

✳ **TABLE 1-27**   **Anatomic Directions Listed in Opposite Pairs**

Directional Term	Definition	Example of Use
Left	To the left of the body or structure being studied (not *your* left, the subject's)	The stomach is to the *left* of the liver.
Right	To the right of the body or structure being studied	The *right* kidney is damaged.
Lateral	Toward the side; away from the midsagittal plane	The eyes are *lateral* to the nose.
Medial	Toward the midsagittal plane; away from the side	The eyes are *medial* to the ears.
Anterior	Toward the front of the body	The nose is on the *anterior* of the head.
Posterior	Toward the back (rear) of the body	The heel is *posterior* to the head.
Superior	Toward the top of the body	The shoulders are *superior* to the hips.
Inferior	Toward the bottom of the body	The stomach is *inferior* to the heart.

Continued

✳ **TABLE 1-27**   **Anatomic Directions Listed in Opposite Pairs—cont'd**

Directional Term	Definition	Example of Use
Dorsal	Along (or toward) the vertebral surface of the body	Her scar is along the *dorsal* surface.
Ventral	Along (or toward) the belly surface of the body	The navel is on the *ventral* surface.
Caudal	Toward the tail (used for four-legged animals)	The neck is *caudal* to the skull.
Cranial	Toward the head (used for four-legged animals)	The neck is *cranial* to the tail.
Proximal	Toward the trunk (describes relative position in a limb or another appendage)	The joint is *proximal* to the toenail.
Distal	Away from the trunk or point of attachment	The hand is *distal* to the elbow.
Visceral	Toward an internal organ; away from the outer wall (describes positions inside a body cavity)	This organ is covered with the *visceral* layer of the membrane.
Parietal	Toward the wall; away from the internal structures	The abdominal cavity is lined with the *parietal* peritoneal membrane.
Deep	Toward the inside of a part; away from the surface (see *internal*)	The thigh muscles are *deep* to the skin.
Superficial	Toward the surface of a part; away from the inside (see *external*)	The skin is a *superficial* organ.
Internal	On the inside of a part (or the body)	The brain is an *internal* organ.
External	On the surface of a part or outside of the part (or the body)	Hairs are *external* structures.
Medullary	Refers to an inner region or to the medulla	The *medullary* portion contains nerve tissue.
Cortical	Refers to an outer region or to the cortex	The *cortical* area produces hormones.
Ipsilateral	On the same side of the body	The left knee is *ipsilateral* to the left ankle.
Contralateral	On the opposite side of the body	The left knee is *contralateral* to the right knee.
Central	Toward the center of a part (or the body)	The *central* nervous system includes the brain and the spinal cord.
Peripheral	Toward the outside boundary of a part (or the body)	Blood is pumped out of the heart and toward the *peripheral* vessels.
Basal	Toward or at the base of a part	The *basal* surface of the lung rests on the diaphragm.
Apical	Toward or at the point (apex) of a part	The *apical* surface of the cell possesses microvilli.

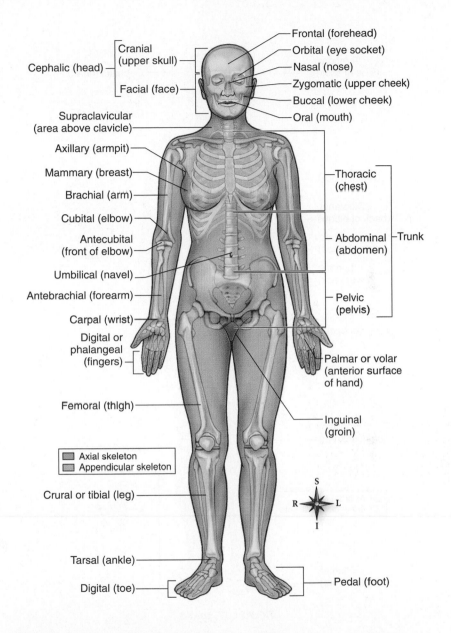

FIGURE 1-17 Specific Body Regions. Note that the body as a whole can be subdivided into two major portions:
    1, Axial (along the middle or axis of the body)
    2, Appendicular (the arms and legs or appendages)
The names of specific body regions follow the Latin form, with the English equivalent given in parentheses.
These names are also listed in Table 1-27.

Continued

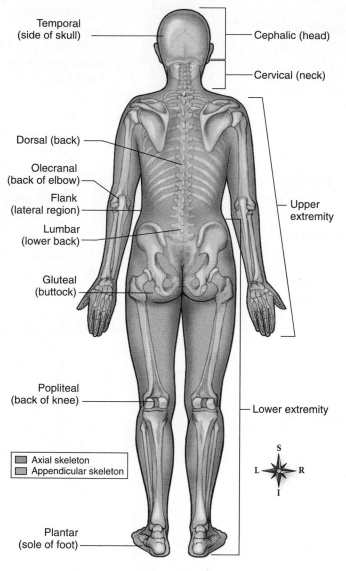

Temporal (side of skull)

Cephalic (head)

Cervical (neck)

Dorsal (back)

Olecranal (back of elbow)

Flank (lateral region)

Lumbar (lower back)

Upper extremity

Gluteal (buttock)

Popliteal (back of knee)

Lower extremity

Axial skeleton
Appendicular skeleton

S
L — R
I

Plantar (sole of foot)

FIGURE 1-17, cont'd

✳ TABLE 1-28   Latin-Based Descriptive Terms for Body Regions*

Body Region	Area or Example
Abdominal (ab-DOM-in-al)	Anterior torso below the diaphragm
Acromial (ah-KRO-me-al)	Shoulder
Antebrachial (an-tee-BRAY-kee-al)	Forearm
Antecubital (an-tee-KYOO-bi-tal)	Depressed area just in front of the elbow
Axillary (AK-si-lair-ee)	Armpit (axilla)
Brachial (BRAY-kee-al)	Upper arm
Buccal (BUK-al)	Cheek (inside)
Calcaneal (cal-CANE-ee-al)	Heel of foot
Carpal (KAR-pal)	Wrist
Cephalic (se-FAL-ik)	Head
Cervical (SER-vi-kal)	Neck
Coxal (COX-al)	Hip
Cranial (KRAY-nee-al)	Skull
Crural (KROOR-al) or tibial (TIBB-ee-al)	Leg
Cubital (KYOO-bi-tal)	Elbow
Cutaneous (kyoo-TANE-ee-us)	Skin (or body surface)
Digital (DIJ-i-tal)	Fingers or toes
Dorsal (DOR-sal)	Back or top
Facial (FAY-shal)	Face
Femoral (FEM-or-al)	Thigh
Frontal (FRON-tal)	Forehead
Gluteal (GLOO-tee-al)	Buttock
Hallux (HAL-luks)	Great toe
Inguinal (ING-gwi-nal)	Groin
Lumbar (LUM-bar)	Lower back between the ribs and the pelvis
Mammary (MAM-er-ee)	Breast
Manual (MAN-yoo-al)	Hand

Continued

✳ **TABLE 1-28**	**Latin-Based Descriptive Terms for Body Regions—cont'd**
Body Region	**Area or Example**
Mental (MEN-tal)	Chin
Nasal (NAY-zal)	Nose
Navel (NAY-val)	Area around the navel or umbilicus
Occipital (ok-SIP-i-tal)	Back of the lower skull
Olecranal (o-LECK-ra-nal)	Back of the elbow
Oral (OR-al)	Mouth
Orbital or ophthalmic (OR-bi-tal or op-THAL-mik)	Eyes
Otic (O-tick)	Ear
Palmar (PAHL-mar)	Palm of the hand
Patellar (pa-TELL-er)	Front of the knee
Pedal (PED-al)	Foot
Pelvic (PEL-vik)	Lower portion of the torso
Perineal (pair-i-NEE-al)	Area (perineum) between the anus and the genitals
Plantar (PLAN-tar)	Sole of the foot
Pollex (POL-ex)	Thumb
Popliteal (pop-li-TEE-al)	Area behind the knee
Pubic (PYOO-bik)	Pubis
Supraclavicular (soo-pra-cla-VIK-yoo-lar)	Area above the clavicle
Sural (SUR-al)	Calf
Tarsal (TAR-sal)	Ankle
Temporal (TEM-por-al)	Side of the skull
Thoracic (tho-RAS-ik)	Chest
Zygomatic (zye-go-MAT-ik)	Cheek

*The left column lists English adjectives that are based on Latin terms and that describe the body parts listed in English in the right column.

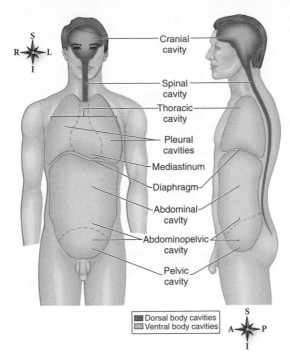

Cranial cavity
Spinal cavity
Thoracic cavity
Pleural cavities
Mediastinum
Diaphragm
Abdominal cavity
Abdominopelvic cavity
Pelvic cavity

■ Dorsal body cavities
□ Ventral body cavities

FIGURE 1-18 Major Body Cavities. The **dorsal body cavities** are in the dorsal (back) part of the body and is subdivided into a **cranial cavity** above and a **spinal cavity** below. The **ventral body cavities** are on the ventral (front) side of the trunk and is subdivided into the **thoracic cavity** above the diaphragm and the **abdominopelvic cavity** below the diaphragm. The **thoracic cavity** is subdivided into the **mediastinum** in the center and **pleural cavities** to the sides. The abdominopelvic cavity is subdivided into the **abdominal cavity** above the pelvis and the **pelvic cavity** within the pelvis.

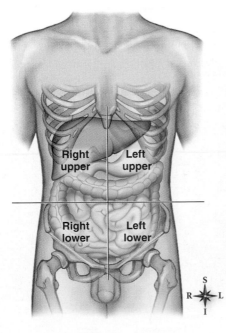

Right upper
Left upper
Right lower
Left lower

FIGURE 1-19 Division of the Abdomen into Four Quadrants. Health professionals frequently divide the abdomen into four quadrants to describe the site of abdominopelvic pain or to locate some type of internal pathology such as a tumor or abscess. Horizontal and vertical line passing through the umbilicus (navel) divide the abdomen into right and left upper quadrants and right and left lower quadrants.

FIGURE 1-20 Nine Regions of the **Abdominopelvic Cavity.** For convenience in locating abdominal organs, anatomists divide the abdomen like a tic-tac-toe grid into nine imaginary regions. Only the most superficial structures of the internal organs are shown here.

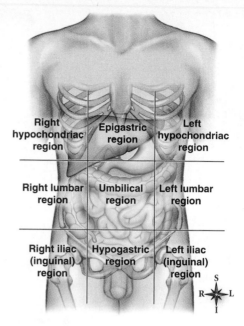

F. Homeostasis

FIGURE 1-21 Diagram of the Body's **Internal Environment.** The human body is like a bag of fluid that is separated from the external environment. Tubes, such as the digestive tract and the respiratory tract, bring the external environment to deeper parts of the bag, where substances may be absorbed into the internal fluid environment or excreted into the external environment. All of the "accessories" somehow help to maintain a constant environment inside the bag, allowing the cells that live there to survive. **Homeostasis** is the name for this maintenance of relative constancy of the body's internal fluid environment. Table 1-28 summarizes the roles of all of the major systems and organs in maintaining homeostasis.

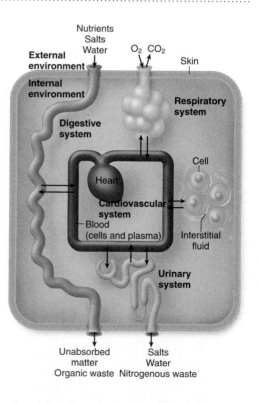

✳ **TABLE 1-29**   **Body Systems**

Functional Category	System	Principal Organs	Primary Functions
Support and movement	Integumentary	Skin	Separates the internal environment from the external environment; protection, temperature regulation, and sensation
	Skeletal	Bones, ligaments	Support, protection, movement, mineral and fat storage, and blood production
	Muscular	Skeletal muscles, tendons	Movement, posture, and heat production
Communication, control, and integration	Nervous	Brain, spinal cord, nerves, sensory organs	Sensation, integration, control, and coordination of other systems; memory
	Endocrine	Pituitary gland, adrenals, pancreas, thyroid, parathyroids, other glands	Control and regulation of other systems
Transportation and defense	Cardiovascular	Heart, arteries, veins, capillaries	Exchange and transport of materials
	Lymphatic	Lymph nodes, lymphatic vessels, spleen, thymus, tonsils	Immunity and fluid balance
	Immune	Many cells and tissues throughout the body, particularly the blood and lymphoid tissue	Immunity and response to injury
Respiration, nutrition, and excretion	Respiratory	Lungs, bronchial tree, trachea, larynx, nasal cavity	Gas exchange (O_2 and CO_2) and acid–base balance
	Digestive	Stomach, small and large intestines, esophagus, liver, mouth, pancreas	Breakdown and absorption of nutrients; elimination of waste
	Urinary	Kidneys, ureters, bladder, urethra	Keeps internal environment in balance by excretion of waste, fluid and electrolyte balance, and acid–base balance
Reproduction and development	Reproductive	*Male:* Testes, vas deferens, prostate, seminal vesicles, penis *Female:* Ovaries, fallopian tubes, uterus, vagina, breasts	Reproduction, continuity of genetic information, and nurturing of offspring

FIGURE 1-22 Basic
**Components of Homeostatic
Control Mechanisms.**
A, Heat regulation by a
furnace controlled by a
thermostat.

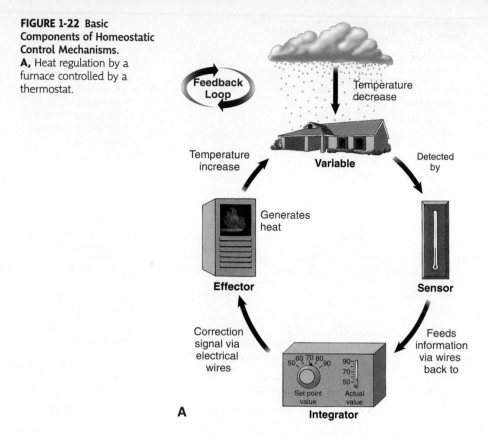

A

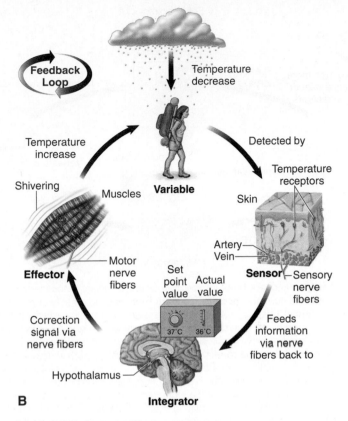

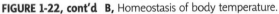

FIGURE 1-22, cont'd B, Homeostasis of body temperature.
Note that, in both **A** and **B,** a stimulus or disturbance of the **controlled variable** (a drop in temperature) activates a **sensor** mechanism (the thermostat or body temperature receptor) that sends input or **feedback** to an **integrator** or control center (the on–off switch or hypothalamus). The integrator compares the actual value of the variable to the **setpoint** value of the variable, which in this case reveals that the temperature has dropped below the setpoint. The integrator then sends regulatory output to an **effector** mechanism (the furnace or contracting muscle). The resulting heat that is produced maintains the temperature in a normal range. Feedback of effector activity to the sensor mechanism completes the control loop.
This is an example of a **negative feedback loop,** because sensory feedback results in a reversal (negation) of the trend away from the setpoint for the variable. Negative feedback loops thus automatically *stabilize* the variable—maintaining homeostasis.

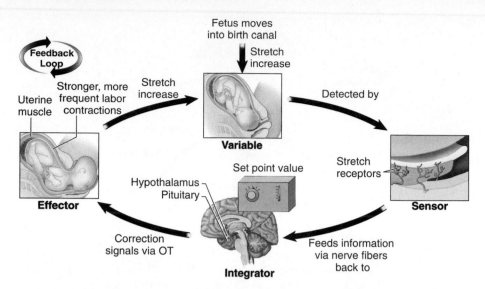

FIGURE 1-23 Positive Feedback Loop. Instead of opposing a change in the internal environment and causing a return to normal, a **positive feedback loop** tends to amplify or reinforce the change that is occurring. This happens when the integrator responds by activating effectors that drive the variable further away from the setpoint. The only way to stop a positive feedback loop from getting out of hand quickly is to break the loop. Ordinarily, positive feedback regulation would be abnormal. But there are some situations, such as childbirth (pictured) or blood clotting, when the rapid amplification of positive feedback is helpful in maintaining health. For example, as delivery begins, the baby is pushed from the *womb* or *uterus* into the *birth canal* or *vagina*. Stretch receptors in the wall of the reproductive tract detect the increased stretch that is caused by movement of the baby. Information regarding increased stretch is fed back to the brain, which triggers the pituitary gland to secrete a hormone called *oxytocin* (OT). OT travels to the uterus and triggers stronger contractions. Stronger contractions push the baby farther along the birth canal, thereby increasing stretch and stimulating the release of more OT. Uterine contractions (labor contractions) quickly get stronger and stronger until the baby is pushed out of the body and the positive feedback loop is broken. OT can also be injected therapeutically by a physician to stimulate labor contractions.

◇ FIELD NOTES

Wallenda Model

My friend, Tino, has an interesting job. He and his wife Olinka—and most of the rest of his family—are in the circus. Performing as *The Flying Wallendas,* Tino's family members have amazed folks around the world with their ability to walk on the high wire. Tino is especially well known for his skill in walking on unusually high wires strung up over particularly high and hazardous areas, like across a waterfall or between skyscrapers. Yikes.

The image of a high-wire artist like Tino Wallenda is a good model for understanding homeostasis in the body—what I like to call the *Wallenda Model of Homeostasis.*

Homeostasis is a kind of relative constancy of the body that is analogous to the kind of relative constancy of position that Tino must maintain on the high wire if he is to survive.

Tino's grandfather, Karl, didn't survive. Karl was walking on a wire between two hotels in very windy conditions several decades ago. As good as Karl was, he couldn't maintain his position on the wire, and he fell to his death. I'm not telling you this to be morbid, but that's part of the usefulness of the model: if you don't maintain homeostatic balance in your body, you'll die. As a matter of fact, that's usually the mechanism involved in a person's death.

When Tino is on the high wire, the position just over the wire is his setpoint. If his "sensors"— such as his eyes (vision receptors), ears (equilibrium receptors), and muscles (stretch receptors)—tell him that he's falling to his left, then the integrators in his brain will instruct his muscles to pull him a little to the right. This is a form of negative feedback: Tino's body is using feedback sensory information to regulate effectors (his muscles) to change his direction back toward the setpoint.

When you watch Tino perform, you'll notice that he sways back and forth and back and forth somewhat unpredictably as he crosses the wire. Likewise, in the body, conditions are constantly being disturbed and feedback mechanisms are being pulled back toward their setpoints. Tino is relatively constant in his position over the wire, just as your body conditions are relatively constant. It takes energy to keep your body's feedback mechanisms working, just as it takes a lot of energy to keep Tino on the wire.

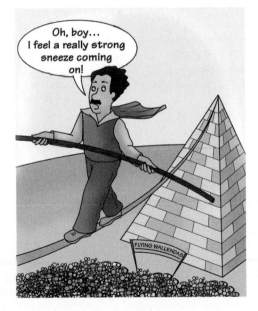

Something else for which the Wallenda family is well known is the pyramid. They stack Wallenda family members, one on top of the other, to form a human pyramid on the high wire. I still can't believe their famous seven-person, three-high pyramid, and I've seen it many times! Imagine how well coordinated each of them needs to be to maintain the pyramid. Likewise, each feedback loop in your body is interdependent on the others. If one feedback loop gets messed up, it's likely to lead to many other problems.

For more about the Wallenda Model of Homeostasis as well as additional models (e.g., the Fishbowl Model, the Engineering Model) and shortcuts for understanding the important concept of homeostasis, see *Mini Lesson: Homeostasis* (my-ap.us/rs3KqV).

2

Support and Movement

Navigation Guide

A. Skin

✳ **TABLE 2-1**   Structure of the Skin

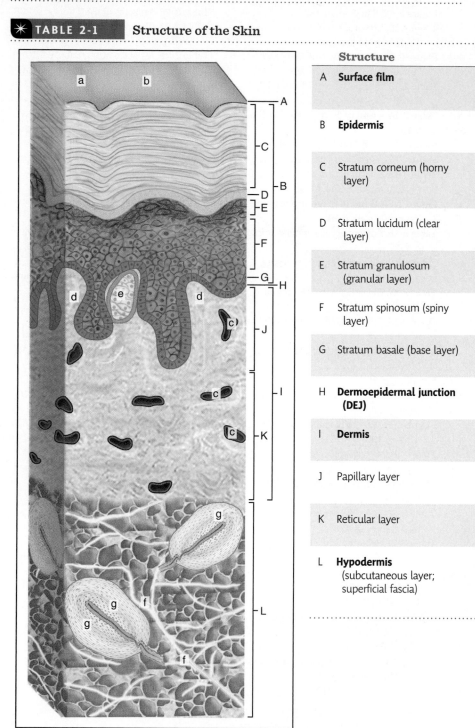

	Structure
A	**Surface film**
B	**Epidermis**
C	Stratum corneum (horny layer)
D	Stratum lucidum (clear layer)
E	Stratum granulosum (granular layer)
F	Stratum spinosum (spiny layer)
G	Stratum basale (base layer)
H	**Dermoepidermal junction (DEJ)**
I	**Dermis**
J	Papillary layer
K	Reticular layer
L	**Hypodermis** (subcutaneous layer; superficial fascia)

Description

Thin film that coats the skin; made up of a mixture of sweat, sebum, desquamated cells/ fragments, and various chemicals; protects the skin

Superficial primary layer of the skin; made up entirely of keratinized stratified squamous epithelium; derived from the ectoderm; also includes hairs, sweat glands, and sebaceous glands

Several layers of flakelike dead cells (or *corneocytes*) mostly made up of dense networks of *keratin* fibers cemented by *glycophospholipids* and forming a tough, waterproof barrier; the keratinized layer *(a)*, the sulcus (groove) *(b)*, and the friction ridge

A few layers of squamous cells filled with *eleidin*, a keratin precursor that gives this layer a translucent quality (not visible in thin skin)

2 to 5 layers of dying, somewhat flattened cells filled with darkly staining keratohyalin granules and multilayered bodies of glycophospholipids; nuclei disappear in this layer

8 to 10 layers of cells pulled by desmosomes into a spiny appearance

Single layer of mostly columnar cells capable of mitotic cell division; it is from this layer that all cells of superficial layers are derived; includes keratinocytes and some melanocytes

The basement membrane; a unique and complex arrangement of adhesive components that glue the epidermis and the dermis together

Deep primary layer of the skin; made up of fibrous tissue; also includes some blood vessels *(c)*, muscles, and nerves; derived from the mesoderm

Loose fibrous tissue with collagenous and elastic fibers; forms nipplelike bumps called *papillae* *(d)*; includes tactile corpuscles, which are touch receptors *(e)*, and other sensory receptors

Tough network (reticulum) of collagenous dense irregular fibrous tissue with some elastic fibers; forms most of the dermis

Loose fibrous (areolar) connective tissue and adipose tissue; under the skin (not part of the skin); includes fibrous bands or *skin ligaments* *(f)* that connect the skin strongly to underlying structures; includes lamellar corpuscles, which are pressure receptors *(g)*, and other sensory receptors

✧ SURVIVAL TIPS

☑ When learning the layers of skin in order, writing the name of each layer on a different index card. Shuffle the cards, and then lay them out on a table in the correct order, checking your results against Table 2-1. Shuffle the deck, and try it again. Keep going, perhaps across several short sessions, until you can do it easily without having to check the table. This is sort of like playing a game of *solitaire*.

☑ Remember that the **hypodermis**, which is also called *superficial fascia* or *subcutaneous tissue*, is *not* part of the skin proper. However, it's discussed along with skin because of its close relationship with the skin and because it's not part of any other organ or system. For practical purposes, it's sometimes spoken of as if it's part of the skin; this may make the technical distinction between the skin and the hypodermis confusing.

✳ TABLE 2-2   Functions of the Skin

Function	Example	Mechanism
Protection	Against microorganisms Against dehydration Against ultraviolet radiation Against mechanical trauma	Surface film/mechanical barrier Keratin Melanin Tissue strength
Sensation	Pain Heat and cold Pressure Touch	Somatic sensory receptors
Permits movement and growth without injury	Body growth and change in body contours during movement	Elastic and recoil properties of the skin and the subcutaneous tissue
Endocrine	Vitamin D production	Activation of precursor compound in skin cells by ultraviolet light
Excretion	Water Urea Ammonia Uric acid	Regulation of sweat volume and content
Immunity	Destruction of microorganisms and interaction with immune system cells (helper T cells)	Phagocytic cells and epidermal dendritic cells
Temperature regulation	Heat loss or retention	Regulation of blood flow to the skin and the evaporation of sweat

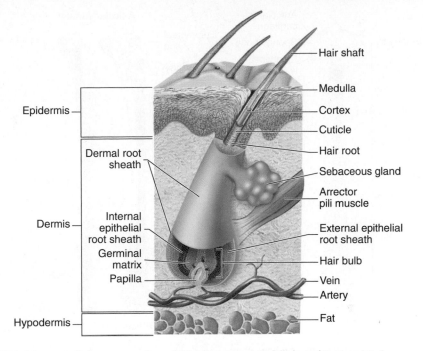

FIGURE 2-1 Hair Follicle. Cross-section of skin showing a hair follicle and its associated structures.

B. Skeletal System and Joints

Gross Structure of a Long Bone

I. **Diaphysis** (dye-AF-i-sis): the main, shaftlike portion

II. **Epiphyses** (eh-PIF-i-seez): the proximal and distal ends of a long bone. Epiphyses have a bulbous shape that provides generous space near joints for muscle attachments and that also gives stability to joints. *Red marrow (myeloid tissue)* fills the spaces within the internal *trabecular (spongy, cancellous) bone*. Early during development, epiphyses are separated from the diaphysis by a layer of cartilage called the *epiphyseal plate*. The cartilage layer is eventually replaced by bone and forms an *epiphyseal line*. The region between the epiphyses and the diaphysis (in a mature bone) or the epiphyseal plate region (in a growing bone) is called the *metaphysis* (meh-TAF-i-sis).

III. **Articular cartilage:** the thin layer of hyaline cartilage that covers the articular or joint surfaces of epiphyses

IV. **Periosteum** (pair-ee-OS-tee-um): the dense, white fibrous membrane that covers bone except at joint surfaces, where articular cartilage forms the covering. Many of the periosteum fibers penetrate the underlying bone and weld these two structures to each other. In addition, muscle tendon fibers interlace with periosteal fibers, thereby anchoring muscles firmly to bone.

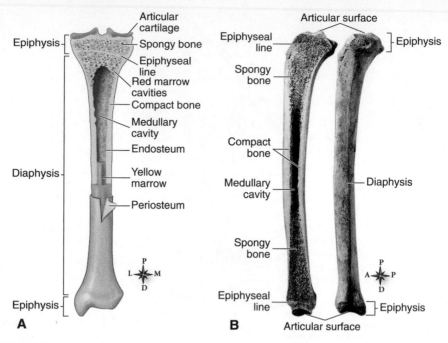

FIGURE 2-2 Gross Structure of a Long Bone.
A, Partial frontal section of a long bone (tibia) showing cancellous and compact bone.
B, Sagittal section of a long bone with a whole long bone (tibia) in lateral view.

 V. **Medullary cavity:** a tubelike hollow space in the diaphysis of a long bone that is also called a *marrow cavity*. In an adult, the medullary cavity is filled with connective tissue that is rich in fat; this substance is called *yellow marrow*.
 VI. **Endosteum** (en-DOS-tee-um): a thin, fibrous membrane that lines the medullary cavity and the trabecular spaces inside long bones

Microscopic Structure of a Long Bone
Compact Bone

 I. Contains many cylinder-shaped structural units called **osteons** or *Haversian systems*
 II. Osteons surround **central** *(osteonal or Haversian)* **canals** that run lengthwise through bone and that are connected by **transverse** *(Volkmann)* **canals**
 III. Osteon structure
   A. Lamellae
     1. **Concentric:** cylinder-shaped layers of calcified matrix around the central canal
     2. **Interstitial:** layers of bone matrix *between* the osteons; leftover from previous osteons
     3. **Circumferential:** few layers of bone matrix that surround all of the osteons; run along the outer circumference of a bone and the inner circumference (the boundary of the medullary cavity) of a bone

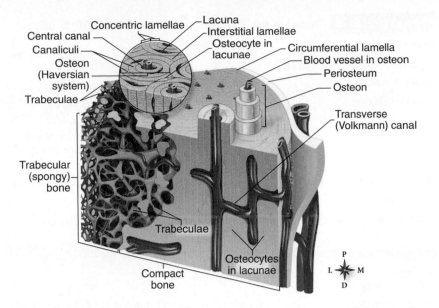

FIGURE 2-3 Microscopic Structure of a Long Bone. Wedge of bone removed from the wall of a long bone diaphysis showing internal **trabecular bone** toward the left and external **compact bone** toward the right.

B. **Lacunae:** small spaces that contain tissue fluid in which bone cells are located between the hard layers of the lamella
C. **Canaliculi:** ultra-small canals that radiate in all directions from the lacunae and connecting them to each other and to the central canal
D. **Central** (osteonal or Haversian) **canal:** extends lengthwise through the center of each osteon; contains blood and lymph vessels
E. **Trabecular bone:** also called spongy bone or cancellous bone
    1. No osteons in cancellous bone; instead, it has **trabeculae**
    2. Lattices of bony branches (trabeculae) are arranged along lines of stress to enhance the bone's strength

Bone Cells

I. **Osteoblasts**
    A. Bone-forming cells found in all bone surfaces
    B. Small cells synthesize and secrete osteoid, which is an important part of the ground substance
    C. Collagen fibrils line up in osteoid and serve as a framework for the deposition of calcium and phosphate
II. **Osteoclasts**
    A. Giant cells with multiple nuclei; many mitochondria and lysosomes
    B. Use acids to dissolve hard bone minerals
III. **Osteocytes**—inactive osteoblasts surrounded by matrix and lying within lacunae

✳ **TABLE 2-3**	Bones of the Typical Adult Skeleton (206 Total)*
Part of Body	**Name of Bone**
Axial Skeleton (80 Bones Total)	
Skull (28 bones total)	
Cranium (8 bones)	Frontal (1), Parietal (2), Temporal (2), Occipital (1), Sphenoid (1), Ethmoid (1)
Face (14 bones)	Nasal (2), Maxillary (2), Zygomatic (malar) (2), Mandible (1), Lacrimal (2), Palatine (2), Inferior nasal conchae (turbinates) (2), Vomer (1)
Ear bones (6 bones)	Malleus (hammer) (2), Incus (anvil) (2), Stapes (stirrup) (2)
Hyoid bone (1)	
Spinal column (26 bones)	Cervical vertebrae (7), Thoracic vertebrae (12), Lumbar vertebrae (5), Sacrum (1), Coccyx (1)
Sternum and ribs (25 bones)	Sternum (1), True ribs (14), False ribs (10)
Appendicular Skeleton (126 Bones Total)	
Upper extremities including shoulder girdle (64 bones)	Clavicle (2), Scapula (2), Humerus (2), Radius (2), Ulna (2), Carpal bones (16), Metacarpal bones (10), Phalanges (28)
Lower extremities including hip girdle (62 bones)	Innominate (2), Fibula (2), Femur (2), Patella (2), Tibia (2), Tarsal bones (14), Metatarsal bones (10), Phalanges (28)

*An inconstant number of small, flat, round bones known as *sesamoid bones* (because of their resemblance to sesame seeds) are found in various tendons in which considerable pressure develops. Because the number of these bones varies greatly among individuals, only two of them—the patellae—have been counted among the 206 bones of the body. Generally, two of them can be found in each thumb (in the flexor tendon near the metacarpophalangeal and interphalangeal joints) and great toe, and several others can be found in the upper and lower extremities. *Sutural bones (wormian bones)*, which are the small islets of bone that are frequently found in some of the cranial sutures, have not been counted in this list of 206 bones because of their variable occurrence. The numeral that follows each bone name is the typical number of that type of bone found in the adult skeleton.

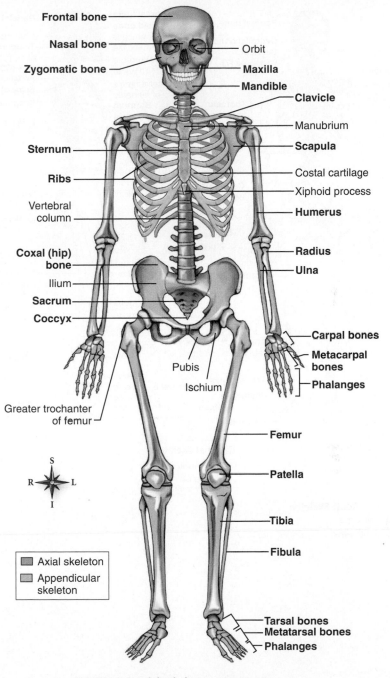

Frontal bone

Nasal bone

Zygomatic bone

Orbit

Maxilla

Mandible

Clavicle

Manubrium

Sternum

Scapula

Ribs

Costal cartilage

Xiphoid process

Vertebral column

Humerus

Coxal (hip) bone

Radius

Ilium

Ulna

Sacrum

Coccyx

Carpal bones

Metacarpal bones

Pubis

Phalanges

Ischium

Greater trochanter of femur

Femur

Patella

Tibia

Fibula

Axial skeleton

Appendicular skeleton

Tarsal bones

Metatarsal bones

Phalanges

FIGURE 2-4 Adult Skeleton, Anterior View.

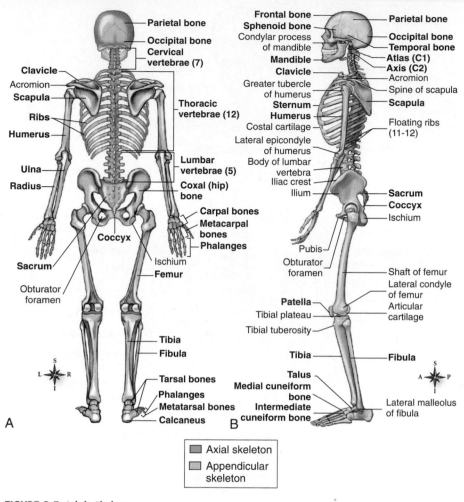

FIGURE 2-5 **Adult Skeleton.**
A, Posterior view.
B, Left lateral view.

✧ FIELD NOTES

Mountains, Hills, and Valleys

Imagine that you're out on a trek through a wilderness that is unknown to you. You have your trusty cell phone, and you use it to occasionally call your friend who is familiar with the territory.

Let's say that your friend says, "Keep going north until you reach the Dardenne River." Therefore, you trek onward, toward the north (you have your compass with you, of course). You reach a large rock outcropping and stop to call your friend. "I think I'm at the Dardenne River," you say, "What now?"

What's wrong with this picture? Obviously, you don't know a rock outcropping from a river; this is *not* great if you're trekking by yourself in the wilderness!

It's the same when "trekking through" the human body; you need to know the *hills* from the *valleys* and the *rivers* from the *oceans*. I'm sure that you're already familiar with what a river is, but do you know what a *foramen* is? Or a *condyle*? What's the difference between a *condyle* and an *epicondyle*?

If you look at Table 2•4, you'll see many of the different features that you may find in the skeleton. If you learn that a foramen is a hole, it'll be pretty easy to find the *optic foramen*; it's a hole in the back of the eye socket through which the optic nerve passes. However, if you don't know what a foramen is, then you'll have to search your reference maps and descriptions; this is a much harder and less accurate way of doing things.

Most students don't take the time to become familiar with the terms listed in Table 2-4. They then discover that finding all of the assigned bone markings will be very difficult and time consuming. However, those students who familiarize themselves with the general types of features find it easy, *fast*, and fun to find the assigned bone markings.

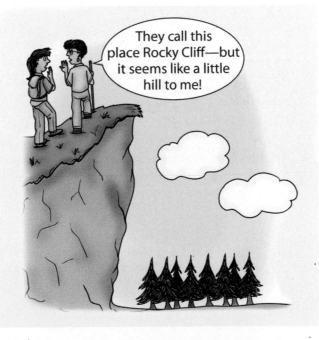

		Descriptions and	
Terms	**Pronunciations**	**Translations**	**Examples**
Angle	ANG-gul	An inside or outside corner	Angle of mandible
			Inferior angle of scapula
Body	BOD-ee	The main or central portion of a bone	Body of sphenoid bone
			Body of vertebra
			Body of sternum
			Body of rib
Condyle	KON-dyle	Rounded bump; usually fits into a fossa on another bone to form a joint (literally "knuckle")	Occipital condyle
			Lateral condyle of femur
			Medial condyle of tibia
Crest	krest	Moderately raised ridge; generally a site for muscle attachment (literally "tuft" or "comb")	Pubic crest of coxal (pelvic) bone
			Intertrochanteric crest of femur
			Crest of tibia
Epicondyle	ep-i-KON-dyle	Bump near a condyle; often gives the appearance of a "bump on a bump"; for muscle attachment (literally "upon a knuckle")	Lateral epicondyle of humerus
			Medial epicondyle of humerus
			Lateral epicondyle of femur
Foramen (*pl.*, foramina or foramens)	foh-RAY-men or FO-ra-men (foh-RAM-in-ah or foh-RAY-menz)	Round hole for vessels and nerves (literally "hole")	Jugular foramen of temporal bone
			Foramen ovale of sphenoid bone
			Obturator foramen of coxal (pelvic) bone
Fossa (*pl.*, fossae)	FOSS-ah (FOSS-ee)	Depression; often receives an articulating bone (literally "ditch")	Mandibular fossa of temporal bone
			Olecranon fossa of humerus
			Intercondylar fossa of femur
Head	hed	Distinct epiphysis on a long bone, separated from the shaft by a narrowed portion or neck	Head of humerus
			Head of radius
			Head of femur

✳ **TABLE 2-4**   Terms Used to Describe Bone Markings

✳ TABLE 2-4   Terms Used to Describe Bone Markings—cont'd

Terms	Pronunciations	Descriptions and Translations	Examples
Line (Latin *linea*)	lyne (LEEN-ee-ah or LIN-ee-ah)	Similar to a crest but not raised as much (is often rather faint)	Superior nuchal line of occipital bone
			Superior temporal line of parietal bone
			Intercondylar line of femur
Neck	nek	A narrowed portion, usually at the base of a head	Neck of rib
			Neck of radius
			Neck of femur
Notch	notch	A V-like "cut" out of the margin or edge of a flat area	Supraorbital notch
			Radial notch of ulna
			Greater sciatic notch of coxal bone
Process	PRAH-ses or PRO-ses	Projection or raised area	Mastoid process of temporal bone
			Spinous process of vertebra
			Coronoid process of ulna
Sinus	SYE-nus	Cavity within a bone (literally "hollow")	Frontal sinus
			Sphenoid sinus
			Maxillary sinus
Spine	spyne	Sharp, pointed process; similar to crested but raised more; for muscle attachment (literally "thorn")	Spine of scapula
			Spine of vertebra
			Ischial spine
Tubercle	TOO-ber-kul	Small tuberosity (see below); small oblong bump (literally "small bump" or "small lump")	Tubercle of rib
			Greater tubercle of humerus
			Adductor tubercle of femur

◇ SURVIVAL TIPS

☑ **Boldface** labels refer to whole bones. The rest are specific features of the bone or skeletal region.

☑ Contrasting colors are added to some of the illustrations to help you distinguish more easily among the bones.

☑ The tables list pronunciations. Use them to practice saying the name of each structure out loud. This seems silly, but it really helps your brain to "get it," and it helps you to retrieve the information from your memory later. See the sidebar titled *Pronunciation* on page 16.

☑ Pay attention to the literal translation of each structure. This will both help you to remember the parts and help to you learn new body parts when you encounter them. See the Field Notes on the facing page.

☑ Be careful about using correct anatomic terminology, which is sometimes different than ordinary usage. For example, the *upper extremity (upper limb)* is not the "arm," as we would say in everyday conversation. Only the part above the elbow is the *arm*; the part below the elbow is the *forearm*. Likewise, the *lower extremity (lower limb)* is not the "leg." The *leg* is the part below the knee; the *thigh* is the part above the knee.

☑ When you use terms like *head, body, shaft,* and so on, you may need to clarify the bone to which you are referring. For example, do you mean head of the *femur,* the head of the *humerus,* the head of the *radius,* or the head of the *ulna*? These references are left off the tables because they are implied by the table headings, so be careful.

☑ You may not need to learn to identify *every* structure listed here for your course. Highlight those required in your course, or cross out those that are not required. However, don't cover up the ones that you don't need right now, because someday you *will* need them.

☑ Don't forget to *practice*! Use skeletal specimens in your lab, library, or learning center when you can. Off campus, use illustrated flash cards or study cards to practice for a few minutes at a time, several times each day. If you don't start practicing *right away*—and keep it up *every day*—you'll find it very difficult to remember all of the parts that you need to identify.

✦ FIELD NOTES

Bone Names Have Meaning

In the last Field Notes entry (see page 143), I stated that, when you know what the name of a bone feature means, you can easily figure out what to look for when first trying to identify it, and it makes it easier to remember structures after you've found them. This principle also applies to the other parts of the names of skeletal structures.

For example, you know from Table 2-4 that *foramen* means "hole." When you see the name *foramen ovale*, you can probably figure out that the terms means "oval hole." Knowing this fact makes the foramen ovale much easier to find among all of the surrounding rounded holes of the skull. When you see the name *foramen lacerum* and when you know that *lacerum* means "jagged" or "lacerated," then this structure is easier to find and much easier to remember.

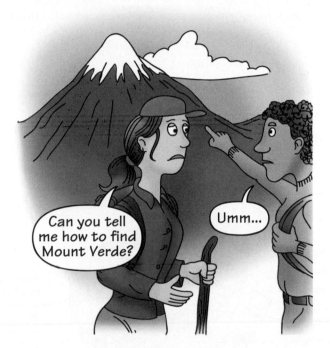

If you're not careful, however, some of these names can mislead you. For example, the *zygomatic arch* at the side of the face is formed by the joining of two processes: the *zygomatic process* and the *temporal process*. One might think that the zygomatic process is part of the zygomatic bone and that the temporal process is part of the temporal bone, but that's not right. They are named for the bones that they *join*, not the bones they belong to! Their full names reveal their true nature: the *zygomatic process of the temporal bone* and the *temporal process of the zygomatic bone*. Be careful!

Continued

✦ FIELD NOTES—cont'd

Some names may seem crazy until you look at the structure. *Sella turcica* means "Turkish chair." What?! But it really *does* look like a little backless chair with flared arms of a style that is often called a Turkish chair. It can be translated as "Turkish saddle," with a raised pommel (front) and cantle (back). Look for some of these other weird names:

- Crista galli: "chicken crest" or "rooster's comb"
- Cribriform plate: "sieve-shaped" plate
- Lateral malleolus: "little hammer on the side"
- Trochlea: "pulley"

Don't forget your directional terms, such as *superior* and *inferior, lateral* and *medial,* and so on. These are used extensively in the naming of bone structures. Review them in Table 1-27 on page 120.

Many of the tables in this section provide the literal translations of the names of skeletal structures. Pay attention to them, because they will help you to both *find* and *remember* the structures.

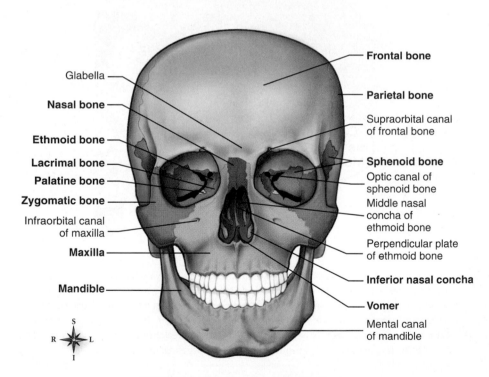

FIGURE 2-6 Anterior View of the Skull.

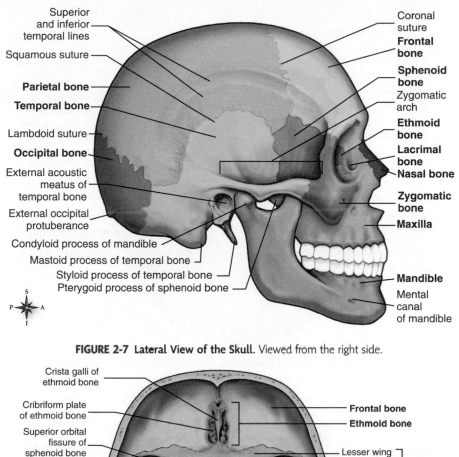

Superior and inferior temporal lines

Squamous suture

Parietal bone

Temporal bone

Lambdoid suture

Occipital bone

External acoustic meatus of temporal bone

External occipital protuberance

Condyloid process of mandible

Mastoid process of temporal bone

Styloid process of temporal bone

Pterygoid process of sphenoid bone

Coronal suture

Frontal bone

Sphenoid bone

Zygomatic arch

Ethmoid bone

Lacrimal bone

Nasal bone

Zygomatic bone

Maxilla

Mandible

Mental canal of mandible

FIGURE 2-7 Lateral View of the Skull. Viewed from the right side.

Crista galli of ethmoid bone

Cribriform plate of ethmoid bone

Superior orbital fissure of sphenoid bone

Optic canal of sphenoid bone

Foramen rotundum of sphenoid bone

Foramen ovale of sphenoid bone

Foramen lacerum of sphenoid bone

Foramen spinosum

Internal acoustic meatus of temporal bone

Jugular foramen

Foramen magnum of occipital bone

Frontal bone

Ethmoid bone

Lesser wing

Greater wing

Sphenoid bone

Sella turcica

Opening of carotid canal

Temporal bone

Petrous part of temporal bone

Hypoglossal canal of occipital bone

Parietal bone

Occipital bone

FIGURE 2-8 Floor of the Cranial Cavity. View from above, with the cap of the skull removed.

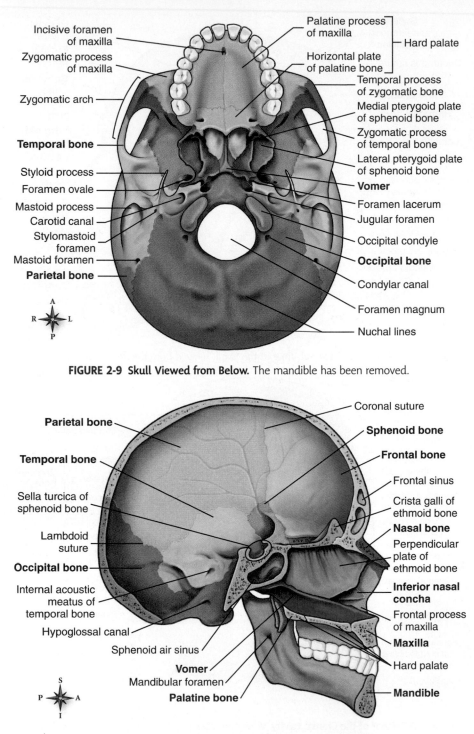

Incisive foramen of maxilla
Zygomatic process of maxilla
Zygomatic arch
Temporal bone
Styloid process
Foramen ovale
Mastoid process
Carotid canal
Stylomastoid foramen
Mastoid foramen
Parietal bone

Palatine process of maxilla
Hard palate
Horizontal plate of palatine bone
Temporal process of zygomatic bone
Medial pterygoid plate of sphenoid bone
Zygomatic process of temporal bone
Lateral pterygoid plate of sphenoid bone
Vomer
Foramen lacerum
Jugular foramen
Occipital condyle
Occipital bone
Condylar canal
Foramen magnum
Nuchal lines

FIGURE 2-9 Skull Viewed from Below. The mandible has been removed.

Parietal bone
Temporal bone
Sella turcica of sphenoid bone
Lambdoid suture
Occipital bone
Internal acoustic meatus of temporal bone
Hypoglossal canal
Sphenoid air sinus
Vomer
Mandibular foramen
Palatine bone

Coronal suture
Sphenoid bone
Frontal bone
Frontal sinus
Crista galli of ethmoid bone
Nasal bone
Perpendicular plate of ethmoid bone
Inferior nasal concha
Frontal process of maxilla
Maxilla
Hard palate
Mandible

FIGURE 2-10 Skull Interior. Midsagittal section of the skull.

✳ TABLE 2-5   Cranial Bones and Their Markings

Bones and Markings	Pronunciations	Translations	Descriptions and Hints
Parietal bone	pah-RYE-i-tal bohn	Wall-related bone	Prominent, bulging bone behind the frontal bone; form the top sides of the cranial cavity
Superior temporal line	soo-PEER-ee-or TEM-poh-ral lyne	Upper line on temple of head	Superior of two very faint curving lines across parietal and frontal bones
Inferior temporal line	in-FEER-ee-or TEM-poh-ral lyne	Lower line on temple of head	Inferior of two very faint curving lines across parietal and frontal bones; sometimes more pronounced than superior line
Temporal bone	TEM-poh-ral bohn	Bone temple of head	Form the lower sides of the cranium and part of the cranial floor; contain the middle and inner ear structures
Squamous portion	SKWAY-muss POR-shun	Scalelike part	Thin, semicircular upper part of the bone
Mastoid portion	MAS-toyd POR-shun	Breastlike part	Rough-surfaced lower part of the bone posterior to the external acoustic meatus
Petrous portion	PET-rus (or PEET-rus) POR-shun	Rocky part	Wedge-shaped process that forms part of the center section of the cranial floor between the sphenoid and occipital bones; looks like a rocky cliff; houses the middle and inner ear structures
Mastoid process	MAS-toyd PRAH-ses	Breastlike projection	Protuberance just behind the ear
Mastoid air cells	MAS-toyd ayr selz	Breastlike air storerooms	Mucosa-lined, air-filled spaces within the mastoid process
External acoustic meatus (or canal)	eks-TER-nal ak-OOS-tik mee-AYT-us (kan-AL)	Outside hearing-related passage	Tube that extends into the temporal bone from the external ear opening to the tympanic membrane
Zygomatic process	zye-goh-MAT-ik PRAH-ses	Projection toward the zygomatic bone	Projection that articulates with the zygomatic bone; posterior part of the zygomatic arch

Continued

✳ **TABLE 2-5**   **Cranial Bones and Their Markings—cont'd**

Bones and Markings	Pronunciations	Translations	Descriptions and Hints
Internal acoustic meatus	in-TER-nal ak-OOS-tik mee-AYT-us	Inside hearing-related passage	Fairly large opening on the posterior surface of the petrous part of the bone, like a cave on a cliff face; transmits the eighth cranial nerve to the inner ear and the seventh cranial nerve on its way to the facial structures
Mandibular fossa	man-DIB-yoo-lar FOSS-ah	Ditch of the jaw	Oval-shaped depression anterior to the external acoustic meatus; forms the socket for the condyle of the mandible
Styloid process	STY-loyd PRAH-ses	Styluslike projection	Slender spike of bone that extends downward and forward from the undersurface of the bone anterior to the mastoid process; often broken off in a dry skull; several neck muscles and ligaments attach to the styloid process
Stylomastoid foramen	sty-loh-MAS-toyd foh-RAY-men (or FO-rah-men)	Styloid–mastoid hole	Tiny opening between the styloid and mastoid processes where the facial nerve emerges from the cranial cavity
Jugular fossa	JUG-yoo-lar FOSS-ah	Throat (vein) ditch	Depression on the undersurface of the petrous part; dilated beginning of the internal jugular vein lodged here
Jugular foramen	JUG-yoo-lar foh-RAY-men (or FO-ra-men)	Throat (vein) hole	Opening in the suture between the petrous part and the occipital bone; transmits the lateral sinus and the ninth, tenth, and eleventh cranial nerves
Carotid canal (or foramen)	kah-ROT-id kah-NAL (foh-RAY-men or FO-ra-men)	Canal (hole) of the carotid (sleep) artery	Channel in the petrous part; best seen from the undersurface of the skull; transmits the internal carotid artery
Frontal bone	FRUN-tel bohn	Forehead (brow) bone	Forehead bone; also forms most of the roof of the orbits (eye sockets) and the anterior part of the cranial floor

✳ TABLE 2-5		Cranial Bones and Their Markings—cont'd	

Bones and Markings	Pronunciations	Translations	Descriptions and Hints
Supraorbital margin	soo-prah-OR-bi-tal MARJ-in	Above eye-socket edge	Curved ridgelike margin just below the eyebrow; forms the upper edge of the orbit
Frontal sinuses	FRUN-tel SYE-nus-ez	Forehead (brow) hollows	Cavities inside the bone just above the supraorbital margin; lined with mucosa; contain air
Frontal tuberosity (tuber or eminence)	FRUN-tel too-ber-AH-sih-tee (TOO-ber or EM-in-ents)	Forehead (brow) bump	Bulge above the eye orbit; most prominent part of forehead
Superciliary arch (ridge)	soo-per-SIL-ee-air-ee arch (rij)	Eyebrow curves	Curved ridge formed by the projection of the frontal sinus; eyebrows lie superficial to this ridge
Supraorbital foramen (sometimes notch)	soo-prah-OR-bi-tal foh-RAY-men (or FO-ra-men) (notch)	Above eye-socket hole	Foramen or notch (can be either) in the supraorbital margin slightly medial to its midpoint; transmits supraorbital nerve and blood vessels
Glabella	glah-BEL-ah	Hairless	Smooth area between the superciliary ridges and above the nose
Occipital bone	ok-SIP-it-al bohn	Back-of-head bone	Forms the posterior part of the cranial floor and walls
Foramen magnum	foh-RAY-men (or FO-ra-men) MAG-num	Huge hole	Hole through which the spinal cord enters the cranial cavity
Occipital condyles	ok-SIP-it-al KON-dylez	Back-of-head knuckles	Convex, oval processes on either side of the foramen magnum; articulate with depressions on the first cervical vertebra
External occipital protuberance	eks-TER-nal ok-SIP-it-al pro-TOOB-er-ents	Outside, back-of-head projecting bumps	Prominent projection on the posterior surface in the midline a short distance above the foramen magnum; can be felt as a definite bump
Superior nuchal line	soo-PEER-ee-or NOO-kel lyne	Upper spinal-cord line	Curved ridge that extends laterally from the external occipital protuberance

Continued

✳ **TABLE 2-5**   **Cranial Bones and Their Markings—cont'd**

Bones and Markings	Pronunciations	Translations	Descriptions and Hints
Inferior nuchal line	in-FEER-ee-or NOO-kel lyne	Lower spinal-cord line	Less well-defined ridge that parallels the superior nuchal line a short distance below it
Internal occipital protuberance	in-TER-nal ok-SIP-it-al pro-TOOB-er-ents	Inside back-of-head projection	Projection in the midline on the inner surface of the bone; grooves for the lateral sinuses extend laterally from this process and the one for the sagittal sinus extends upward from it
Sphenoid bone	SFEE-noyd bohn	Wedgelike bone	Keystone of the cranial floor that forms its midportion; resembles a bat with wings outstretched and legs extended downward posteriorly; lies behind and slightly above the nose and throat; forms part of the floor and sidewalls of the orbit
Body	BOD-ee	Main part	Hollow, cubelike central portion
Greater wings	GRAYT-er wingz	Larger wings	Lateral projections from the body; form part of the outer wall of the orbit
Lesser wings	LESS-er wingz	Smaller wings	Thin, triangular projections from the upper part of the sphenoid body; form the posterior part of the roof of the orbit
Sella turcica	SEL-lah TER-si-kah (or TER-ki-kah)	Turkish chair or saddle	Saddle-shaped depression on the upper surface of the sphenoid body; contains the pituitary gland
Sphenoid sinuses	SFEE-noyd SYE-nus-ez	Hollows of sphenoid bone	Irregular, mucosa-lined, air-filled spaces within the central part of the sphenoid
Pterygoid process	TER-i-goid PRAH-ses	Winglike projection	Downward, double-plate, lateral projection where the body and the greater wing unite; comparable to the extended legs of a bat if the entire bone is likened to this animal; forms part of the lateral nasal wall

✳ **TABLE 2-5**　　**Cranial Bones and Their Markings**

Bones and Markings	Pronunciations	Translations	Descriptions and Hints
Optic canal	OP-tik kah-NAL	Vision (nerve) canal	Opening into the orbit at the root of the lesser wing; transmits the optic nerve
Superior orbital fissure	soo-PEER-ee-or OR-bi-tal FISH-ur	Upper split (crack) in eye socket	Slitlike opening of the sphenoid into the orbit lateral to the optic foramen; transmits the third, fourth, and part of the fifth cranial nerves
Inferior orbital fissure	in-FEER-ee-or OR-bi-tal FISH-ur	Lower split (crack) in eye socket	Slitlike opening between the sphenoid and the maxilla into the orbit; transmits the infraorbital and zygomatic nerves
Foramen rotundum	foh-RAY-men (or FO-ra-men) roh-TUN-dum	Round hole	Opening in the greater wing that transmits the maxillary division of the fifth cranial nerve
Foramen ovale	foh-RAY-men (or FO-ra-men) oh-VAL-ee	Oval hole	Opening in the greater wing that transmits the mandibular division of the fifth cranial nerve
Foramen lacerum	foh-RAY-men (or FO-ra-men) LASS-er-um	Lacerated hole	Opening at the junction of the sphenoid, temporal, and occipital bones; transmits a branch of the ascending pharyngeal artery
Foramen spinosum	foh-RAY-men (or FO-ra-men) spi-NO-sum	Spiny (thorny) hole	Opening in the greater wing that transmits the middle meningeal artery to supply the meninges
Ethmoid bone	ETH-moyd bohn	Sievelike bone	Complex irregular bone that helps make up the anterior portion of the cranial floor, the medial wall of the orbits, the upper parts of the nasal septum, and the sidewalls and part of the nasal roof; lies anterior to the sphenoid and posterior to the nasal bones
Cribriform plate	KRIB-ri-form playt	Sieve-shaped plate	Olfactory nerves pass through numerous holes in this meshlike horizontal plate

Continued

✳ **TABLE 2-5**   Cranial Bones and Their Markings—cont'd

Bones and Markings	Pronunciations	Translations	Descriptions and Hints
Crista galli	KRIS-tah GAL-ee (or GAW-lee)	Chicken (cock) comb	Upward projection from the middle of the cribriform plate; meninges (membranes around the brain) attach to this process
Perpendicular plate	per-pen-DIK-yoo-ler playt	Right-angle plate	Hangs downward into the nasal cavity to form the upper part of the nasal septum
Ethmoid sinuses (cells)	ETH-moyd SYE-nus-ez (selz)	Hollows (storerooms) of ethmoid bone	Honeycombed, mucosa-lined, air spaces within the lateral masses of the bone
Superior and middle nasal conchae (*sing.*, concha) or turbinates	soo-PEER-ee-or and MID-ul NAY-zal KONG-kee (KONG-kah) or TUR-bih-naytz	Upper and middle seashells (spinning tops)	Form part of the lateral walls of the nose
Ethmoidal labyrinth	eth-MOYD-al LAB-i-rinth	Sievelike maze	Hollow lateral masses of the ethmoid; contain many air spaces (ethmoid cells or sinuses); the inner surface forms the superior and middle conchae

✳ **TABLE 2-6**   Facial Bones and Their Markings

Bones and Markings	Pronunciations	Translations	Descriptions and Hints
Vomer bone	VOH-mer bohn	Plowshare bone	Forms the lower and posterior part of the nasal septum; shaped like the wedgelike blade of a plough
Ala (*pl.*, alae)	AY-la or AL-ah (AY-lee or AL-ee)	Wing	Flared, winglike process; articulates with sphenoid and palatine bones
Maxilla (maxillary bone)	mak-SIH-lah (MAK-si-lair-ee bohn)	Upper jawbone	Upper jaw bones; form part of the floor of the orbit, the anterior part of the roof of the mouth, the floor of the nose, and part of the sidewalls of the nose

*TABLE 2-6		Facial Bones and Their Markings	
Bones and Markings	**Pronunciations**	**Translations**	**Descriptions and Hints**
Alveolar process	al-VEE-oh-lar PRAH-ses	Trough (socket)-like projection	Archlike process that holds the tooth sockets
Maxillary sinus	MAK-si-lair-ee SYE-nus	Upper jawbone hollow	Large, air-filled cavity within the body of the maxilla; lined with mucous membrane; largest of the paranasal sinuses
Zygomatic process	zye-goh-MAT-ik PRAH-ses	Projection related to zygomatic (cheek) bone	Extension (corner) that articulates with the zygomatic bone
Palatine process	PAL-ah-tyne PRAH-ses	Projection related to palate (roof of mouth)	Horizontal plate that projects inward from the alveolar process; forms the anterior and larger part of the hard palate
Infraorbital margin	in-frah-OR-bi-tal MARJ-in	Below-eye-socket edge	Curved ridgelike margin that forms the lower edge of the orbit
Infraorbital foramen	in-frah-OR-bi-tal foh-RAY-men (or FO-ra-men)	Below-eye-socket hole	Hole on the external surface orbit; transmits vessels and nerves
Lacrimal groove	LAK-ri-mal groov	Tear-related groove	Groove on the inner surface; joined by a similar groove on the lacrimal bone to form a bony space for the nasolacrimal duct
Zygomatic bone (malar bone)	zye-goh-MAT-ik bohn (MAY-ler or MAY-lar bohn)	Yoke-related (cheek-related) bone	Cheekbones; form part of the floor and sidewall of the eye orbit
Infraorbital margin	in-frah-OR-bi-tal MARJ-in	Below-eye-socket edge	Curved, ridgelike margin that forms the lower edge of the orbit
Temporal process	TEM-poh-ral PRAH-ses	Projection toward the temporal bone	Projection that articulates with the temporal bone
Zygomatic arch	zye-goh-MAT-ik arch	Curve of the cheekbone	Curve formed by the union of the temporal process of and zygomatic bone and the zygomatic process of the temporal bone

Continued

✳ **TABLE 2-6**   Facial Bones and Their Markings—cont'd

Bones and Markings	Pronunciations	Translations	Descriptions and Hints
Palatine bone	PAL-ah-tyne bohn	Palate (mouth roof) bone	Form the posterior part of the hard palate, the floor and part of the sidewalls of the nasal cavity, and the floor of the orbit
Horizontal plate	hor-i-ZON-tal playt	Flat sheet like the horizon	Joined to the palatine processes of the maxillae to complete part of the hard palate
Lacrimal bone	LAK-ri-mal bohn	Tear-related bone	Thin, platelike bones; posterior and lateral to the nasal bones in the medial wall of the eye orbit; help form the sidewall of the nasal cavity (often missing in a dry skull specimen)
Lacrimal groove	LAK-ri-mal groov	Tear-related groove	Depression for nasolacrimal (tear) duct; has widened, inferior lacrimal fossa
Nasal bone	NAY-zal bohn	Nose-related bone	Pair of small bones that form the upper part of the bridge of the nose
Inferior nasal conchae (*sing.,* **concha**) or **turbinates**	in-FEER-ee-or NAY-zal KONG-kee (KONG-kah) or TUR-bih-naytz	Lower, nose-related seashell (spinning-top-like)	Thin scroll of bone that forms a shelf along the inner surface of the sidewall of the nasal cavity; lies above the roof of the mouth
Mandible	MAN-di-bal	Jawbone	Lower jawbone; largest and strongest bone of the face
Body	BOD-ee	Main part	Main part of the bone; forms the chin
Ramus	RAY-mus	Branch	Process, one on either side, that projects upward from the posterior part of the body
Condylar process (mandibular condyle)	KON-dil-er PRAH-ses (man-DIB-yoo-lar KON-dyle)	Knucklelike projection	Part of each ramus that articulates with the mandibular fossa of the temporal bone
Neck	nek	Narrowing below the head	Constricted part just below the condyle

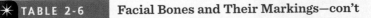

TABLE 2-6   Facial Bones and Their Markings—con't

Bones and Markings	Pronunciations	Translations	Descriptions and Hints
Alveolar process	al-VEE-oh-lar PRAH-ses	Trough (socket)-like projection	Teeth are set into this arch
Mandibular foramen	man-DIB-yoo-lar foh-RAY-men (or FO-ra-men)	Hole of jawbone	Opening on the inner surface of the ramus; transmits nerves and vessels to the lower teeth
Mental foramen	MEN-tal foh-RAY-men (or FO-ra-men)	Chin hole	Opening on the outer surface below the space between the two bicuspids; transmits the terminal branches of the nerves and vessels that enter the bone through the mandibular foramen; dentists inject anesthetics through these foramina
Coronoid process	KOR-uh-noyd PRAH-ses	Crownlike projection	Projection upward from the anterior part of each ramus; the temporal muscle inserts here
Angle	ANG-gul	Corner	Juncture of the posterior and inferior margins of the ramus

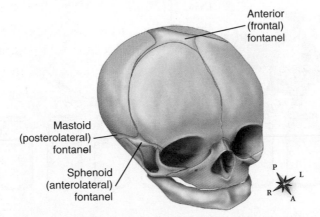

FIGURE 2-11 Skull at Birth. Fontanels or "soft spots" are visible.

⬦ FIELD NOTES

Use Mnemonics to Help You Learn Bone Structures

In Special Survival Skills: The Student Laboratory (see page 60), I suggested using silly sentences—mnemonic devices—to help you learn body structures. This is especially helpful for learning the structures of the skeleton. The best mnemonics have the following qualities:

- **Visual:** They should conjure up a vivid mental image
- **Silly:** The more outlandish, silly, or risqué that they are, the better
- **Personal:** They work better if they relate to something or somebody you know
- **Simple:** If they are too complicated, they don't work well

The best ones are those that you make up yourself. To get some ideas, check out *Mnemonics for A&P* (my-ap.us/12WL7BI).

The cartoon shown here is one I made up to learn some of the major foramina (holes) of the cranial floor in the skull (when viewed from above, with cap removed). I used to work with owls, so this is rather *personal*—and *goofy*. Notice also that not just the first letters match up to the list of foramina; for some, whole words or syllables are similar.

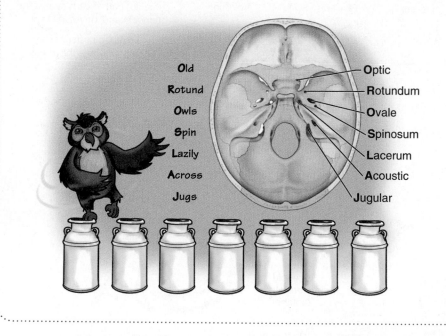

Old	Optic
Rotund	Rotundum
Owls	Ovale
Spin	Spinosum
Lazily	Lacerum
Across	Acoustic
Jugs	Jugular

✳ TABLE 2-7	Special Features of the Skull		
Bones and Markings	**Pronunciations**	**Translations**	**Description and Hints**
Sutures	SOO-churz	Seams	Immovable joints between the skull bones
Squamous (squamosal)	SKWAY-muss (skwa-MOS-al)	Scalelike	Line of articulation along the top curved edge of the temporal bone
Coronal	ko-RO-nal	Crown-related	Joint between the parietal bones and the frontal bone
Lambdoid(al)	LAM-doyd(-al)	Lambda (λ)-like	Joint between the parietal bones and the occipital bone
Sagittal	SAJ-i-tal	Arrow-related	Joint between the right and left parietal bones
Fontanels	FON-tah-nelz	Little fountains	"Soft spots" where ossification is incomplete at birth; allow for some compression of the skull during birth; also important for determining the position of the head before delivery; six such areas are located at the angles of the parietal bones
Anterior (or frontal)	an-TEER-ee-or (FRUN-tel)	Front (forehead/ brow)	At the intersection of the sagittal and coronal sutures (i.e., the juncture of the parietal bones and the frontal bone); diamond shaped; largest of the fontanels; usually closed by 11.2 years of age
Posterior (or occipital)	pohs-TEER-ee-or (ok-SIP-it-al)	Rear (back of head)	At the intersection of the sagittal and lambdoid sutures (i.e., the juncture of the parietal bones and the occipital bone); triangular; usually closed by the second month of life
Sphenoid (or anterolateral)	SFEE-noyd (an-ter-oh-LAT-er-al)	Wedgelike (front-side)	At the juncture of the frontal, parietal, temporal, and sphenoid bones
Mastoid (or posterolateral)	MAS-toyd (pos-ter-oh-LAT-er-al)	Breastlike (rear-side)	At the juncture of the parietal, occipital, and temporal bones; usually closed by the second year of life

Continued

✳ **TABLE 2-7**   **Special Features of the Skull—cont'd**

Bones and Markings	Pronunciations	Translations	Description and Hints
Air sinuses	ayr SYE-nus-ez	Air hollows	Spaces or cavities within bones; those that communicate with the nose are called *paranasal sinuses* (frontal, sphenoidal, ethmoidal, and maxillary); mastoid cells communicate with the middle ear rather than the nose, so they are not included among the paranasal sinuses
Sutural bones (wormian or **intrasutural bones)**	bohnz (bohnz)	Seam-related (after Ole Worm, Danish anatomist; within suture) bones	Small islets of bone in sutures; these vary greatly from person to person
Auditory ossicles	AW-di-toh-ree OS-ik-ulz	Little bones of hearing	Tiny bones in the middle ear cavity within the temporal bones; resemble, respectively, a miniature hammer, an anvil, and a stirrup
Malleus	MAL-ee-us	Hammer	
Incus	IN-kus	Anvil	
Stapes	STAY-peez	Stirrup	

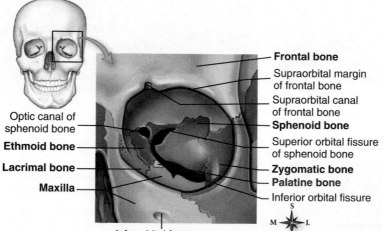

FIGURE 2-12 Bones of the Eye Orbit. Left eye orbit.

✳ **TABLE 2-8**   Bones of the Eye Orbits

Bone	Location in Orbit	Bone	Location in Orbit
Frontal bone	Roof of the orbit	Zygomatic bone	Lateral wall
Ethmoid bone	Medial wall	Maxilla	Floor
Lacrimal bone	Medial wall	Palatine bone	Floor
Sphenoid bone	Lateral wall		

✳ **TABLE 2-9**   **Bones of the Nasal Septum** Partition in the midline of the nasal cavity; separates the cavity into right and left halves

Features	Descriptions and Hints
Perpendicular plate of the ethmoid bone	Forms the upper part of the septum
Vomer	Forms the lower, posterior part of the septum
Cartilage	Forms the anterior part of the septum

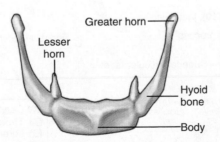

FIGURE 2-13 Hyoid Bone. This bone is located just above the larynx (voice box) and anterior to the cervical vertebrae. It does not articulate with any other bone.

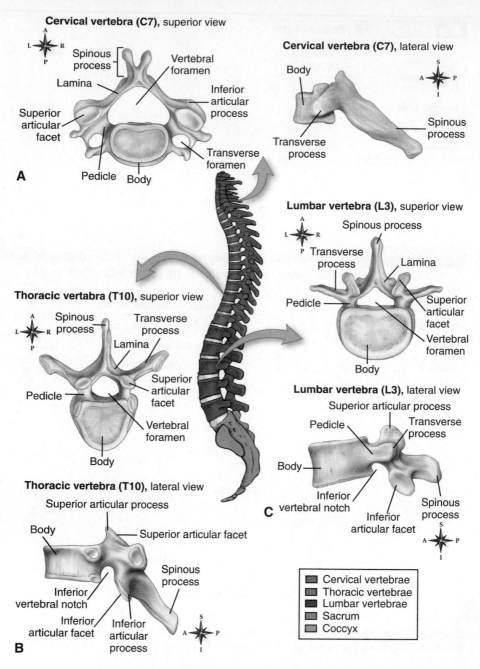

Cervical vertebra (C7), superior view

Spinous process
Lamina
Vertebral foramen
Inferior articular process
Superior articular facet
Pedicle
Body
Transverse foramen

A

Cervical vertebra (C7), lateral view

Body
Transverse process
Spinous process

Thoracic vertabra (T10), superior view

Spinous process
Transverse process
Lamina
Pedicle
Superior articular facet
Vertebral foramen
Body

Thoracic vertebra (T10), lateral view

Superior articular process
Body
Superior articular facet
Spinous process
Inferior vertebral notch
Inferior articular facet
Inferior articular process

B

Lumbar vertebra (L3), superior view

Spinous process
Transverse process
Lamina
Pedicle
Superior articular facet
Vertebral foramen
Body

Lumbar vertebra (L3), lateral view

Superior articular process
Pedicle
Transverse process
Body
Inferior vertebral notch
Spinous process
Inferior articular facet

C

Cervical vertebrae
Thoracic vertebrae
Lumbar vertebrae
Sacrum
Coccyx

FIGURE 2-14 Vertebrae.

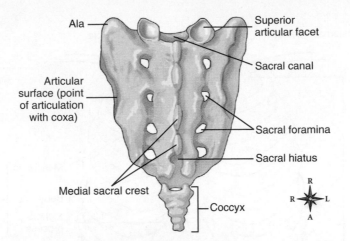

FIGURE 2-15 Sacrum. Posterior view.

◆ FIELD NOTES

The Vertebral Pagoda

Many skeletal structures resemble other objects. Such similarities can be used as mnemonic aids to help you identify and remember your required skeletal structures. For example, when a vertebra is viewed from above, I think it resembles a far-eastern pagoda or a pavilion set atop a flat-faced boulder.

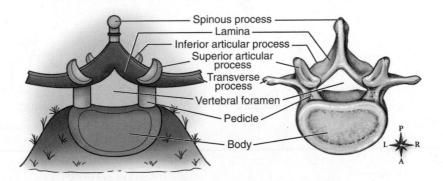

The curving roof resembles the lamina, the peak resembles the *spinous process*, the *pedicles* are like the supporting columns, the *articular processes* are like gutters, the lip of the roof resembles a *transverse process*, the space under the roof is the *vertebral foramen*, and the boulder is the *body* of the vertebra. The roof and columns of the pagoda form the *neural arch*.

Sometimes, a translation of a structure's name hints at a useful image. For example, *pedicle* can be translated as "foot stalk" or "little foot," and *lamina* can be translated as "thin plate"—which can help you to visualize and remember them.

What other resemblances can you see? A typical *cervical vertebra*, when viewed posteriorly, looks a little bit like the face of an aardvark or anteater. Likewise, *thoracic vertebrae* look like giraffe heads, and each *lumbar vertebra* looks sort of like a moose head. When you notice such resemblances, use them as memory aids!

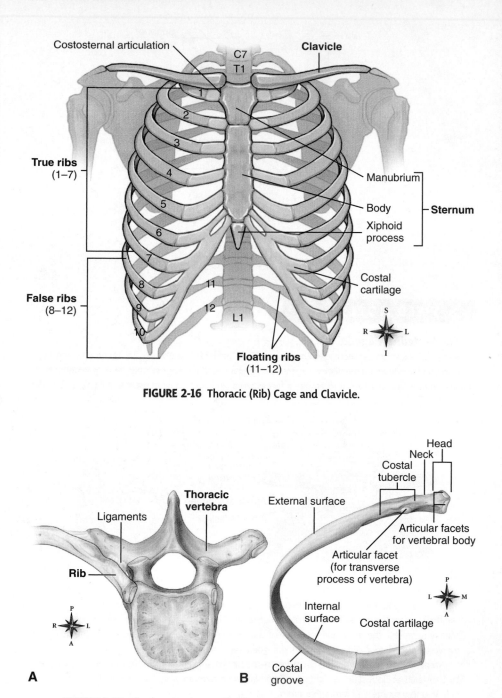

FIGURE 2-16 Thoracic (Rib) Cage and Clavicle.

FIGURE 2-17 Rib. **A,** Articulation of rib and vertebra. **B,** Structure of left fifth rib.

| TABLE 2-10 | Hyoid, Vertebrae, and Thoracic Bones and Their Markings |

Bones and Markings	Pronunciations	Translations	Descriptions and Hints
Hyoid bone	HYE-oyd bohn	U-like	U-shaped bone in the neck between the mandible and the upper part of the larynx; distinctive as the only bone in the body that does not form a joint with any other bone; suspended by ligaments from the styloid processes of the temporal bones
Body	BOD-ee	Main part	Central part (apex of the U)
Lesser horn	LESS-er horn	Smaller animal horn	Tiny, anterior horn on each lateral end of the body
Greater horn	GRAYT-er horn	Larger animal horn	Posterior horns (arms of the U)
Vertebral column	VER-teh-bral (or ver-TEE-bral) KAHL-um	Pillar of joints	Not actually a column but rather a flexible, segmented, curved rod; forms the axis of the body; the head is balanced above, the ribs and viscera are suspended in front, and the lower extremities are attached below; encloses the spinal cord
			General features: Anterior part of each vertebra (except for the first two cervical) consists of the body; posterior part of the vertebrae consists of the neural arch, which in turn consists of two pedicles, two laminae, and seven processes that project from the laminae
Body	BOD-ee	Main part	Flat, round, main part that is located anteriorly; supporting or weight-bearing part of the vertebra
Pedicles	PED-i-kul	Foot stalks	Short projections that extend posteriorly from the body
Lamina	LAM-i-nah	Thin plate	Posterior part of the vertebra to which the pedicles join and from which the processes project

Continued

✳ **TABLE 2-10** Hyoid, Vertebrae, and Thoracic Bones and Their Markings—cont'd

Bones and Markings	Pronunciations	Translations	Descriptions and Hints
Neural arch	NOOR-al arch	Nerve-related curve	Formed by the pedicles and the laminae; protects the spinal cord posteriorly; the congenital absence of one or more neural arches is known as *spina bifida* (the cord may protrude right through the skin)
Spinous process	SPY-nus PRAH-ses	Spiny (thornlike) projection	Sharp process that projects inferiorly from the laminae in the midline
Transverse processes	tranz-VERS PRAH-ses-ez	Turned-across projections	Right and left lateral projections from the laminae
Superior articulating processes	soo-PEER-ee-or ar-TIK-yoo-layt-ing PRAH-ses-ez	Upper joining projections	Project upward from the laminae; have smooth *superior articular facets*
Inferior articulating processes	in-FEER-ee-or ar-TIK-yoo-layt-ing PRAH-ses-ez	Lower joining projections	Project downward from the laminae; articulate with the superior articulating processes of the vertebrae below; have smooth *inferior articular facets*
Spinal (vertebral) foramen	SPY-nal foh-RAY-men (or FO-ra-men)	Spinal cord hole	Hole in the center of the vertebra formed by the union of the body, the pedicles, and the laminae; when the vertebrae are superimposed on top of one another, the spinal foramina form the spinal cavity that houses the spinal cord
Intervertebral foramina	in-ter-VER-teh-bral (or in-ter-ver-TEE-bral) foh-RAM-in-ah	Holes between vertebrae	Opening between the vertebrae through which the spinal nerves emerge
Cervical vertebrae C_1 **(atlas)** C_2 **(axis)** C_3 C_4 C_5 C_6 C_7	SER-vi-kal VER-teh-bray (VER-teh-bree)	Joints of the neck	First or upper seven vertebrae; the foramen in each transverse process is for the transmission of the vertebral artery and vein and the plexus of nerves; short bifurcated spinous processes (except on the seventh vertebra, where it is extra long) and may be felt as a protrusion when the head is bent forward; the bodies of these vertebrae are small, whereas the spinal foramina are large and triangular

✳ TABLE 2-10	Hyoid, Vertebrae, and Thoracic Bones and Their Markings—cont'd		
Bones and Markings	**Pronunciations**	**Translations**	**Descriptions and Hints**
Atlas	AT-las	Supporter (in Greek mythology, Atlas supported the heavens [later mistaken as earth's globe])	First cervical vertebra; lacks a body and a spinous process; superior articulating processes are concave ovals that act as rockerlike cradles for the condyles of the occipital bone; named *atlas* because it supports the head as Atlas supports the world in Greek mythology
Axis (epistropheus)	AK-sis (ep-i-STROH-fee-us)	Axle or pivot (thing upon which something turns)	Second cervical vertebra, so named because the atlas rotates about this bone during rotating movements of the head; the *dens* or odontoid process is a peglike projection that extends upward from the body of the axis that forms a pivot for the rotation of the atlas
Thoracic vertebrae T1 T2 T3 T4 T5 T6 T7 T8 T9 T10 T11 T12	thoh-RASS-ik VER-teh-bray (VER-teh-bree)	Joints of the chest (thorax)	Next 12 vertebrae; 12 pairs of ribs are attached to these vertebrae; these are stronger, with more massive bodies than the cervical vertebrae; no transverse foramina; two sets of facets for articulation with the corresponding rib: one on the body and the second on the transverse process; the upper thoracic vertebrae have elongated spinous processes
Lumbar vertebrae L1 L2 L3 L4 L5	LUM-bar VER-teh-bray (VER-teh-bree)	Joints of the loin	Next five vertebrae; strong and massive; superior articulating processes directed medially instead of upward; inferior articulating processes directed laterally instead of downward; short, blunt spinous processes

Continued

✳ TABLE 2-10   Hyoid, Vertebrae, and Thoracic Bones and Their Markings—cont'd

Bones and Markings	Pronunciations	Translations	Descriptions and Hints
Sacrum	SAY-krum	Sacred bone (possibly used in animal sacrifices)	Five separate vertebrae (S1 through S5) until the individual reaches about 25 years of age, then they fuse to form one wedge-shaped bone
Sacral promontory	SAY-kral PRAH-mon-tor-ee	Jutting mountaintop of the sacrum	Protuberance from the anterior upper border of the sacrum into the pelvis; of obstetrical importance because its size limits the anteroposterior diameter of the pelvic inlet
Sacral canal	SAY-kral kah-NAL	Passage of the sacrum	Inferior part of the vertebral (spinal) canal
Anterior (sacral) foramina	an-TEER-ee-or (SAY-kral) foh-RAM-in-ah	Holes on the front (of the sacrum)	Pairs of holes along the anterior (pelvic) surface of the sacrum for the passage of the spinal nerves; sometimes called the *pelvic foramina*
Posterior (sacral) foramina	pohs-TEER-ee-or (SAY-kral) foh-RAM-in-ah	Holes on the back (of the sacrum)	Pairs of holes along the posterior (dorsal) surface of the sacrum for the passage of the spinal nerves; sometimes called the *dorsal foramina*
Sacral hiatus	SAY-kral hye-AY-tus	Gap of sacrum	Gap in the posterior wall of the sacral canal in the bottom segment(s) of the sacrum
Superior articular facet	soo-PEER-ee-or	Upper joint face	Flat joint surface on each side of the superior entrance to the sacral canal
Medial sacral crest	MEE-dee-al SAY-kral krest	Ridge of the sacrum toward the middle	Bumpy ridge along the middle of the posterior surface; similar to spinous processes of the vertebrae
Intermediate sacral crest	in-ter-MEE-dee-it SAY-kral krest	Ridge of the sacrum midway toward the middle	Bumpy ridge just medial to the posterior foramina
Lateral sacral crest	LAT-er-al SAY-kral krest	Ridge of the sacrum toward the side	Bumpy ridge just lateral to the posterior foramina

✳ TABLE 2-10	Hyoid, Vertebrae, and Thoracic Bones and Their Markings—cont'd		
Bones and Markings	**Pronunciations**	**Translations**	**Descriptions and Hints**
Apex	AY-peks	Tip	Inferior tip of the sacrum
Auricular surface	ah-RIK-yoolar SUR-fess	Surface like a little ear	Ear-shaped surface that articulates with the ilium of the pelvic bone
Coccyx	KOK-sis	Cuckoo (beak)	Four or five separate vertebrae in a child but fused into one in an adult
Spinal curves	SPY-nal kervz	Bends	Curves have great structural importance because they increase the carrying strength of the vertebral column and make balance possible in an upright position (if the column was straight, the weight of the viscera would pull the body forward); they absorb jolts from walking (a straight column would transmit jolts straight to the head) and protect the column from fracture
Primary curves	PRY-mair-ee kervz	First-order bends	Column curves at birth from the head to the sacrum with the convexity posteriorly; after the child stands, the convexity persists only in the thoracic and sacral regions, which are therefore called *primary curves*
Thoracic curve	thoh-RASS-ik kerv	Bend of the chest	
Sacral curve	SAY-kral kerv	Bend of the sacrum	
Secondary curves	SEK-on-dair-ee kervz	Second-order bends	Concavities in the cervical and lumbar regions; the cervical concavity results from the infant's attempts to hold the head erect at 2 to 4 months of age; the lumbar concavity results from balancing efforts when learning to walk at 10 to 18 months of age
Cervical curve	SER-vi-kal kerv	Bend of the neck	
Lumbar curve	LUM-bar kerv	Bend of the loin	
Sternum	STER-num	Breastbone	Breastbone; a flat, dagger-shaped bone; the sternum, ribs, and thoracic vertebrae together form a bony cage known as the *thorax*
Body	BOD-ee	Main part	Large, central part of the sternum
Manubrium	mah-NOO-bree-um	Handle	Flaring, upper part of the sternum

Continued

✳ **TABLE 2-10** Hyoid, Vertebrae, and Thoracic Bones and Their Markings—cont'd

Bones and Markings	Pronunciations	Translations	Descriptions and Hints
Xiphoid process	ZYE-foyd PRAH-ses	Swordfishlike projection	Projection of cartilage at the lower border of the bone
Ribs			
Types of Ribs			
True ribs	troo ribz	True ribs	Upper seven pairs; fasten to the sternum via the costal cartilages
False ribs	fals ribz	False ribs	False ribs do not attach to the sternum directly; the upper three pairs of false ribs attach by means of the costal cartilage of the seventh ribs
Floating ribs	FLOHT-ing ribz	Floating ribs	The last two pairs of the false ribs do not attach to the sternum at all and are therefore called "floating" ribs
Parts of Ribs			
Head	hed	Head	Projection at the posterior end of a rib; articulates (via *articular facets*) with the corresponding thoracic vertebra and the one above, except the last three pairs, which join the corresponding vertebrae only
Neck	nek	Narrowing below the head	Constricted portion just below the head
Tubercle	TOO-ber-kul	Small bump	Small knob just below the neck; articulates with the transverse process of the corresponding thoracic vertebra; missing in the lowest three ribs
Body (shaft)	BOD-ee (shaft)	Main part (long cylinder)	Main (elongated) part of a rib
Costal cartilage	KOS-tal KAR-ti-lij	Gristle of the rib	Cartilage at the sternal end of the true ribs; attaches the ribs (except the floating ribs) to the sternum
Costal groove	KOS-tal groov	Rib groove	Thin groove on the inferior border of the rib for the intercostal artery

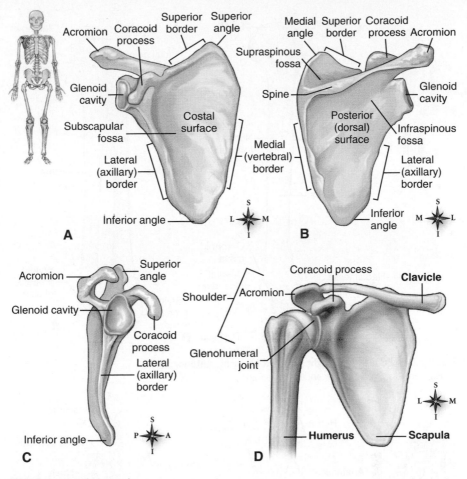

FIGURE 2-18 Right Scapula.
A, Anterior view.
B, Posterior view.
C, Lateral view.
D, Posterior view showing articulation with clavicle.

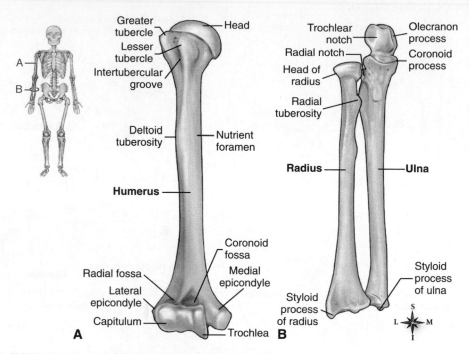

FIGURE 2-19 Bones of the Right Arm and Forearm, Anterior View.
A, Humerus (arm). **B,** Radius and ulna (forearm).

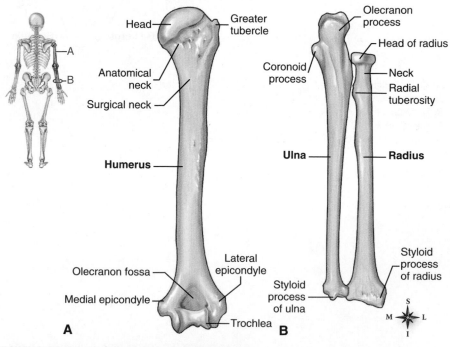

FIGURE 2-20 Bones of the Right Arm, Posterior View.
A, Humerus (arm). **B,** Radius and ulna (forearm).

✳ TABLE 2-11   Upper Extremity Bones and Their Markings

Bones and Markings	Pronunciations	Translations	Descriptions and Hints
Clavicle	KLAV-i-kul	Little key or bolt	Collar bones; the shoulder girdle is joined to the axial skeleton by the articulation of the clavicles with the sternum (the scapula does not form a joint with the axial skeleton)
Sternal end	STER-nel end	End near sternum	Thick end near the sternum
Acromial end	ah-KRO-mee-al end	End near acromion (of scapula)	Oval end near the acromion of the scapula
Body (shaft)	BOD-ee (shaft)	Main part (long cylinder)	Central shaft
Scapula	SKAP-yoo-lah	Shoulder	Shoulder blades; the scapulae and clavicles together make up the shoulder girdle
Borders			
Superior border	soo-PEER-ee-or BOHR-der	Upper	Upper margin
Medial (vertebral) border	MEE-dee-al (VER-teh-bral or ver-TEE-bral) BOHR-der	Middle	Margin toward the vertebral column
Lateral (axillary) border	LAT-er-al (AK-sil-lair-ee) BOHR-der	Side (armpit)	Lateral margin, toward the axilla
Angles	ANG-gulz	Corners	The three corners of the scapula
Inferior angle	in-FEER-ee-or ANG-gul	Lower corner	Corner where the lateral and medial borders meet at the bottom of the scapula
Lateral angle	LAT-er-al ANG-gul	Side corner	Corner where the lateral and superior borders meet at the glenoid cavity
Superior (medial) angle	soo-PEER-ee-or (MEE-dee-al) ANG-gul	Upper (middle) corner	Corner where the medial and superior borders meet at the top of the scapula
Spine	spyne	Thorn	Sharp ridge that runs diagonally across the posterior surface of the shoulder blade
Acromion	ah-KRO-mee-un	Shoulder extremity	Slightly flaring projection at the lateral end of the scapular spine; may be felt at the tip of the shoulder; articulates with the clavicle

Continued

✳ TABLE 2-11	Upper Extremity Bones and Their Markings—cont'd		
Bones and Markings	**Pronunciations**	**Translations**	**Descriptions and Hints**
Coracoid process	KOH-rah-koyd PRAH-ses	Projection like a crow (beak)	Projection on the anterior surface from the upper border of the bone; may be felt in the groove between the deltoid and pectoralis major muscles, about 1 inch below the clavicle
Supraspinous fossa	soo-pra-SPY-nus FOSS-ah	Depression above the spine	Concavity formed above the spine's attachment to the body of the scapula
Infraspinous fossa	in-fra-SPY-nus FOSS-ah	Depression below the spine	Concavity formed below the spine's attachment to the body of the scapula
Subscapular fossa	sub-SKAP-yoo-lar FOSS-ah	Depression below the scapula	Concave surface on the "underside" of the scapula against the rib cage
Glenoid cavity	GLEE-noyd KAV-i-tee	Hollow like an eye socket	Arm socket
Humerus	HYOO-mer-us	Arm	Long bone of the arm
Head	hed	Head	Smooth, hemispherical enlargement at the proximal end of the humerus
Anatomical neck	an-ah-TOM-i-kal nek	Structural narrowing below the head	Oblique groove just below the head
Greater tubercle	GRAYT-er TOO-ber-kul	Larger little bump	Rounded projection lateral to the head on the anterior surface
Lesser tubercle	LESS-er TOO-ber-kul	Smaller little bump	Prominent projection on the anterior surface just below the anatomical neck
Intertubercular groove (sulcus)	in-ter-too-BER-kyool-ar groov (SUL-kus)	Groove between little bumps	Deep groove between the greater and lesser tubercles; the long tendon of the biceps muscle lodges here
Surgical neck	SERJ-ik-al nek	Narrowing below head of clinical interest	Region just below the tubercles; so named because of its liability to fracture

TABLE 2-11   **Upper Extremity Bones and Their Markings—cont'd**

Bones and Markings	Pronunciations	Translations	Descriptions and Hints
Deltoid tuberosity	DEL-toyd too-ber-AH-sih-tee	Delta (Δ)-like bump	V-shaped, rough area about midway down the shaft where the deltoid muscle inserts
Radial groove (sulcus)	RAY-dee-al groov (SUL-kus)	Groove related to the radius	Groove that runs obliquely downward from the deltoid tuberosity; lodges the radial nerve
Lateral epicondyle	LAT-er-al ep-i-KON-dyle	Side knuckle-end	Rough projections at the lateral side of the distal end
Medial epicondyle	MEE-dee-al ep-i-KON-dyle	Middle knuckle-end	Rough projections at the medial side of the distal end
Capitulum	kah-PITCH-uh-lum	Little head	Rounded knob below the lateral epicondyle; articulates with the radius; sometimes called the *radial head of the humerus*
Trochlea	TROK-lee-ah	Pulley	Projection with a deep depression through the center, similar to the shape of a pulley; articulates with the ulna
Olecranon fossa	oh-LEK-rah-non FOSS-ah	Ditch for the head (cranium) of elbow	Depression on the posterior surface just above the trochlea; receives the olecranon of the ulna when the forearm extends
Coronoid fossa	KOR-uh-noyd FOSS-ah	Ditch for the crownlike (process)	Depression on the anterior surface above the trochlea; receives the coronoid process of the ulna during flexion of the forearm
Body (shaft)	BOD-ee (shaft)	Main part (long cylinder)	Central shaft
Radius	RAY-dee-us	Staff or spoke	Bone of the thumb side of the forearm
Head	hed	Head	Disk-shaped process that forms the proximal end of the radius; articulates with the capitulum of the humerus and with the radial notch of the ulna
Neck	nek	Neck	Narrowing just distal to the head

Continued

> ✳ **TABLE 2-11** **Upper Extremity Bones and Their Markings—cont'd**

Bones and Markings	Pronunciations	Translations	Descriptions and Hints
Radial tuberosity	RAY-dee-al too-ber-AH-sih-tee	Bump of the staff (radius)	Roughened projection on the ulnar side, a short distance below the head; the biceps muscle inserts here
Styloid process	STY-loyd PRAH-ses	Styluslike projection	Protuberance at the distal end on the lateral surface (with the forearm in the anatomical position)
Body (shaft)	BOD-ee (shaft)	Main part (long cylinder)	Central shaft
Ulna	UL-nah	Elbow	Bone of the little finger side of the forearm; longer than the radius
Olecranon	oh-LEK-rah-non	Head (cranium) of elbow	Scooplike process that joins the trochlea of the humerus at the elbow
Coronoid process	KOR-uh-noyd PRAH-ses	Crownlike projection	Projection on the anterior surface of the proximal end of the ulna; the trochlea of the humerus fits snugly between the olecranon and the coronoid processes
Trochlear notch	TROK-lee-ar notch	V-cut for the pulley	Curved notch between the olecranon and the coronoid process into which the trochlea fits; also called the *semilunar notch*
Radial notch	RAY-dee-al notch	V-cut for the staff (radius)	Curved notch that is lateral and inferior to the trochlear (semilunar) notch; the head of the radius fits into this concavity
Head	hed	Head	Rounded process at the distal end; does not articulate with the wrist bones but rather with the fibrocartilaginous disk
Styloid process	STY-loyd PRAH-ses	Projection	Sharp protuberance at the distal end; can be seen from outside on the posterior surface
Carpal bones	KAR-pal bohnz	Bones of wrist	Wrist bones; arranged in two rows (proximal and distal) at the proximal end of the hand

TABLE 2-11   Upper Extremity Bones and Their Markings—cont'd

Bones and Markings	Pronunciations	Translations	Descriptions and Hints
Pisiform (lentiform)	PY-zi-form (LEN-ti-form)	Pea-shaped (lens-shaped)	First (medial/thumbside) bone of the proximal row; looks like a slightly flattened pea sticking out from the triquetrum on the palmar side
Triquetrum (triangular, cuneiform, or pyramidal)	try-KWET-rum or try-KWEET-rum (try-ANG-yoo-lar, KYOO-neh-form, or pih-RAM-id-al)	Three-cornered (three-angled, wedge-shaped, or pyramidlike)	Second bone of the proximal row; looks like a triangle from the dorsal view; only bone connected to the pisiform
Lunate (semilunar)	LOON-ayt (sem-ee-LOON-er)	Moonlike (half-moon–like)	Third bone of the proximal row; its crescent outline resembles a half moon
Scaphoid (navicular)	SKAF-oyd (na-VIK-yoo-lar)	Boat-shaped	Fourth bone of the proximal row; the curving largest bone of the row; resembles a small boat
Hamate (unciform)	HAY-mayt or HAM-ayt (UN-si-form)	Hook-shaped	First (medial/thumbside) bone of the distal row; wedgelike bone has large "hook" on the palmar side; dorsal outline resembles a ham
Capitate	KAP-ee-tayt or KAP-i-tayt	Having a head	Second bone of the distal row; largest of all of the carpals; has a "head" that fits into the curve of the scaphoid and the lunate
Trapezoid (lesser multangular)	TRAP-eh-zoyd (LESS-er mul-TANG-yoo-lar)	Tablelike (smaller many-angled)	Third bone of the distal row; smallest bone of the row; wedge-like, pointing toward the palmar side
Trapezium (greater multangular)	tra-PEEZ-ee-um (GRAYT-er mul-TANG-yoo-lar)	Table (larger many-angled)	Fourth bone of the distal row; trapezoid outline with a deep groove on the palmar side
Metacarpal bones	met-ah-KAR-pal bohnz	Bones after the wrist	Long bones that form the supporting framework of the palm of the hand; numbered from the medial (thumb) side; each has a *base*, a *shaft*, and a *head*
I	won	Roman 1	
II	too	Roman 2	
III	three	Roman 3	
IV	fohr	Roman 4	
V	fyve	Roman 5	

Continued

✳ TABLE 2-11	Upper Extremity Bones and Their Markings—cont'd		
Bones and Markings	**Pronunciations**	**Translations**	**Descriptions and Hints**
Phalanges (*sing.,* **phalanx**)	fah-LAN-jeez (fah-LANKS)	Ranks of soldiers	Miniature long bones of the fingers; there are three in each finger and two in each thumb; numbered from the medial/thumb side; each has a *base*, a *shaft*, and a *head;* lined up like a military parade formation
Proximal (I, II, III, IV, V)	PROK-si-mal	Near (Roman 1, 2, 3, 4, 5)	
Middle (II, III, IV, V)	MID-dul	Middle (Roman 2, 3, 4, 5)	
Distal (I, II, III, IV, V)	DIS-tal	Distant (Roman 1, 2, 3, 4, 5)	

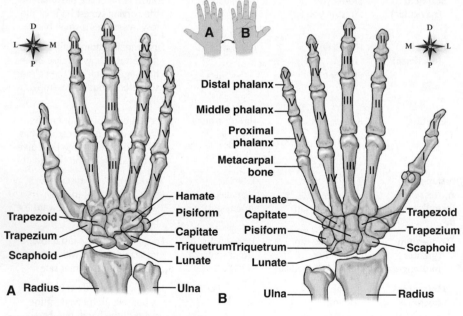

FIGURE 2-21 Bones of the Hand and Wrist.
A, Palmar view of the right hand and wrist.
B, Dorsal view of the right hand and wrist.

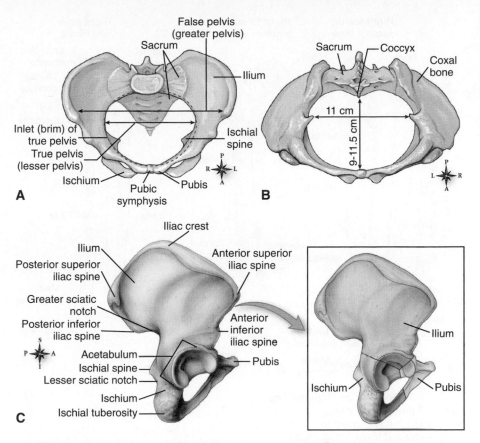

FIGURE 2-22 Pelvic Girdle. The **pelvic girdle** *(pelvis)* is a ring of three bones: the sacrum and both pelvic bones.
A, Superior view. Note that the brim of the true pelvis *(dotted line)* marks the boundary between the superior false pelvis *(pelvis major)* and the inferior true pelvis *(pelvis minor)*.
B, Posterior view.
C, Lateral view of the right pelvic bone. The inset shows major divisions.
A comparison of the male and female pelvises is shown in Figure 2-25.

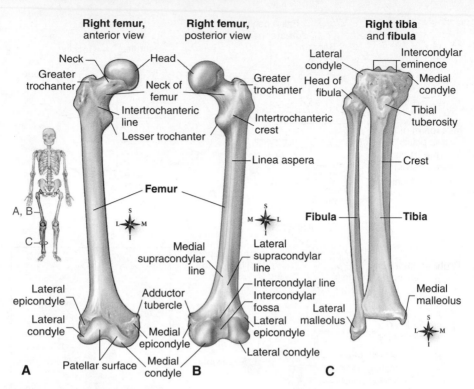

FIGURE 2-23 Bones of the Thigh and Leg.
A, Right femur, anterior surface.
B, Right femur, posterior surface.
C, Right tibia and fibula, anterior surface.

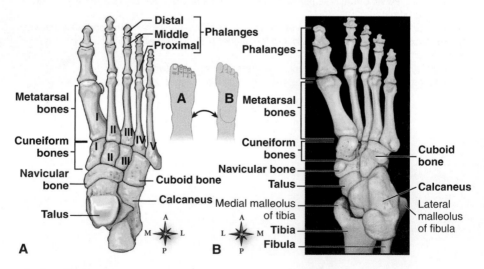

FIGURE 2-24 The Foot.
A, Superior view.
B, Inferior view.

✳ TABLE 2-12		Lower Extremity Bones and Their Markings	
Bones and Markings	Pronunciations	Translations	Descriptions and Hints
Coxal bone (pelvic bone or coxa)	KOK-sal bohn (PEL-vik bohn or KOK-sah)	Hip bone (basin bone or hip)	Large hip bone (pelvic bone); with the sacrum and the coccyx, forms the basinlike pelvic cavity; lower extremities are attached to the axial skeleton by the coxal bones
Ilium	IL-ee-um	Flank	Upper, flaring portion (this is a separate bone during early development)
Ischium	ISS-kee-um	Hip joint	Lower, posterior portion (this is a separate bone during early development)
Pubis (pl., pubes)	PYOO-bis (PYOO-beez)	Groin	Medial, anterior section (this is a separate bone during early development)
Acetabulum	ass-eh-TAB-yoo-lum	Vinegar cup	Hip socket; formed by the union of the ilium, the ischium, and the pubis
Iliac crest	IL-ee-ak krest	Flank ridges	Upper, curving boundary of the ilium
Iliac spines	IL-ee-ak spynez	Flank thorns	Sharp projections at the "corners" of the ilium
Anterior superior spine	an-TEER-ee-or soo-PEER-ee-or spyne	Front upper thorn	Prominent projection at the anterior end of the iliac crest; can be felt externally as the "point" of the hip
Anterior inferior spine	an-TEER-ee-or in-FEER-ee-or spyne	Front lower thorn	Less prominent projection a short distance below the anterior superior spine
Posterior superior spine	pohs-TEER-ee-or soo-PEER-ee-or spyne	Back upper thorn	At the posterior end of the iliac crest
Posterior inferior spine	pohs-TEER-ee-or in-FEER-ee-or spyne	Back lower thorn	Just below the posterior superior spine
Greater sciatic notch	GRAYT-er sye-AT-ik notch	Larger V-cut of hip	Large notch on the posterior surface of the ilium just below the posterior inferior spine
Ischial tuberosity	ISS-kee-al too-ber-AH-sih-tee	Hip bump	Large, rough, quadrilateral process that forms the inferior part of the ischium; in an erect sitting position, the body rests on these tuberosities

Continued

✳ **TABLE 2-12**   **Lower Extremity Bones and Their Markings—cont'd**

Bones and Markings	Pronunciations	Translations	Descriptions and Hints
Ischial spine	ISS-kee-al spyne	Hip thorn	Pointed projection just above the tuberosity
Lesser sciatic notch	LESS-er sye-AT-ik notch	Smaller V-cut of hip	Small notch on the posterior surface of the ischium just below the ischial spine (well below the greater sciatic notch of the ilium)
Pubic symphysis	PYOO-bik SIM-fi-sis	Groin fibrocartilage joint	Cartilaginous, amphiarthrotic joint between the pubic bones
Superior pubic ramus	soo-PEER-ee-or PYOO-bik RAY-mus	Upper branch of groin	Part of the pubis that lies between the symphysis and the acetabulum; forms the upper part of the obturator foramen
Inferior pubic ramus	in-FEER-ee-or PYOO-bik RAY-mus	Lower branch of groin	Part that extends down from the symphysis and unites with the ischium
Pubic arch	PYOO-bik arch	Curve of groin	Curve formed by the two inferior rami
Subpubic angle	sub-PYOO-bik ANG-gul	Corner under groin	Inside angle formed under the inferior pubic rami; generally larger in women than in men
Pubic crest	PYOO-bik krest	Ridge (comb) of groin	Upper margin of the superior ramus
Pubic tubercle	PYOO-bik TOO-ber-kul	Small bump of groin	Rounded process at the end of the crest
Obturator foramen	OB-tyoor-ayt-or foh-RAY-men (or FO-ra-men)	Hole of the hole-obstructor (obturator muscles)	Large hole in the anterior surface of the coxal bone; formed by the pubis and the ischium; largest foramen in the body
Pelvic inlet (or brim)	PEL-vik IN-let (brim)	Entrance (rim) of basin	Boundary of the aperture that leads into the true pelvis; formed by the pubic crests, the iliopectineal lines, and the sacral promontory; the size and shape of this inlet have obstetrical importance because, if any of its diameters are too small, the infant's skull cannot enter the true pelvis (or the lesser pelvis) for natural birth

TABLE 2-12 Lower Extremity Bones and Their Markings—cont'd

Bones and Markings	Pronunciations	Translations	Descriptions and Hints
True pelvis (or greater pelvis)	troo PEL-vis (GRAYT-er PEL-vis)	True basin	Space below the pelvic brim; true "basin," with bone and muscle walls and a muscle floor; the pelvic organs are located in this space
False pelvis (or lesser pelvis)	fals PEL-vis (LESS-er PEL-vis)	False basin	Broad, shallow space above the pelvic brim or the pelvic inlet; the name "false pelvis" is misleading, because this space is actually part of the abdominal cavity rather than the pelvic cavity
Pelvic outlet	PEL-vik OWT-let	Exit of basin (drain)	Irregular circumference that marks the lower limits of the true pelvis; bounded by the tip of the coccyx and two ischial tuberosities
Pelvic girdle (or bony pelvis)	PEL-vik GERD-ul (BOHN-ee PEL-vis)	Basinlike belt	Complete bony ring; composed of two coxal (pelvic) bones, the sacrum, and the coccyx; forms a firm base by which the trunk rests on the thighs and for the attachment of the lower extremities to the axial skeleton
Femur	FEE-mur		Thigh bone; the largest, strongest bone of the body
Head	hed	Head	Rounded upper end of the bone; fits into the acetabulum
Neck	nek	Narrowing below the head	Constricted portion just below the head
Greater trochanter	GRAYT-er troh-KAN-ter (or TROH-kan-ter)	Bigger runner	Protuberance located inferiorly and laterally to the head
Lesser trochanter	LESS-er troh-KAN-ter (or TROH-kan-ter)	Smaller runner	Small protuberance located inferiorly and medially to the greater trochanter
Intertrochanteric line	in-ter-troh-KAN-ter-ik lyne	Line between runners	Line that extends between the greater and lesser trochanter
Linea aspera	LEEN-ee-ah (or LIN-ee-ah) ASS-per-ah	Rough line	Prominent ridge that extends lengthwise along the concave posterior surface

Continued

✳ **TABLE 2-12**   **Lower Extremity Bones and Their Markings—cont'd**

Bones and Markings	Pronunciations	Translations	Descriptions and Hints
Supracondylar lines (ridges)	soo-prah-KON-dil-er lynz (RIJ-ez)	Above-knuckle ridges	Two ridges formed by the division of the linea aspera at its lower end; the medial supracondylar ridge extends inward to the inner condyle and the lateral ridge to the outer condyle
Medial condyle	MEE-dee-al KON-dyle	Middle knuckle	Large, rounded bulge at the distal end of the femur; on the medial aspect
Lateral condyle	LAT-er-al KON-dyle	Side knuckle	Large, rounded bulge at the distal end of the femur; on the lateral aspect
Medial epicondyle	MEE-dee-al ep-i-KON-dyle	Middle knuckle-end	Blunt projection from the side of the medial condyle
Lateral epicondyle	LAT-er-al ep-i-KON-dyle	Side knuckle-end	Blunt projection from the side of the lateral condyle
Adductor tubercle	ad-DUK-ter TOO-ber-kul	Small bump of the bringer-in (muscles)	Small projection just above the medial condyle; marks the termination of the medial supracondylar ridge
Trochlea	TROK-lee-ah	Pulley	Smooth depression between the condyles on the anterior surface; articulates with the patella
Intercondylar fossa (notch)	in-trah-KON-dil-er FOSS-ah (notch)	Between-knuckle ditch	Deep depression between the condyles on the posterior surface; the cruciate ligaments, which help to bind the femur to the tibia, lodge in this notch
Body (shaft)	BOD-ee (shaft)	Main part (long cylinder)	Central shaft
Intertrochanteric crest	in-ter-troh-kan-TAYR-ik krest	Ridge between trochanters (large bumps)	Raised ridge on the posterior surface that runs between the greater and lesser trochanter
Intercondylar line	in-ter-KON-dil-er lyne	Line between knuckles	Ridge on the posterior surface between the bases of the condyles
Patella	pah-TEL-ah	Little pan (kneecap)	Kneecap; the largest sesamoid bone of the body; embedded in the tendon of the quadriceps femoris muscle
Tibia	TIB-ee-ah	Shinbone	Shin bone

❋ TABLE 2-12	Lower Extremity Bones and Their Markings—cont'd		
Bones and Markings	**Pronunciations**	**Translations**	**Descriptions and Hints**
Medial condyle	MEE-dee-al KON-dyle	Middle knuckle	Bulging medial prominence at the proximal end of the tibia; the surface is concave for articulation with the femur
Lateral condyle	LAT-er-al KON-dyle	Side knuckle	Concave prominence lateral to the medial condyle
Intercondylar eminence	in-ter-KON-dil-er EM-in-ents	Raised thing between knuckles	Upward projection on the articular surface between the condyles
Crest	krest	Ridge (comb)	Sharp ridge on the anterior surface
Tibial tuberosity	TIB-ee-al too-ber-AH-sih-tee	Bump of the shinbone	Projection in the midline on the anterior surface
Medial malleolus (*pl.*, malleoli)	MEE-dee-al MAL-lee-o-lus	Little hammer toward the middle	Rounded downward projection at the distal end of the tibia; forms the prominence on the medial surface of the ankle
Body (shaft)	BOD-ee (shaft)	Main part (long cylinder)	Central shaft
Fibula	FIB-yoo-lah	Clasp	Long, slender bone of the lateral side of the leg
Head	hed	Head	Proximal enlargement
Neck	nek	Narrowing below the head	Constricted portion just below the head
Lateral malleolus (*pl.*, malleoli)	LAT-er-al MAL-lee-o-lus (mal-LEE-o-lee or mal-LEE-o-lye)	Little hammer to the side	Rounded prominence at the distal end of the fibula; forms the prominence on the lateral surface of the ankle
Body (shaft)	BOD-ee (shaft)	Main part (long cylinder)	Central shaft
Tarsal bones	TAR-sal bohnz	Ankle bones	Bones that form the heel and proximal or posterior half of the foot
Calcaneus	kal-KAY-nee-us	Heel bone	Heel bone
Talus	TAY-lus	Anklebone or knucklebone	Uppermost of the tarsal bones; articulates with the tibia and the fibula; boxed between the medial and lateral malleoli
Navicular (scaphoid)	na-VIK-yoo-lar (SKAF-oyd)	Boat-shaped	Curved bone anterior and slightly medial to talus and posterior to the cuneiform bones; looks like a little boat

Continued

✳ **TABLE 2-12**   **Lower Extremity Bones and Their Markings—cont'd**

Bones and Markings	Pronunciations	Translations	Descriptions and Hints
Cuboid	KYOO-boyd	Like a cube	Looks like a cube from the top but really more of a pyramid (the base is medial); on the lateral side of the foot, anterior to the calcaneus and posterior to metatarsals IV and V
Medial cuneiform (I)	MEE-dee-al KYOO-neh-form	Wedge-shaped (bone) toward the middle (Roman 1)	Looks like a cube from the top but really more of a wedge; between navicular and metatarsal I
Intermediate cuneiform (II)	in-ter-MEE-dee-it KYOO-neh-form	Wedge-shaped (bone) in the middle (Roman 2)	Looks like a cube from the top but really more of a wedge; between navicular and metatarsal II
Lateral cuneiform (III)	LAT-er-al KYOO-neh-form	Wedge-shaped (bone) to the side (Roman 3)	Looks like a cube from the top but really more of a wedge; between navicular and metatarsal III
Arches of foot	ARCH-ez ov foot	Curves of foot	Curves of the bones of the foot and ankle that, along with muscles and other soft tissues, properly support the mass of the skeleton
Longitudinal arches	lon-jih-TOO-di-nal ARCH-ez	Lengthwise curves	Tarsal and metatarsal bones so arranged as to form an arch from the front to the back of the foot
Medial arch	MEE-dee-al arch	Toward middle	Formed by the calcaneus, the talus, the navicular, the cuneiforms, and three medial metatarsal bones
Lateral arch	LAT-er-al arch	To the side	Formed by the calcaneus, the cuboid, and two lateral metatarsal bones
Transverse (or metatarsal) arch	tranz-VERS (met-ah-TAR-sal) arch	Turned-across (or after-the-ankle) curve	Metatarsal and distal row of tarsal bones (cuneiforms and cuboid) articulated so as to form an arch across the foot; bones are kept in two arched positions by means of powerful ligaments in the sole of the foot and by muscles and tendons

⁂ **TABLE 2-12**   Lower Extremity Bones and Their Markings—cont'd

Bones and Markings	Pronunciations	Translations	Descriptions and Hints
Metatarsal bones	met-ah-TAR-sal bohnz	Bones after the ankle	Long bones of the anterior portion of the foot; numbered from the medial/thumb side; each has a *base,* a *shaft,* and a *head*
I	won	Roman 1	
II	too	Roman 2	
III	three	Roman 3	
IV	fohr	Roman 4	
V	fyve	Roman 5	
Phalanges (*sing.,* phalanx)	fah-LAN-jeez (fah-LANKS)	Ranks of soldiers	Miniature long bones of the toes; two in each great toe and three in the other toes; numbered from the medial/thumb side; each has a *base,* a *shaft,* and a *head*
Proximal (I, II, III, IV, V)	PROK-si-mal	Near (Roman 1, 2, 3, 4, 5)	
Middle (II, III, IV, V)	MID-dul	Middle (Roman 2, 3, 4, 5)	
Distal (I, II, III, IV, V)	DIS-tal	Distant (Roman 1, 2, 3, 4, 5)	

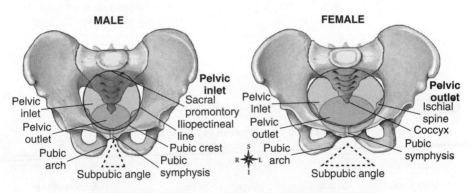

FIGURE 2-25 Comparison of Male and Female Bony Pelvises.

✳ **TABLE 2-13**　Comparison of Male and Female Skeletons

Portion of Skeleton	Male	Female
General form	Bones heavier and thicker	Bones lighter and thinner
	Muscle attachment sites more massive	Muscle attachment sites less distinct
	Joint surfaces relatively large	Joint surfaces relatively small
Skull	Forehead shorter vertically	Forehead more elongated vertically
	Mandible and maxillae relatively smaller	Mandible and maxillae relatively larger
	Facial area rounder, with less pronounced features	Facial area more pronounced
	Processes less pronounced	Processes more prominent
Pelvis		
Pelvic cavity	Narrower in all dimensions	Wider in all dimensions
	Deeper	Shorter and roomier
	Pelvic outlet relatively small	Pelvic outlet relatively large
Sacrum	Long and narrow, with a smooth concavity (sacral curvature); sacral promontory more pronounced	Short, wide, and flat concavity more pronounced in a posterior direction; sacral promontory less pronounced
Coccyx	Less movable	More movable and follows the posterior direction of the sacral curvature

✳ **TABLE 2-14**　Primary Joint Classifications

Functional Name	Structural Name	Degree of Movement Permitted	Example
Synarthroses	Fibrous	Immovable	Sutures of the skull
Amphiarthroses	Cartilaginous	Slightly movable	Pubic symphysis
Diarthroses	Synovial	Freely movable	Shoulder joint

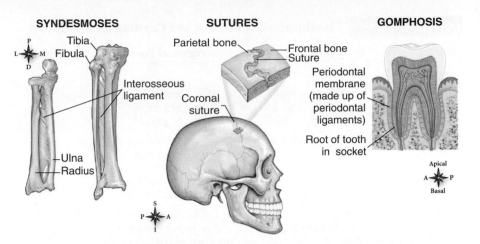

FIGURE 2-26 Fibrous Joints. Examples of the major types of fibrous joints.

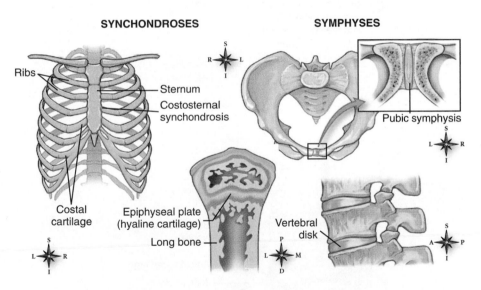

FIGURE 2-27 Cartilaginous Joints. Examples of the major types of cartilaginous joints.

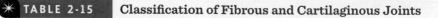

✳ **TABLE 2-15** **Classification of Fibrous and Cartilaginous Joints**

Types	Examples	Structural Features	Movement
Fibrous Joints			
Syndesmoses	Joints between the distal ends of the radius and the ulna	Fibrous bands (ligaments) connect articulating bones	Slight
Sutures	Joints between the skull bones	Teethlike projections of articulating bones interlock with a thin layer of fibrous tissue that connects them	None
Gomphoses	Joints between the roots of the teeth and the jaw bones	Fibrous tissue connects the roots of the teeth to the alveolar processes	None
Cartilaginous Joints			
Synchondroses	Costal cartilage attachments of the first rib to the sternum; epiphyseal plate between the diaphysis and the epiphysis of a growing long bone	Hyaline cartilage connects articulating bones	Slight
Symphyses	Pubic symphysis; joints between the bodies of vertebrae	Fibrocartilage between articulating bones	Slight

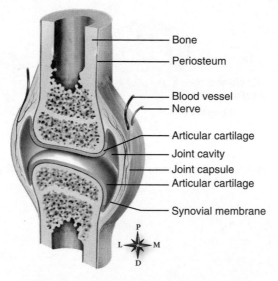

- Bone
- Periosteum
- Blood vessel
- Nerve
- Articular cartilage
- Joint cavity
- Joint capsule
- Articular cartilage
- Synovial membrane

FIGURE 2-28 General Structure of a Synovial Joint.

✳ TABLE 2-16	Structures of Synovial Joints
Structure	**Description**
Joint capsule	Sleevelike extension of the periosteum of each of the articulating bones; the capsule forms a complete casing around the ends of the bones, thereby binding them to each other
Synovial membrane	Moist, slippery membrane that lines the inner surface of the joint capsule; it attaches to the margins of the articular cartilage and it also secretes synovial fluid, which lubricates and nourishes the inner joint surfaces
Articular cartilage	Thin layer of hyaline cartilage that covers and cushions the articular surfaces of the bones
Joint cavity	Small space between the articulating surfaces of the two bones of the joint; the absence of tissue between articulating bone surfaces permits extensive movement (synovial joints are therefore diarthroses or freely movable joints)
Menisci (articular disks)	Pads of fibrocartilage located between the articulating ends of bones in some diarthroses; usually these pads divide the joint cavity into two separate cavities (e.g., the knee joint contains two large menisci)
Ligaments	Strong cords of dense, white fibrous tissue at most synovial joints; ligaments grow between the bones and lash them even more firmly together than is possible with the joint capsule alone
Bursae	Some synovial joints contain a closed, pillowlike structure called a **bursa** that consists of a synovial membrane filled with synovial fluid; bursae tend to be associated with bony prominences (e.g., knee, elbow), where they function to cushion the joint and facilitate the movement of tendons
Joint capsule	Sleevelike extension of the periosteum of each of the articulating bones; the capsule forms a complete casing around the ends of the bones, thereby binding them to each other

UNIAXIAL JOINTS

A   HINGE JOINT
Elbow joint

B   PIVOT JOINT
Dens of axis rotating against atlas
Head of radius rotating against ulna

BIAXIAL JOINTS

C   SADDLE JOINT
Carpometacarpal joint of thumb

D   CONDYLOID JOINT
Atlantooccipital joint

MULTIAXIAL JOINTS

E   BALL-AND-SOCKET JOINT
Shoulder joint
Hip joint

F   GLIDING JOINT
Articular processes between vertebrae

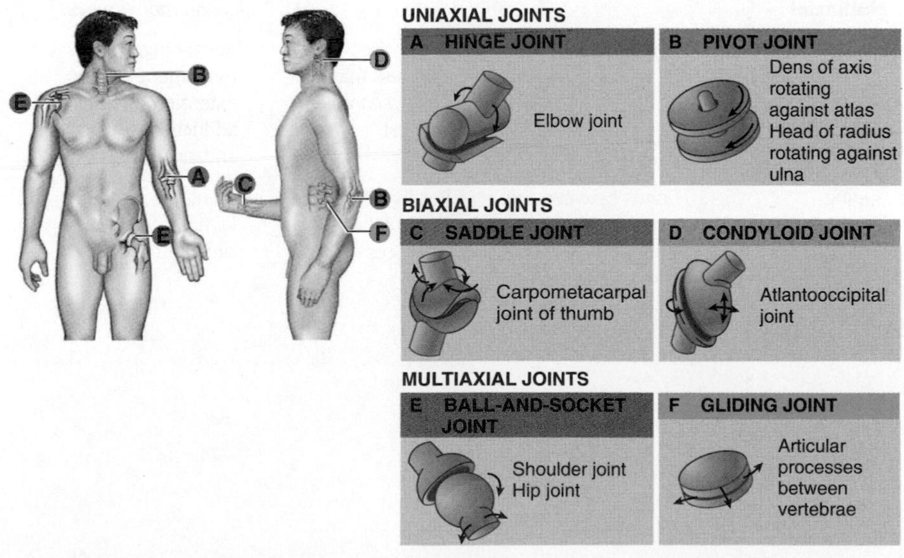

FIGURE 2-29 Types of Synovial Joints. In these simplified cartoons, notice that the shapes of the articulating bones dictate the type of movement that is permitted at each joint.

✳ TABLE 2-17   Classification of Synovial Joints

Types	Examples	Structure	Movement
Uniaxial			Around one axis; in one place
Hinge	Elbow joint	Spool-shaped process that fits into a concave socket	Flexion and extension only
Pivot	Joint between the first and second cervical vertebrae	Arch-shaped process that fits around a peglike process	Rotation
Biaxial			Around two axes that are perpendicular to each other; in two planes
Saddle	Thumb joint between the first metacarpal and the carpal bone	Saddle-shaped bone that fits into a socket that is concave–convex–concave	Flexion and extension in one plane; abduction and adduction in the other plane; opposing the thumb to the fingers
Condyloid (ellipsoidal)	Joint between the radius and the carpal bones	Oval condyle that fits into an elliptical socket	Flexion and extension in one plane; abduction and adduction in the other plane
Multiaxial			Around many axes
Ball and socket	Shoulder joint and hip	Ball-shaped process that fits into a concave socket	Widest range of movement: flexion, extension, abduction, adduction, rotation, and circumduction
Gliding	Joints between the articular facets of adjacent vertebrae; joints between the carpal and tarsal bones	Relatively flat articulating surfaces	Gliding movements without any angular or circular movements

✳ TABLE 2-18	Examples of Specific Joints		
Name	**Articulating Bones**	**Type**	**Movements**
Atlantoepistropheal	Anterior arch of the atlas rotates about the dens of the axis (epistropheus)	Synovial (pivot)	Pivoting or partial rotation of the head
Vertebral	Between bodies of the vertebrae	Cartilaginous (symphyses)	Slight movement between any two vertebrae but considerable motility for the column as a whole
	Between articular processes	Synovial (gliding)	Gliding
Sternoclavicular	Medial end of the clavicle with the manubrium of the sternum	Synovial (gliding)	Gliding
Acromioclavicular	Distal end of the clavicle with the acromion of the scapula	Synovial (gliding)	Gliding; elevation, depression, protraction, and retraction
Thoracic	Heads of ribs with bodies of vertebrae	Synovial (gliding)	Gliding
	Tubercles of ribs with transverse processes of vertebrae	Synovial (gliding)	Gliding
Shoulder	Head of the humerus in the glenoid cavity of the scapula	Synovial (ball and socket)	Flexion, extension, abduction, adduction, rotation, and circumduction of the upper part of the arm
Elbow	Trochlea of the humerus with the semilunar notch of the ulna; head of the radius with the capitulum of the humerus	Synovial (hinge)	Flexion and extension
	Head of the radius in the radial notch of the ulna	Synovial (pivot)	Supination and pronation of the forearm and the hand; rotation of the forearm on the upper extremity
Wrist	Scaphoid, lunate, and triquetral bones articulate with the radius and the articular disk	Synovial (condyloid)	Flexion, extension, abduction, and adduction of the hand
Carpal	Between various carpal bones	Synovial (gliding)	Gliding

Continued

✳ TABLE 2-18   **Examples of Specific Joints—cont'd**

Name	Articulating Bones	Type	Movements
Hand	Proximal end of the first metacarpal bone with the trapezium	Synovial (saddle)	Flexion, extension, abduction, adduction, and circumduction of the thumb and opposition to the fingers
	Distal end of the metacarpal bones with the proximal end of the phalanges	Synovial (hinge)	Flexion, extension, limited abduction, and adduction of the fingers
	Between the phalanges	Synovial (hinge)	Flexion and extension of the finger sections
Sacroiliac	Between the sacrum and the two ilia	Synovial (gliding)	None or slight
Pubic symphysis	Between the two pubic bones	Cartilaginous (symphysis)	Slight, particularly during pregnancy and delivery
Hip	Head of the femur in the acetabulum of the coxal bone	Synovial (ball and socket)	Flexion, extension, abduction, adduction, rotation, and circumduction
Knee	Between the distal end of the femur and the proximal end of the tibia	Synovial (hinge)	Flexion and extension; slight rotation of the tibia
Tibiofibular (proximal)	Head of the fibula with the lateral condyle of the tibia	Synovial (gliding)	Gliding
Ankle	Distal end of the tibia and fibula with the talus	Synovial (hinge)	Flexion (dorsiflexion) and extension (plantarflexion)
Foot	Between the tarsal bones	Synovial (gliding)	Gliding; inversion and eversion
	Between the metatarsal bones and the phalanges	Synovial (hinge)	Flexion, extension, slight abduction, and adduction
	Between the phalanges	Synovial (hinge)	Flexion and extension

TABLE 2-19	Major Types of Joint Movements	
Movement	**Example**	**Description**
Flexion (to flex a joint)		Reduces the angle of the joint, as when bending the elbow
Extension (to extend a joint)		Increases the angle of a joint, as when straightening a bent elbow
Rotation (to rotate a joint)		Spins one bone relative to another, as when rotating the head at the neck joint
Circumduction (to circumduct a joint)		Moves the distal end of a bone in a circle while keeping the proximal end relatively stable, as when moving the arm in a circle and thus circumducting the shoulder joint
Abduction (to abduct a joint)		Increases the angle of a joint to move a part away from the midline, as when moving the arm up and away from the side of the body
Adduction (to adduct a joint)		Decreases the angle of a joint to move a part toward the midline, as when moving the arm in and down toward the side of the body
Hyperextension		Increasing the angle of a joint beyond its usual anatomical position, as when tilting the neck backward; can also refer to abnormally extending a part and causing injury
Plantarflexion		Bends the ankle to point the toes and foot downward

Continued

✳ TABLE 2-19   Major Types of Joint Movements—cont'd

Movement	Example	Description
Dorsiflexion		Bends the ankle to point the toes and foot upward
Supination		Twists the forearm to move the hand to a thumb-outward (lateral) position; also applies to a similar twisting movement of the leg
Pronation		Twists the forearm to move the hand to a thumb-inward (medial) position; also applies to a similar twisting movement of the leg
Inversion		Bends the ankle to move the sole of the foot inward (medially)
Eversion		Bends the ankle to move the sole of the foot outward (laterally)
Protraction		Moves a part forward, as when thrusting the mandible anteriorly
Retraction		Moves a part backward, as when pulling the mandible inward (posteriorly)
Elevation		Moves a part upward, as when raising the mandible to close the mouth
Depression		Moves a part downward, as when lowering the mandible to open the mouth

C. Muscles

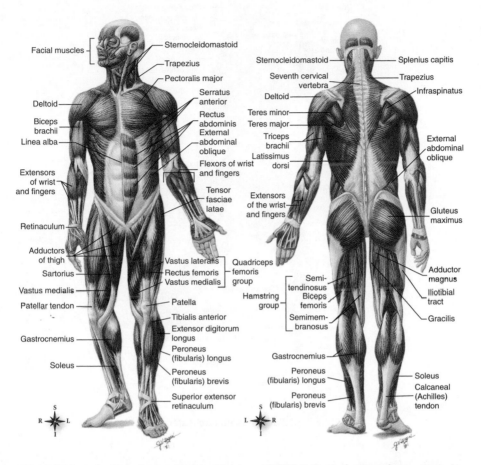

FIGURE 2-30 Body Musculature, Anterior View.

FIGURE 2-31 Body Musculature, Posterior View.

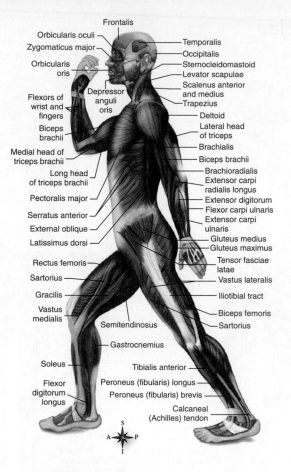

FIGURE 2-32 Body Musculature, Lateral View.

⬥ FIELD NOTES

Uncle Red, Freckles, and Muscles

I always loved holiday gatherings with my mom's extended family. I often saw relatives, relatives of relatives, and friends of relatives that I didn't otherwise get to visit. One of those folks was Uncle Red. That wasn't his real name; honestly, I still don't know his real name. He was called "Red" because he had brilliant red hair. It's what you noticed about him first. Whenever he came to a holiday party, he always brought his dog Freckles. Freckles was called that because he was a spaniel with lots of red dots on his white fur that made him look, well, freckled!

The problem for me was that, when they arrived everyone, would call out, "Red and Freckles are here!" In would strut the happy dog, followed by his master; I always thought that the dog was Red—he *was* red in parts—and that the man was Freckles, because he did indeed have prominent

◇ FIELD NOTES—cont'd

red freckles on his face. I'm still not sure I have it right, but my mom insists that the man was Red and the dog was Freckles.

My point is that, even though this one case confused me (and still does), most of the time such names are very helpful (as we learned in the previous Field Notes entries about identifying bone features by name; see pages 143 and 147). We often use one or two physical features to give a nickname a person, an animal, or a building. We use a similar system when naming bones and muscles.

Looking at muscle names, you'll notice that they work like the nicknames that we give people. Just as names like Big Al, Uncle Red, or Pastor Eddie tell you something about the way these people look or what they do, muscle names provide similar information. However, because muscle names are Latin in origin, you'll need to know that, for example, *maximus* means "big," *minimus* means "small," and *adductor* means "an agent that pulls toward the midline of the body." Check out *Muscle Names* (my-ap.us/Xqx2lS) for more tips.

The next several tables list translations of muscle names. If you take the time to become familiar with them, you'll find the muscle names easy to remember, because they'll make sense to you. You'll also find that it will be easy to find these muscles in the body and to figure out their actions.

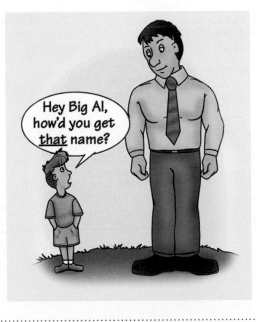

✳ **TABLE 2-20**   Selected Muscles Grouped by Function

Part Moved	Example of Flexor	Example of Extensor	Example of Abductor	Example of Adductor
Head	Sternocleidomastoid	Semispinalis capitis		
Upper arm	Pectoralis major	Trapezius, latissimus dorsi	Deltoid	Pectoralis major with latissimus dorsi
Forearm	With forearm supinated: biceps brachii; with forearm pronated: brachialis; with semisupination or semipronation: brachioradialis	Triceps brachii		
Hand	Flexor carpi radialis and ulnaris; palmaris longus	Extensor carpi radialis, longus, and brevis; extensor carpi ulnaris	Flexor carpi radialis	Flexor carpi ulnaris
Thigh	Iliopsoas, rectus femoris (of quadriceps femoris group)	Gluteus maximus	Gluteus medius and gluteus minimus	Adductor group
Leg	Hamstrings	Quadriceps femoris group		
Foot	Tibialis anterior	Gastrocnemius, soleus	Evertors, peroneus longus, peroneus brevis	Invertor, tibialis anterior
Trunk	Iliopsoas, rectus abdominis	Erector spinae		

✳ TABLE 2-21　Selected Muscles Grouped by Shape

Name	Meaning	Example
Deltoid	Triangular	Deltoid
Gracilis	Slender	Gracilis
Trapezius	Trapezoid	Trapezius
Serratus	Notched	Serratus anterior
Teres	Round	Pronator teres
Rhomboid	Rhomboidal	Rhomboid major
Orbicularis	Round or circular	Orbicularis oris
Pectinate	Comblike	Pectineus
Piriformis	Wedge-shaped	Piriformis
Platys	Flat	Platysma
Quadratus	Square	Quadratus femoris
Lumbrical	Wormlike	Lumbricals

✳ TABLE 2-22　Selected Muscles Grouped by Number of Heads and Direction of Fibers

Name	Meaning	Example
Number of Heads		
Biceps	Two heads	Biceps brachii
Triceps	Three heads	Triceps brachii
Quadriceps	Four heads	Quadriceps
Digastric	Two bellies	Digastric
Direction of Fibers		
Oblique	Diagonal	External oblique rectus
Rectus	Straight	Rectus abdominis
Transverse	Transverse	Transversus abdominis
Circular	Around	Orbicularis oris
Spiral	Oblique	Supinator

✳ **TABLE 2-23** **Selected Muscles Grouped by Size**

Name	Meaning	Example
Major	Large	Pectoralis major
Maximus	Largest	Gluteus maximus
Minor	Small	Pectoralis minor
Minimus	Smallest	Gluteus minimus
Longus	Long	Adductor longus
Brevis	Short	Extensor pollicis brevis
Latissimus	Very wide	Latissimus dorsi
Longissimus	Very long	Longissimus
Magnus	Very large	Adductor magnus
Vastus	Vast or huge	Vastus medialis

◆ **SURVIVAL TIPS**

☑ Use the names in the preceding tables to help you deduce the characteristics of the muscles listed in the tables that follow. Translations of the names have been included to help you.

☑ Because muscle names are often so descriptive when you know their translations, they are easily adapted to visual mnemonics that will help you to remember them.

☑ The names of muscles can be difficult to pronounce. Use the pronunciation keys listed in the following tables to say each one *out loud*. It sounds silly, but in addition to helping you learn how to say them when you need to use them, this actually acts as a mnemonic aid to help you to remember them!

☑ Flash cards are especially useful when memorizing muscles.

◇ SURVIVAL TIPS—cont'd

☑ The **origin** and **insertion** are the points of attachment of each skeletal muscle. If you pay attention to them, it will help you to figure out where the muscle is located. That's important, because labels on diagrams and models only show *one* point along a muscle, not the entire muscle.

☑ The attachment points also help you to deduce each muscle's primary action: the *insertion* point is usually pulled toward the *origin* point. In the figure, you can see that the **biceps brachii** muscle pulls its insertion in the forearm toward its origin in the shoulder, thereby flexing the elbow joint. Diarthrotic joints like the elbow each act as a **fulcrum** (turning point) to allow muscles to move bones in useful ways.

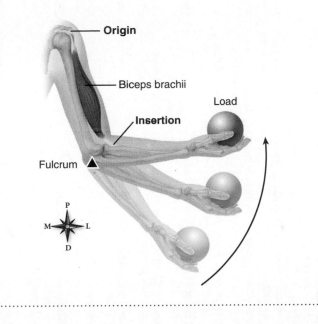

✳ TABLE 2-24   Muscles of Facial Expression and Mastication

Muscle	Pronunciation	Translation	Origin	Insertion	Function	Nerve Supply
Muscles of Facial Expression						
Occipitofrontalis (part of epicranius)	ok-sip-i-toh-fron-TAL-is (epi-CRAY-nee-us)	Back and front of head (upon the head)				
Frontal belly	FRUN-tel BEL-ee	Forehead (brow) swelling	Epicranial aponeurosis	Tissues of eyebrows and bridge of nose	Raises eyebrows; wrinkles forehead horizontally	Cranial nerve VII
Occipital belly	ok-SIP-it-al BEL-ee	Back-of-head swelling	Occipital bone (highest nuchal line)	Epicranial aponeurosis	Draws scalp backward	Cranial nerve VII
Corrugator supercilii	KOR-uh-gay-tor soo-per-SIL-ee-eye	Wrinkler above eyelashes	Frontal bone (superciliary ridge)	Skin of eyebrow	Wrinkles forehead vertically	Cranial nerve VII
Orbicularis oculi	or-bik-yoo-LAIR-is OK-yoo-lye	Little circle [around] eye	Encircles eyelid		Closes eye	Cranial nerve VII
Zygomaticus major	zye-goh-MAT-ik-us MA-jer	Greater [muscle] of zygomatic [bone]	Zygomatic bone	Angle of mouth	Laughing (elevates angle of mouth)	Cranial nerve VII
Orbicularis oris	or-bik-yoo-LAR-is OR-is	Little circle [around] mouth	Encircles mouth		Draws lips together	Cranial nerve VII
Buccinator	BUK-sih-NAY-tor	Trumpeter	Maxillae	Skin of sides of mouth	Facilitates smiling; blowing, as when playing the trumpet	Cranial nerve VII
Depressor anguli oris	dee-PRESS-er ANG-yoo-lee OR-is	Presser-down [muscle] of corner of mouth	Mandible	Angle of mouth	Draws ends of mouth downward, as when frowning	Cranial nerve IV
Muscles of Mastication						
Masseter	mah-SEE-ter	Chewer	Zygomatic arch	Mandible (external surface)	Elevates mandible to close jaw	Cranial nerve V
Temporalis	tem-poh-RAL-is	Temple (of head) [muscle]	Temporal bone	Mandible	Elevates mandible to close jaw	Cranial nerve V
Pterygoids (lateral and medial)	TERi-goidz (LAT-er-al and MEE-dee-al)	Winglike (side and middle)	Undersurface of skull	Mandible (medial surface)	Grates teeth	Cranial nerve V

✳ TABLE 2-25 Muscles That Move the Head

Muscle	Pronunciation	Translation	Origin	Insertion	Function	Nerve Supply
Sternocleidomastoid	STERN-oh-KLYE-doh-MAS-toyd	Sternum-clavicle-mastoid process	Sternum	Temporal bone (mastoid process)	Flexes head and neck (prayer muscle)	Accessory nerve
			Clavicle		One muscle alone that rotates head toward opposite side; spasm of this muscle alone or in association with trapezius is called *torticollis* or *wryneck*	
Semispinalis capitis	sem-ee-spy-NAYl-is KAP-i-tis	Half spine (muscle) of the head	Vertebrae (transverse processes of the upper six thoracic, articular processes of the lower four cervical)	Occipital bone (between the superior and inferior nuchal lines)	Extends head and neck; bends it laterally	First five cervical nerves
Splenius capitis	SPLEH-nee-us KAP-i-tis	Head patch	Ligamentum nuchae	Temporal bone (mastoid process)	Extends head and neck	Second, third, and fourth cervical nerves
			Vertebrae (spinous processes of the upper three or four thoracic)	Occipital bone	Bends and rotates head toward the same side as when contracting a muscle	
Longissimus capitis	lon-JIS-i-mus KAP-i-tis	Longest head (muscle)	Vertebrae (transverse processes of the upper six thoracic, articular processes of the lower four cervical)	Temporal bone (mastoid process)	Extends head and neck; bends and rotates the head toward the contracting side	Multiple innervation

★ **TABLE 2-26**   **Muscles of the Thorax**

Muscle	Pronunciation	Translation	Origin	Insertion	Function	Nerve Supply
External intercostals	eks-TER-nal in-ter-KOS-tal	Outer (muscle) between the ribs	Rib (lower border; forward fibers)	Rib (upper border of rib below origin)	Elevate ribs	Intercostal nerves
Internal intercostals	in-TER-nal in-ter-KOS-tal	Inner (muscle) between the ribs	Rib (inner surface, lower border; backward fibers)	Rib (upper border of rib below origin)	Depress ribs	Intercostal nerves
Diaphragm	DYE-ah-fram	Across-enclosure	Lower circumference of thorax (of ribcage)	Central tendon of diaphragm	Enlarges thorax, thereby causing inspiration	Phrenic nerves

✳ **TABLE 2-27** Muscles of the Abdominal Wall

Muscle	Pronunciation	Translation	Origin	Insertion	Function	Nerve Supply
External oblique	eks-TER-nal oh-BLEEK	Outer slanted (muscle)	Ribs (lower eight)	Pelvis (iliac crest and pubis by way of the inguinal ligament)	Compresses abdomen	Lower seven intercostal nerves and iliohypogastric nerves
				Linea alba by way of an aponeurosis	Rotates trunk laterally	
Internal oblique	in-TER-nal oh-BLEEK	Inner slanted (muscle)	Pelvis (iliac crest and iliopsoas fascia)	Ribs (lower three)	The important postural function of all abdominal muscles is to pull the front of the pelvis upward, thereby flattening the lumbar curve of the spine; when these muscles lose their tone, common figure faults of protruding abdomen and lordosis develop	Last three intercostal nerves; iliohypogastric and ilioinguinal nerves
			Lumbodorsal fascia	Linea alba		
Transversus abdominis	tranz-VERS-us ab-DAH-min-us	Belly-crossing (muscle)	Ribs (lower six)	Pubic bone	Same as external oblique	Last three intercostal nerves; iliohypogastric and ilioinguinal nerves
			Pelvis (iliac crest, iliopsoas fascia)	Linea alba		
			Lumbodorsal fascia	Ribs (costal cartilage of the fifth, sixth, and seventh ribs)	Same as external oblique	Last five intercostal nerves; iliohypogastric and ilioinguinal nerves
Rectus abdominis	REK-tus ab-DOM-i-nis	Straight belly (muscle)	Pelvis (pubic bone and pubic symphysis)	Sternum (xiphoid process)	Same as external oblique; because abdominal muscles compress the abdominal cavity, they aid in straining, defecation, forced expiration, and childbirth; abdominal muscles are antagonists of the diaphragm, relaxing as the diaphragm contracts and vice versa; flexes trunk	Last six intercostal nerves
Quadratus lumborum	kwah-DRAT-is lum-BOR-um	Four-sided lumbar (muscle)	Iliolumbar ligament; iliac crest	Last rib; transverse process of vertebrae L1 through L4	Flexes vertebral column laterally; depresses last rib	Lumbar

✳ TABLE 2-28   Muscles of the Back

Muscle	Pronunciation	Translation	Origin	Insertion	Function	Nerve Supply
Erector spinae group	eh-REK-tor SPINE-ee	Spine straightener				
Iliocostalis group	ILL-ee-oh-KOS-tal-is	(Pelvic) ilium to rib (muscle)	Various regions of the pelvis and the ribs	Ribs and vertebra (superior to the origin)	Extends and laterally flexes the vertebral column	Spinal, thoracic, or lumbar nerves
Longissimus group	lon-JIS-i-mus	Very long (longest)	Cervical and thoracic vertebrae, ribs	Mastoid process, upper cervical vertebrae, or upper lumbar vertebrae	Extends head, neck, or vertebral column	Cervical or thoracic and lumbar nerves
Spinalis group	spy-NAY-lis	Spine (muscle)	Lower cervical or lower thoracic and upper lumbar vertebrae	Upper cervical or middle and upper thoracic vertebrae (superior to the origin)	Extends the neck or vertebral column	Cervical or thoracic nerves
Transversospinalis group	tranz-VERS-o-spy-NAY-lis	Transverse (vertebral) spine (muscle)				
Semispinalis group	sem-ee-spy-NAY-lis	Half spine (muscle)	Transverse processes of vertebrae T2 through T11	Spinous processes of vertebrae C2 through T4	Extends the neck or the vertebral column	Cervical or thoracic nerves
Multifidus group	mul-TIF-i-dus	Split into many parts	Transverse processes of the vertebrae; sacrum and ilium	Spinous processes of the next superior vertebrae	Extends and rotates the vertebral column	Spinal nerves
Rotatores group	roh-tah-TOR-eez	Turner (muscles)	Transverse processes of the vertebrae	Spinous processes of the next superior vertebrae	Extends and rotates the vertebral column	Spinal nerves
Splenius	SPLEH-nee-us	Patch	Spinous processes of vertebrae C7 through T1 or T3 through T6	Lateral occipital/mastoid or transverse processes of vertebrae C1 through C4	Rotates and extends the neck and flexes the neck laterally	Cervical nerves
Interspinales group	in-ter-spy-NAH-leez	Between spines	Spinous processes of the vertebrae	Spinous processes of the next superior vertebrae	Extends the back and the neck	Spinal nerves

✳ TABLE 2-29   Muscles of the Pelvic Floor

Muscles	Pronunciation	Translation	Origin	Insertion	Function	Nerve Supply
Levator ani	leh-VAY-tor A-nye	Anus lifter	Pubis and spine of the ischium	Coccyx	Together with the coccygeus muscles forms the floor of the pelvic cavity and supports the pelvic organs	Pudendal nerve
Ischiocavernosus	is-kee-oh-KAV-er-no-sus	(Pelvic) ischium to the crus (cross) of the penis's cavernosum	Ischium	Penis or clitoris	Compresses the base of the penis or clitoris	Perineal nerve
Bulbospongiosus	bul-boh-spun-jee-OH-ses	Spongy bulb (base of penis)				
Male			Bulb of the penis	Perineum and bulb of the penis	Constricts the urethra and erects the penis	Pudendal nerve
Female			Perineum	Base of the clitoris	Erects the clitoris	Pudendal nerve
Deep transverse perineal	deep tranz-VERS pair-in-EE-al	Deep across (muscle) around the excretion (openings)	Ischium	Central tendon (median raphe)	Supports the pelvic floor	Pudendal nerve
Urethral sphincter	yoo-REE-thral SFINGK-ter	Urethra tightener	Pubic ramus	Central tendon (median raphe)	Constricts the urethra	Pudendal nerve
External anal sphincter	eks-TER-nal AY-nal SFINGK-ter	Outer anus tightener	Coccyx	Central tendon (median raphe)	Closes the anal canal	Pudendal and S4

✱ **TABLE 2-30**   Muscles That Act on the Shoulder Girdle

Muscle	Pronunciation	Translation	Origin	Insertion	Function	Nerve Supply
Trapezius	trah-PEE-zee-us	Table-shaped (muscle)	Occipital bone (protuberance)	Clavicle	Raises or lowers the shoulders and shrugs them	Spinal accessory; second, third, and fourth cervical nerves
			Vertebrae (cervical and thoracic)	Scapula (spine and acromion)	Extends the head and neck when the occiput acts as the insertion	
Pectoralis minor	pek-toh-RAL-is MYE-ner	Lesser chest (muscle)	Ribs (second to fifth)	Scapula (coracoid)	Pulls the shoulder girdle down and forward	Medial and lateral anterior thoracic nerve
Serratus anterior	ser-RAY-tus an-TEER-ee-or	Front saw-tooth (muscle)	Ribs (upper eight or nine)	Scapula (anterior surface, vertebral border)	Pulls the shoulder down and forward; abducts and rotates it upward	Long thoracic nerve
Levator scapulae	leh-VAY-tor SCAP-yoo-lee	Scapula lifter	C1 through C4 transverse processes	Scapula (superior angle)	Elevates and retracts the scapula and abducts the neck	Dorsal scapular nerve
Rhomboid	ROM-boyd	Rhombus (equilateral parallelogram)				
Major	MA-jer	Greater	T1 through T4	Scapula (medial border)	Retracts, rotates, and fixes the scapula	Dorsal scapular nerve
Minor	MYE-ner	Lesser	C6 through C7	Scapula (medial border)	Retracts, rotates, elevates, and fixes the scapula	Dorsal scapular nerve

✳ TABLE 2-31 Muscles That Move the Arm

Muscle	Pronunciation	Translation	Origin	Insertion	Function	Nerve Supply
Axial*	AK-see-all	Related to the axis				
Pectoralis major	pek-toh-RAL-is MA-jer	Greater chest (muscle)	Clavicle (medial half); sternum; costal cartilages of the true ribs	Humerus (greater tubercle)	Flexes the arm and adducts the arm anteriorly; draws it across the chest	Medial and lateral anterior thoracic nerves
Latissimus dorsi	lat-ISS-im-is DOR-sye	Very wide back (muscle)	Spines of the lower thoracic, lumbar, and sacral vertebrae; ilium (crest); lumbodorsal fascia	Humerus (intertubercular groove)	Extends the arm and adducts the arm posteriorly	Thoracodorsal nerve
Scapular*	SKAP-yoo-lar	Related to shoulder				
Deltoid	DEL-toyd	Trianglelike	Clavicle; scapula (spine and acromion)	Humerus (lateral side about halfway down at the deltoid tubercle)	Abducts the arm; assists with the flexion and extension of the arm	Axillary nerve
Coracobrachialis	KOR-uh-ko-BRAY-kee-al-is	Coracoid process of the arm (muscle)	Scapula (coracoid process)	Humerus (middle third, medial surface)	Adduction; assists with the flexion and medial rotation of the arm	Musculocutaneous nerve
Supraspinatus[†]	SOO-prah-spy-nah-tus	Above spine (muscle)	Scapula (supraspinous fossa)	Humerus (greater tubercle)	Assists with the abduction of the arm	Suprascapular nerve
Teres minor[†]	TER-eez MYE-ner	Lesser rounded (muscle)	Scapula (axillary border)	Humerus (greater tubercle)	Rotates the arm outward	Axillary nerve
Teres major	TER-eez MA-jer	Greater rounded (muscle)	Scapula (lower part, axillary border)	Humerus (upper part, anterior surface)	Assists with the extension, adduction, and medial rotation of the arm	Lower subscapular nerve
Infraspinatus[†]	IN-frah-spy-nah-tus	Below the spine	Scapula (infraspinatus border)	Humerus (greater tubercle)	Rotates the arm outward	Suprascapular nerve
Subscapularis[†]	sub-SKAP-yoo-lar-is	Under the scapula (muscle)	Scapula (subscapular fossa)	Humerus (lesser tubercle)	Medial rotation	Suprascapular nerve

*Axial muscles originate on the axial skeleton. Scapular muscles originate on the scapula.
[†]Muscles of the rotator cuff (i.e., the SITS muscles).

✳ **TABLE 2-32** Muscles That Move the Forearm

Muscle	Pronunciation	Translation	Origin	Insertion	Function	Nerve Supply
Flexors	FLEK-serz	Benders				
Biceps brachii	BYE-seps BRAY-kee-eye	Two-headed arm (muscle)	Supraglenoid tuberosity and coracoid of the scapula	Radius (tuberosity at the proximal end)	Flexes the supinated forearm; supinates the forearm and hand	Musculocutaneous nerve
Brachialis	BRAY-kee-al-is	Arm (muscle)	Humerus (distal half, anterior surface)	Ulna (front of the coronoid process)	Flexes the pronated forearm	Musculocutaneous nerve
Brachioradialis	BRAY-kee-oh-ray-dee-AL-is	Arm and radius (muscle)	Humerus (above the lateral epicondyle)	Radius (styloid process)	Flexes the semipronated or semisupinated forearm; supinates the forearm and hand	Radial nerve
Extensor	ek-STEN-ser	Stretcher				
Triceps brachii	TRY-seps BRAY-kee-eye	Three-headed arm (muscle)	Scapula (infraglenoid tuberosity); humerus (posterior surface: lateral head attached above the radial groove and the medial head attached below)	Ulna (olecranon)	Extends the lower arm	Radial nerve
Pronators	PRO-nay-terz	Forward twister				
Pronator teres	PRO-nay-ter TAIR-eez	Rounded forward-twister	Humerus (medial epicondyle); ulna (coronoid process)	Radius (middle third of the lateral surface)	Pronates and flexes the forearm	Median nerve
Pronator quadratus	PRO-nay-ter kwah-DRAT-is	Four-sided forward-twister	Ulna (distal fourth, anterior surface)	Radius (distal fourth, anterior surface)	Pronates the forearm	Median nerve
Supinator	SOO-pin-ayt-er	Back-layer				
Supinator	SOO-pin-ayt-er	Back-layer	Humerus (lateral epicondyle); ulna (proximal fifth)	Radius (proximal third)	Supinates the forearm	Radial nerve

✳ **TABLE 2-33** Muscles That Move the Wrist, Hand, and Fingers

Muscle	Pronunciation	Translation	Origin	Insertion	Function	Nerve Supply
Extrinsic	eks-TRIN-sik	Outside				
Flexor carpi radialis	FLEK-ser KAR-pye ray-dee-AL-is	Wrist bender at radius	Humerus (medial epicondyle)	Base of second metacarpal	Flexes the hand and the forearm	Median nerve
Palmaris longus	PAL-mar-is LONG-us	Long palm (muscle)	Humerus (medial epicondyle)	Fascia of the palm	Flexes the hand	Median nerve
Flexor carpi ulnaris	FLEK-ser KAR-pye ul-NAIR-is	Wrist bender at ulna	Humerus (medial epicondyle); Ulna (proximal two thirds)	Pisiform bone; Third, fourth, and fifth metacarpals	Flexes the hand; Adducts the hand	Ulnar nerve
Extensor carpi radialis longus	ek-STEN-ser KAR-pye ray-dee-AL-is LONG-us	Long wrist stretcher at radius	Humerus (ridge above the lateral epicondyle)	Base of the second metacarpal	Extends the hand and abducts the hand (moves toward the thumb side when the hand is supinated)	Radial nerve
Extensor carpi radialis brevis	ek-STEN-ser KAR-pye ray-dee-AL-is BREV-is	Short wrist stretcher at radius	Humerus (lateral epicondyle)	Bases of the second and third metacarpals	Extends the hand	Radial nerve
Extensor carpi ulnaris	ek-STEN-ser KAR-pye ul-NAIR-is	Wrist stretcher at ulna	Humerus (lateral epicondyle); ulna (proximal three fourths)	Base of the fifth metacarpal	Extends the hand and adducts the hand (moves toward the little finger side when the hand is supinated)	Radial nerve
Flexor digitorum profundus	FLEK-ser diji-TOH-rum pro-FUN-dis	Deep finger bender	Ulna (anterior surface)	Distal phalanges (fingers 2 through 5)	Flexes the distal interphalangeal joints	Median and ulnar nerves
Flexor digitorum superficialis	FLEK-ser diji-TOH-rum soo-per-fish-ee-AL-is	Superficial finger bender	Humerus (medial epicondyle), radius, and ulna (coronoid process)	Tendons of the fingers	Flexes the fingers	Median nerve
Extensor digitorum	ek-STEN-ser diji-TOH-rum	Finger stretcher	Humerus (lateral epicondyle)	Phalanges (fingers 2 through 5)	Extends the fingers	Radial nerve

Continued

✳ TABLE 2-33   Muscles That Move the Wrist, Hand, and Fingers—cont'd

Muscle	Pronunciation	Translation	Origin	Insertion	Function	Nerve Supply
Intrinsic	in-TRIN-sik	Inside				
Opponens pollicis	oh-POH-nenz POL-i-sis (or POL-i-kiss)	Thumb opposer	Trapezium	Thumb metacarpal	Opposes the thumb to the fingers	Median nerve
Abductor pollicis brevis	ab-DUK-ter POL-ih-sis (or POL-ih-kiss) BREV-is	Short bringer-away muscle of thumb	Trapezium	Proximal phalanx of the thumb	Abducts the thumb	Median nerve
Adductor pollicis	ad-DUK-ter POL-ih-sis (or POL-ih-kiss)	Bringer-in muscle of thumb	Second and third metacarpals; trapezoid and capitate	Proximal phalanx of the thumb	Adducts the thumb	Ulnar nerve
Flexor pollicis brevis	FLEK-ser POL-ih-sis (or POL-ih-kiss) BREV-is	Short thumb bender	Flexor retinaculum	Proximal phalanx of the thumb	Flexes the thumb	Median and ulnar nerves
Abductor digiti minimi	ab-DUK-ter DIJ-ih-tye MIN-ih-mye	Small finger bringer-away (muscle)	Pisiform	Base of the proximal phalanx of the fifth finger	Abducts and flexes the fifth finger	Ulnar nerve
Flexor digiti minimi brevis	FLEK-ser DIJ-ih-tye MIN-ih-mye BREV-is	Small, short finger bender	Hamate	Proximal and middle phalanx of the fifth finger	Flexes the fifth finger	Ulnar nerve
Opponens digiti minimi	oh-POH-nenz DIJ-ih-tye MIN-ih-mye	Small finger opposer	Hamate and flexor retinaculum	Fifth metacarpal	Opposes the fifth finger slightly	Ulnar nerve
Interosseous (palmar and dorsal)	in-ter-OS-see-us (PALM-er and DOR-sal)	Between-bone (muscle) (back and palm-side)	Metacarpals	Proximal phalanges	Adducts the second, fourth, and fifth fingers (palmar); abducts the second, third, and fourth fingers (dorsal)	Ulnar nerve
Lumbricals	LUM-bri-kulz	Wormlike	Tendons of the flexor digitorum profundus	Phalanges (2 through 5)	Flexes the proximal phalanges (2 through 5); extends the middle and distal phalanges (2 through 5)	Median nerve (phalanges 2 and 3); ulnar nerve (phalanges 4 and 5)

★ TABLE 2-34 Muscles That Move the Thigh

Muscles	Pronunciation	Translation	Origin	Insertion	Function	Nerve Supply
Iliopsoas (iliacus, psoas major, and psoas minor)	ILL-ee-oh-SOH-is (ih-LYE-ah-kus, SO-is MAY-jer, and SO-is MYE-ner)	Iliacus (ilium of pelvic bone) and psoas (lumbar) (muscles)	Ilium (iliac fossa)	Femur (lesser trochanter)	Flexes the thigh	Femoral and second to fourth lumbar nerves
			Vertebrae (bodies of twelfth thoracic to fifth lumbar)		Flexes the trunk (when the femur acts as the origin)	
Rectus femoris	REK-tus FEM-uh-ris (or fem-OR-is)	Straight thigh (muscle)	Ilium (anterior, inferior spine)	Tibia (by way of the patellar tendon)	Flexes the thigh and extends the leg	Femoral nerve
Gluteal group	GLOO-tee-al	Butt (buttocks)				
Gluteus maximus	GLOO-tee-us MAK-sim-us	Large butt (muscle)	Ilium (crest and posterior surface); sacrum and coccyx (posterior surface); sacrotuberous ligament	Femur (gluteal tuberosity) and iliotibial tract	Extends the thigh and rotates outward	Inferior gluteal nerve
Gluteus medius	GLOO-tee-us MEE-dee-us	Medium butt (muscle)	Ilium (lateral surface)	Femur (greater trochanter)	Abducts the thigh and rotates outward; stabilizes the pelvis on the femur	Superior gluteal nerve
Gluteus minimus	GLOO-tee-us MIN-ih-mus	Small butt (muscle)	Ilium (lateral surface)	Femur (greater trochanter)	Abducts the thigh; stabilizes the pelvis on the femur; rotates the thigh medially	Superior gluteal nerve
Tensor fasciae latae	TEN-sor FASH-ee (or FASH-ee-ay) LAT-tee	Puller-of-side bundle	Ilium (anterior part of the crest)	Tibia (by way of the iliotibial tract)	Abducts the thigh and tightens the iliotibial tract	Superior gluteal nerve
Adductor group	ad-DUK-ter	Bringer in				
Adductor brevis	ad-DUK-ter BREV-is	Short bringer-in (muscle)	Pubic bone	Femur (linea aspera)	Adducts the thigh	Obturator nerve
Adductor longus	ad-DUK-ter LONG-us	Long bringer-in (muscle)	Pubic bone	Femur (linea aspera)	Adducts the thigh	Obturator nerve
Adductor magnus	ad-DUK-ter MAG-nus	Great bringer-in (muscle)	Pubic bone	Femur (linea aspera)	Adducts the thigh	Obturator nerve
Gracilis	GRASS-ih-lis	Slender (muscle)	Pubic bone (just below the symphysis)	Tibia (medial surface behind the sartorius)	Adducts the thigh and flexes and adducts the leg	Obturator nerve

✳ TABLE 2-35 Muscles That Move the Leg

Muscle	Pronunciation	Translation	Origin	Insertion	Function	Nerve Supply
Quadriceps femoris group	KWAH-drih-seps FEM-uh-ris (or fem-OR-is)	Four-headed thigh group				
Rectus femoris	REK-tus FEM-uh-ris (or fem-OR-is)	Straight thigh (muscle)	Ilium (anterior inferior spine)	Tibia (by way of the patellar tendon)	Flexes the thigh and extends the leg	Femoral nerve
Vastus lateralis	VAS-tus lat-er-AL-is	Vast (enormous) on-the-side (muscle)	Femur (linea aspera)	Tibia (by way of the patellar tendon)	Extends the leg	Femoral nerve
Vastus medialis	VAS-tus mee-dee-AL-is	Vast (enormous) toward-the-middle (muscle)	Femur	Tibia (by way of the patellar tendon)	Extends the leg	Femoral nerve
Vastus intermedius	VAS-tus in-ter-MEE-dee-us	Vast (enormous) in-between (muscle)	Femur (anterior surface)	Tibia (by way of the patellar tendon)	Extends the leg	Femoral nerve
Sartorius	sar-TOR-ee-us	Tailor (muscle)	Coxal (anterosuperior iliac spines)	Tibia (medial surface of the upper end of the shaft)	Adducts and flexes the leg; permits crossing of the legs tailor fashion	Femoral nerve
Hamstring Group						
Biceps femoris	BYE-seps FEM-uh-ris	Two-headed thigh (muscle)	Ischium (tuberosity)	Head of the fibula	Extends the thigh and flexes the leg	Common fibular nerve (branch of the sciatic nerve)
			Femur (linea aspera)	Tibia (lateral condyle)	Flexes the leg	Tibial nerve
Semitendinosus	sem-ee-ten-din-OH-sis	Half tendon (muscle)	Ischium (tuberosity)	Tibia (proximal end, medial surface)	Extends the thigh and flexes the leg	Tibial nerve
Semimembranosus	sem-ee-mem-brah-NO-sis	Half membrane (muscle)	Ischium (tuberosity)	Tibia (medial condyle)	Extends the thigh and flexes the leg	Tibial nerve

✳ **TABLE 2-36**   **Muscles That Move the Foot**

Muscle	Pronunciation	Translation	Origin	Insertion	Function	Nerve Supply
Extrinsic	eks-TRIN-sik	Outside				
Tibialis anterior	tib-ee-AL-is an-TEER-ee-or	Front shinbone (muscle)	Tibia (lateral condyle of the upper body)	Tarsal (first cuneiform); metatarsal (base of first)	Flexes and inverts the foot	Common and deep peroneal nerves
Gastrocnemius	GAS-trok-NEE-mee-us	Belly of leg	Femur (condyles)	Tarsal (calcaneus by way of the Achilles tendon)	Extends the foot and flexes the leg	Tibial nerve (branch of the sciatic nerve)
Soleus	SOH-lee-us	Sole (of foot) (muscle)	Tibia (underneath the gastrocnemius); fibula	Tarsal (calcaneus by way of the Achilles tendon)	Extends the foot (plantarflexion)	Tibial nerve
Fibularis longus (peroneus longus)	fib-yoo-LAIR-is LONG-us (per-oh-NEE-us LONG-us)	Long fibula (long boot) (muscle)	Tibia (lateral condyle) Fibula (head and shaft)	First cuneiform Base of the first metatarsal	Extends the foot (plantarflexion) Everts the foot	Common peroneal nerve
Fibularis brevis (peroneus brevis)	fib-yoo-LAIR-is BREV-is (per-oh-NEE-us BREV-is)	Short fibula (short boot) (muscle)	Fibula (lower two thirds of the lateral surface of the shaft)	Fifth metatarsal (tubercle, dorsal surface)	Everts and flexes the foot	Superficial peroneal nerve
Fibularis tertius (peroneus tertius)	fib-yoo-LAIR-is TER-shee-us (per-oh-NEE-us TER-shee-us)	Third fibula (third boot) (muscle)	Fibula (distal third)	Bases of the fourth and fifth metatarsals	Flexes and everts the foot	Deep peroneal nerve
Extensor digitorum longus	ek-STEN-ser dij-i-TOH-rum LONG-gus	Long toe stretcher	Tibia (lateral condyle); fibula (anterior surface)	Second and third phalanges (four lateral toes)	Dorsiflexion of the foot and extension of the toes	Deep peroneal nerve

Continued

✴ TABLE 2-36   Muscles that Move the Foot—cont'd

Muscle	Pronunciation	Translation	Origin	Insertion	Function	Nerve Supply
Intrinsic	in-TRIN-sik	Inside				
Lumbricals	LUM-bri-kulz	Wormlike	Tendons of the flexor digitorum longus	Phalanges (2 through 5)	Flex the proximal phalanges; extend the middle and distal phalanges	Lateral and medial plantar nerve
Flexor digiti minimi brevis	FLEK-ser DIJ-ih-tye MIN-ih-mye BREV-is	Small, short toe bender	Fifth metatarsal	Proximal phalanx of the fifth toe	Flexes the fifth (small) toe	Lateral plantar nerve
Flexor hallucis brevis	FLEK-ser HAL-oos-is (or HAL-uh-kiss) BREV-is	Short big-toe bender	Cuboid; medial and lateral cuneiform	Proximal phalanx of the first (great) toe	Flexes the first (great) toe	Medial and lateral plantar nerve
Flexor digitorum brevis	FLEK-ser diji-TOH-rum BREV-is	Short toe bender	Calcaneus; plantar fascia	Middle phalanges of the toes (2 through 5)	Flexes toes 2 through 5	Medial plantar nerve
Abductor digiti minimi	ab-DUK-ter DIJ-ih-tye MIN-ih-mye	Small toe bringer-away (muscle)	Calcaneus	Proximal phalanx of the fifth (small) toe	Abducts and flexes the fifth (small) toe	Lateral plantar nerve
Abductor hallucis	ab-DUK-ter HAL-oos-is (or HAL-uh-kiss)	Big-toe bringer-away (muscle)	Calcaneus	First (great) toe	Abducts the first (great) toe	Medial plantar nerve

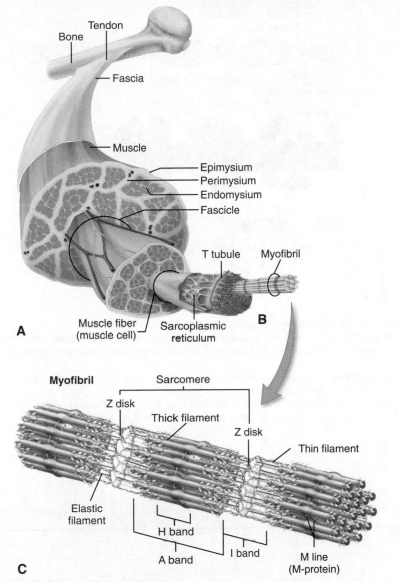

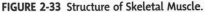

FIGURE 2-33 Structure of Skeletal Muscle.
A, A skeletal muscle organ, which is composed of bundles of contractile muscle fibers held together by connective tissue. The **epimysium** is the connective tissue wrapping of the whole muscle organ. The **perimysium** wraps small bundles of muscle fibers called **fascicles.** The **endomysium** wraps individual muscle fibers. The wrappings converge to form a **tendon,** which connects to bone or another muscle. **Fascia** is the connective tissue outside of the muscle organ. **B,** Greater magnification of single fiber showing smaller fibers—**myofibrils**—in the sarcoplasm. **C,** Myofibril magnified further to show **thick myofilaments** and **thin myofilaments.** The **sarcomere** is a structural unit between **Z disks** (Z lines).

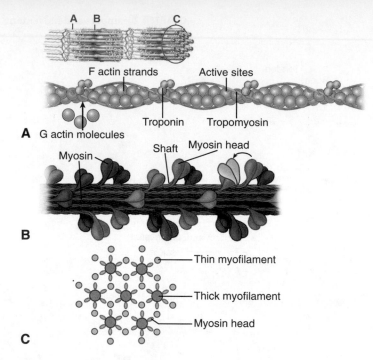

FIGURE 2-34 Structure of Myofilaments.
A, Thin myofilament made up of a double **F-actin** strand composed of **G-actin** molecules. Note also that **tropomyosin** strands, which are held in place by **troponin** molecules, block actin's active sites.
B, Thick myofilament made up of **myosin** molecules having movable **heads** that can bind to actin's active sites, when available.
C, Cross-section of several thick and thin myofilaments showing the relative positions of myofilaments and the myosin heads that will form **cross bridges** between them.

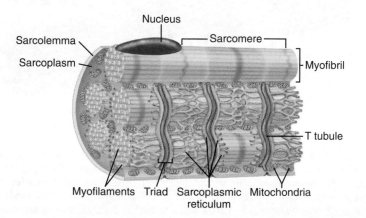

FIGURE 2-35 Unique Features of the Skeletal Muscle Fiber. Notice especially the **T tubules,** which are extensions of the **sarcolemma** (plasma membrane), and the **sarcoplasmic reticulum (SR),** a type of *smooth endoplasmic reticulum* that forms networks of tubular canals and sacs that contain stored **calcium ions.** A **triad** is a triplet of adjacent tubules: a terminal *(end)* sac of the SR, a T tubule, and another terminal sac of the SR. Cylindrical sections of the cytoskeleton called **myofibrils** are made up of thick and thin myofilaments. Numerous **mitochondria** in the muscle fiber *(muscle cell)* transfer energy to **adenosine triphosphate (ATP)** to supply the high energy consumption of muscular contraction.

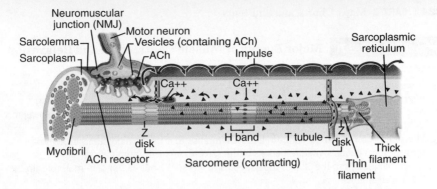

FIGURE 2-36 Excitation and Contraction of Skeletal Muscle Fiber. A nerve impulse travels to the neuromuscular junction (NMJ), where vesicles of **acetylcholine (ACh)** are released and trigger **ACh receptors** in the **sarcolemma.** Resulting **excitation** of the sarcolemma initiates a new impulse (action potential) that travels across the sarcolemma and through the **T tubules,** where it triggers adjacent sacs of the **sarcoplasmic reticulum** to release a flood of **calcium ions (Ca^{++})** into the sarcoplasm. Ca^{++} is then free to bind to **troponin** molecules in the thin filaments. This binding, in turn, initiates the chemical reactions that produce a **contraction** (see Figure 2-37). The linkage of excitation and contraction is called **excitation–contraction coupling.**

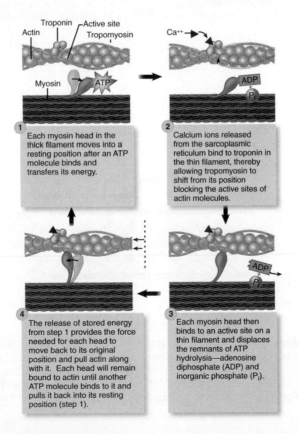

1. Each myosin head in the thick filament moves into a resting position after an ATP molecule binds and transfers its energy.

2. Calcium ions released from the sarcoplasmic reticulum bind to troponin in the thin filament, thereby allowing tropomyosin to shift from its position blocking the active sites of actin molecules.

3. Each myosin head then binds to an active site on a thin filament and displaces the remnants of ATP hydrolysis—adenosine diphosphate (ADP) and inorganic phosphate (P$_i$).

4. The release of stored energy from step 1 provides the force needed for each head to move back to its original position and pull actin along with it. Each head will remain bound to actin until another ATP molecule binds to it and pulls it back into its resting position (step 1).

FIGURE 2-37 Actin–Myosin Reaction. Contraction is produced by myosin heads grasping actin at active sites and pulling the thin filaments toward the center of the sarcomere to produce the contraction of the myofibrils (Figure 2-38). When calcium is removed from troponin and ATP binds to myosin, the reaction stops and the resting state is restored.

✴ TABLE 2-37   Major Events of Muscle Contraction and Relaxation

Excitation and Contraction

1. A nerve impulse reaches the end of a motor neuron and triggers the release of the neurotransmitter acetylcholine (ACh).
2. ACh diffuses rapidly across the gap of the neuromuscular junction and binds to ACh receptors on the motor endplate of the muscle fiber.
3. The stimulation of ACh receptors initiates an impulse that travels along the sarcolemma, through the T tubules, and to the sacs of the sarcoplasmic reticulum (SR).
4. Ca^{++} is released from the SR into the sarcoplasm, where it binds to troponin molecules in the thin myofilaments.
5. Tropomyosin molecules in the thin myofilaments shift and thereby expose actin's active sites.
6. Energized myosin cross bridges of the thick myofilaments bind to actin and use their energy to pull the thin myofilaments toward the center of each sarcomere. This cycle repeats itself many times per second, as long as adenosine triphosphate is available.
7. As the filaments slide past the thick myofilaments, the entire muscle fiber shortens.

Relaxation

1. After the impulse is over, the SR begins actively pumping Ca^{++} back into its sacs.
2. As Ca^{++} is stripped from troponin molecules in the thin myofilaments, tropomyosin returns to its position and blocks actin's active sites.
3. Myosin cross bridges are prevented from binding to actin and thus can no longer sustain the contraction.
4. Because the thick and thin myofilaments are no longer connected, the muscle fiber may return to its longer, resting length.

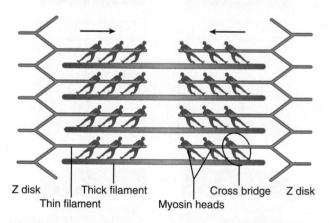

Z disk   Thick filament   Cross bridge   Z disk
Thin filament   Myosin heads

FIGURE 2-38 Sliding Filament Model. This cartoon illustrates the concept of muscle contraction as a sort of tug-of-war game in which the myosin heads (shown here as little people) hold onto thin filament "ropes" to form cross bridges. As the myosin heads pull on the thin filaments, the Z disks (Z lines) get closer together, thereby shortening the sarcomere. Likewise, the short length of a sarcomere may be held in position by the continued effort of the myosin heads.

✦ FIELD NOTES

The Muscle Love Story

The molecular processes of the muscle fiber that produce the contraction of a muscle are still not completely understood. Therefore, it's no wonder that beginning A&P students sometimes have a hard time understanding this. Analogies are a good way to learn physiologic processes. Here is my favorite analogy for muscle contraction, in the form of a love story:

The story begins in the Land of the Muscle Fiber, where several interesting characters live. Myosin is in love with the girl next door, Actin. The problem is that some of the villagers want to keep Myosin and Actin apart (young lovers are never a likely match, according to others, are they?). A group of women, each called Troponin, constantly try to keep Myosin from getting to his true love Actin by holding up poles made of tropomyosin. These tropomyosin poles could be easily knocked out of the way by the brave and strong Myosin, but all those Troponin girls are very strong, too, and they keep the tropomyosin in its blocking position.

Every good love story needs tension like that—something keeping the lovers apart. In addition, there is a good subplot: the Troponin girls are in love, too. They all pine away for their true loves, all of whom are named Calcium. The problem for them is worse than for Actin and Myosin. All of the Calciums are under guard in the SR (sarcoplasmic reticulum). The SR happens to be a sort of prison yard on the banks of the rivers, which the villagers call "T tubules." Given their situation, it's very unlikely that any of the Troponins will ever be visited by a distant Calcium imprisoned in the SR. Poor things.

However, one day an odd thing happens, as it always does in these stories. A stranger (of course) called Acetylcholine is sent by the governing nervous system. Acetylcholine, or ACh to his friends, hits the sarcolemma, which is the wall around the village. That launches a traveling voltage fluctuation. You and I would call it an action potential, but the villagers think of it as a lightning strike.

Well, that voltage travels right along the sarcolemma. When it gets to each of the T tubules, it travels right down the T tubules and thus crisscrosses the village. As it travels down each T tubule, the voltage zaps the SR, which sure does startle the guards. The guards are so stunned that they let many of the Calciums escape and run all over the village. Oh my!

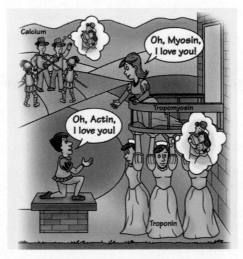

Continued

The Troponins, of course, can hardly believe it! They dreamt last night that they were surrounded by Calciums, and lo, it has happened! The Calciums and the Troponins embrace; in the heat of passion, they twist around a little, and the Troponins completely forget about holding up the tropomyosin poles.

Well, that gives Myosin the chance that he and Actin have been waiting for! He moves across the barrier, and Myosin and Actin immediately start, well, getting passionate with each other. Myosin is very excited and just keeps Actin moving along. (I'd get into sliding filaments here, but it's a family book, OK? You get the picture.) We have contraction because Actin is being actively pulled along by Myosin, who is using a lot of energy.

In the meantime, back at the SR, the guards have recovered and are now rounding up the Calciums and taking them back to the SR where they belong. As each Troponin tearfully bids her Calcium goodbye, she realizes that she was not paying attention to her job and gets back to it. The next time Myosin is ready to cross over to Actin, he can't—he's again blocked by the tropomyosin poles, which are being held in place by the Troponins.

Thus, the little village returns to its relaxed state, if you can call it that. It's just a matter of time until it all happens again: all of the old attractions are still there, and someday ACh will ride into town and stir up another electrical storm.

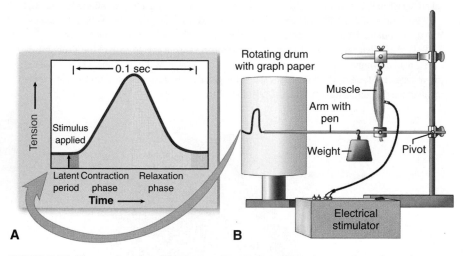

FIGURE 2-39 Myography of Muscle Contraction. Myography is the recording of muscle contractions.
A, A **twitch contraction** is a brief, jerky contraction in response to a single stimulus. The **myogram** shows three distinct phases: *(1) the latent period, (2) the contraction phase,* and *(3) the relaxation phase.*
B, A classic **myograph** setup that shows what the myogram represents. Note that an artificial electric stimulus (not a nerve stimulus) is needed to produce the twitch contraction; such single, isolated stimuli do not normally occur in the body.

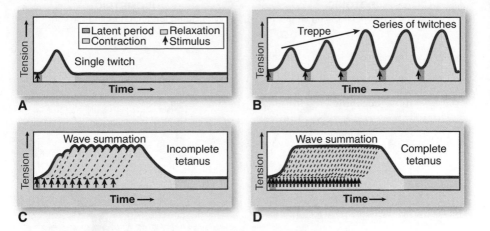

FIGURE 2-40 Myograms of Various Types of Muscle Contractions.
A, A single **twitch contraction.**
B, The **treppe** phenomenon or *staircase effect* is a steplike increase in the force of contraction over the first few in a series of twitches.
C, Incomplete tetanus occurs when a rapid succession of stimuli produces *twitches* that seem to add together (**wave summation**) to produce a rather sustained contraction.
D, Complete tetanus is a smoother sustained contraction that is produced by the summation of "twitches" that occur so close together that the muscle cannot relax at all.

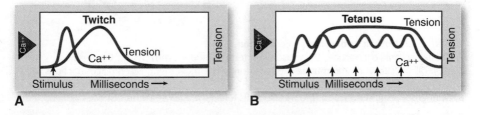

FIGURE 2-41 Role of Calcium in Twitch and Tetanus.
A, A single, sudden increase in calcium (Ca^{++}) availability triggers the twitch contraction.
B, Repeated stimuli maintain a high level of calcium, thereby permitting sustained (tetanic) contraction.

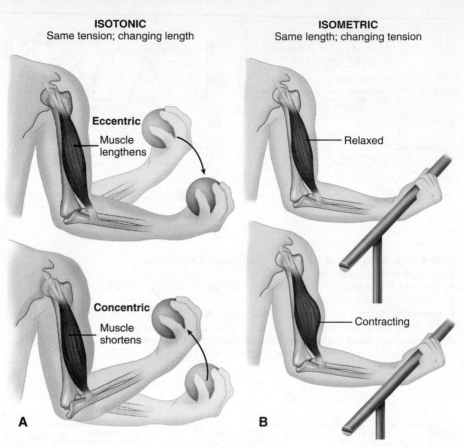

ISOTONIC
Same tension; changing length

Eccentric
Muscle lengthens

Concentric
Muscle shortens

ISOMETRIC
Same length; changing tension

Relaxed

Contracting

A

B

FIGURE 2-42 Isotonic and Isometric Contraction.
A, During isotonic contraction, the muscle shortens to produce movement. Concentric contractions occur when the muscle shortens during the movement. Eccentric contractions occur when the contracting muscle lengthens.
B, During isometric contraction, the muscle pulls forcefully against a load but does not shorten.

✳ TABLE 2-38 Characteristics of Muscle Tissues

	Skeletal	Cardiac	Smooth
Principal location	Skeletal muscle organs	Wall of heart	Walls of many hollow organs
Principal functions	Movement of bones, heat production, posture	Pumping of blood	Movement in walls of hollow organs (peristalsis, mixing of fluids)
Type of control	Voluntary	Involuntary	Involuntary
Structural Features			
Striations	Present	Present	Absent
Nucleus	Many near the sarcolemma	Single (sometimes double); near the center of the cell	Single; near the center of the cell
T tubules	Narrow; form triads with the SR	Large diameter; form dyads with the SR; regulate Ca^{++} entry into the sarcoplasm	Absent
Sarcoplasmic reticulum	Extensive; stores and releases Ca^{++}	Less extensive than in skeletal muscle	Very poorly developed
Cell junctions	No gap junctions	Intercalated disks	Single-unit*: many gap junctions Multiunit: few gap junctions
Contraction style	Rapid twitch contractions of motor units usually summate to produce sustained tetanic contractions; must be stimulated by a neuron	Syncytium of fibers compress the heart chambers in slow, separate contractions (does not exhibit tetanus or fatigue); exhibits autorhythmicity	Single-unit: electrically coupled sheets of fibers contract autorhythmically and produce peristalsis or mixing movements Multiunit: individual fibers contract when stimulated by a neuron

*Also referred to as *visceral smooth muscle tissue*.
SR, Sarcoplasmic reticulum.

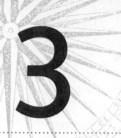

CHAPTER THREE

Communication, Control, and Integration

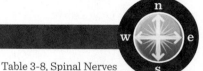

Navigation Guide

A. Nervous System

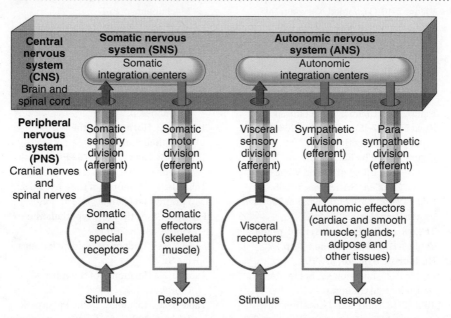

FIGURE 3-1 Organizational Plan of the Nervous System. This diagram summarizes the scheme used by most neurobiologists to study the nervous system. Both the **somatic nervous system (SNS)** and the **autonomic nervous system (ANS)** include components of the **central nervous system (CNS)** and **peripheral nervous system (PNS)**. *Somatic sensory pathways* conduct information toward integrators in the CNS, and *somatic motor pathways* conduct information toward somatic effectors. In the ANS, *visceral sensory pathways* conduct information toward CNS integrators, whereas the *sympathetic* and *parasympathetic pathways* conduct information toward autonomic effectors.

◆ SURVIVAL TIP

☑ The nervous system can seem daunting if you don't know how it's organized. Before taking another step, stop and become familiar with the layout of the nervous system. All the rest will then make sense, and it won't be so difficult.

☑ An easy way to become familiar with the organization of the nervous system is to put all of the parts illustrated in Figure 3-1 on separate index cards. Shuffle the cards, and then try to arrange them properly on a table. When you are done, check your arrangement against Figure 3-1. Keep practicing until you can do it easily and without peeking—only then are you ready to move forward.

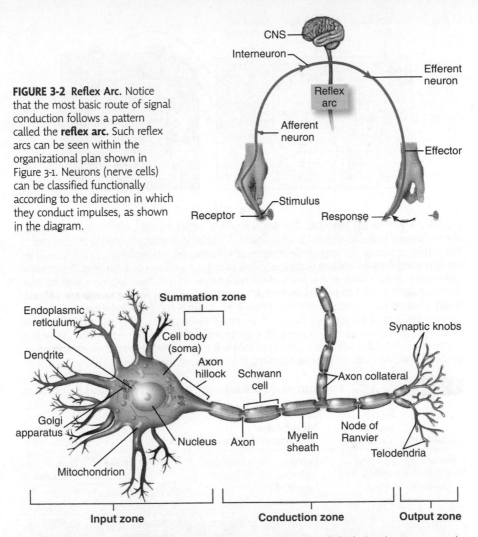

FIGURE 3-2 Reflex Arc. Notice that the most basic route of signal conduction follows a pattern called the **reflex arc.** Such reflex arcs can be seen within the organizational plan shown in Figure 3-1. Neurons (nerve cells) can be classified functionally according to the direction in which they conduct impulses, as shown in the diagram.

FIGURE 3-3 Structure of a Typical Neuron. Neurons consist of a **cell body** (*perikaryon* or *soma*) and at least two processes (nerve fibers): one **axon** and one or more **dendrites.** The dendrites and cell body act primarily as an *input zone,* receiving nerve stimulation and initiating nerve impulses in response. The axon extends from a tapered portion of the cell body called the **axon hillock.** The axon hillock acts as a *summation zone* by adding together all of the nerve impulses arriving from the cell body and dendrites and then deciding whether to send the impulse any further. Axons conduct impulses away from the cell body and are the *conduction zone.* An axon often has one or more side branches *(axon collaterals).* The distal tips of axons form branches called *telodendria* that each terminate in a **synaptic knob** in the neuron. These end structures act as an output zone where **vesicles** of *neurotransmitters* are released.

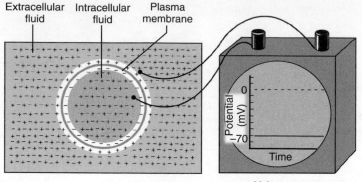

Voltmeter

FIGURE 3-4 Membrane Potential. The diagram on the left represents a cell maintaining a very slight difference in the concentration of oppositely charged ions across its plasma membrane. The voltmeter records the magnitude of electrical difference over time, which, in this case, does not fluctuate from −70 mV (the voltage recorded over time is shown as a red line). The negative sign represents the charge on the *inside* of the membrane. At rest, there are more **sodium ions (Na⁺)** outside the cell than **potassium ions (K⁺)** inside the cell. This **resting membrane potential (RMP)** is maintained by the normal concentration gradients of Na⁺ and K⁺, the permeability of the membrane, and the action of the *Na⁺-K⁺ pumps*. If Na⁺ channels open, sodium ions will rush inward (down their concentration gradient), thereby making the inside more positive (the voltage will increase). If K⁺ channels open, potassium ions will rush outward (down their concentration gradient), thereby making the inside more negative (dropping the voltage).

✴ TABLE 3-1   Sodium and Potassium Channel Types and Functions

Channel	Effect on Ion Transport*	Effect on Membrane Potential	Type	Trigger	Response
Sodium (Na⁺) channels	Na⁺ ions diffuse into the cell	Increase (more positive)	Stimulus-gated	Sensory stimulus	Rapid response
				Chemical stimulus (neurotransmitter)	Rapid response
			Voltage-gated	Increase in membrane potential (to threshold potential [−59 mV] or beyond)	Rapid response
Potassium (K⁺) channels	K⁺ ions diffuse out the of cell	Decrease (more negative)	Stimulus-gated	Sensory stimulus	Rapid response
				Chemical stimulus (neurotransmitter)	Rapid response
			Voltage-gated	Increase in membrane potential (to threshold potential [−59 mV] or beyond)	Slow response

*This reflects the net diffusion of ions down their respective concentration gradients.

✴ **TABLE 3-2**   **Types of Membrane Potentials**

Membrane Potential	Polarization	Typical Voltage*	Summation	Conduction	Description
Resting membrane potential (RMP)	Polarized	−70 mV	Not applicable	Not applicable	Membrane voltage when the neuron is not excited and not conducting an impulse
Local potential	Depolarized (excitatory; EPSP)	Graded; varies; greater than −70 mV	Yes	Decremental	Temporary fluctuation in a local region of the membrane in response to a sensory or nerve stimulus; may be an upward or downward fluctuation in voltage; loses amplitude as it spreads along the membrane
	Hyperpolarized (inhibitory; IPSP)	Graded; varies; less than −70 mV	Yes	Decremental	
Threshold potential	Depolarized	−59 mV	Yes	Triggers action potential	Minimum local depolarization needed to trigger voltage-gated channels that produce the action potential
Action potential	Depolarized	+30 mV	No	Nondecremental	Temporary maximum depolarization of membrane voltage that travels to the end of the axon without losing amplitude

*Example used in this chapter; actual values in body vary depending on many diverse factors. *EPSP,* Excitatory postsynaptic potential; *IPSP,* inhibitory postsynaptic potential.

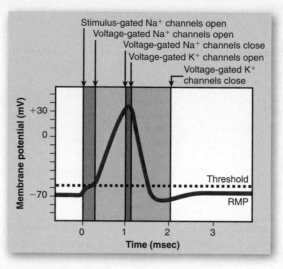

FIGURE 3-5 The Action Potential. Changes in membrane potential in a local area of a neuron's membrane result from changes in membrane permeability, as listed in the steps of Table 3-3.

✳ TABLE 3-3	Steps of the Mechanism That Produces an Action Potential

Step	Description
1	A stimulus triggers stimulus-gated Na^+ channels to open and allow inward Na^+ diffusion. This causes the membrane to depolarize.
2	As the threshold potential is reached, voltage-gated Na^+ channels open.
3	As more Na^+ enters the cell through voltage-gated Na^+ channels, the membrane depolarizes even further.
4	The magnitude of the action potential peaks (at +30 mV) when voltage-gated Na^+ channels close.
5	Repolarization begins when voltage-gated K^+ channels open, allowing outward diffusion of K^+.
6	After a brief period of hyperpolarization, the resting potential is restored by the sodium-potassium pump and the return of ion channels to their resting state.

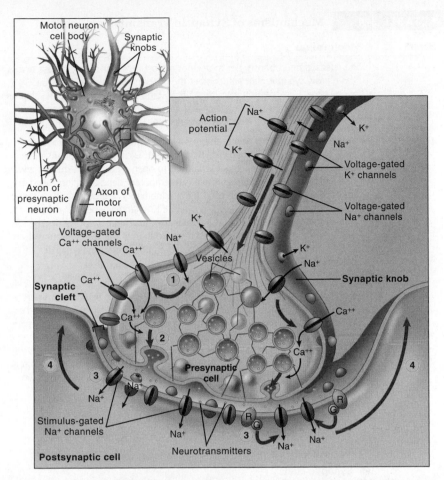

FIGURE 3-6 The Chemical Synapse. Details of a **synaptic knob** (axon terminal), a **presynaptic neuron**, the plasma membrane of a **postsynaptic neuron**, and a **synaptic cleft** are shown.

✳ TABLE 3-4	Mechanisms of Synaptic Transmission
Step*	**Mechanism**
1	When an action potential reaches a synaptic knob, voltage-gated calcium channels in its membrane open and allow calcium ions (Ca^{++}) to diffuse into the knob rapidly. Many voltage-gated Ca^{++} channels are present in the membrane of the neuron's output zone (see Figure 3-3).
2	The increase in intracellular Ca^{++} concentration triggers the movement of neurotransmitter vesicles to the plasma membrane of the synaptic knob. Once there, they fuse with the membrane and release their neurotransmitter by exocytosis. Thousands of neurotransmitter molecules spurt out of the open vesicles into the synaptic cleft.

Continued

✳ TABLE 3-4	Mechanisms of Synaptic Transmission—cont'd
Step*	**Mechanism**
3	The released neurotransmitter molecules almost instantaneously diffuse across the narrow synaptic cleft and contact the postsynaptic neuron's plasma membrane. Here, neurotransmitters briefly bind to receptor molecules that are also gated channels (Figure 3-7) or that are coupled to gated channels (Figure 3-8). Binding of neurotransmitters triggers the channels to open.
4	The opening of ion channels in the postsynaptic membrane may produce a local potential called a **postsynaptic potential**. Excitatory neurotransmitters cause both Na⁺ channels and K⁺ channels to open. Because Na⁺ rushes inward faster than K⁺ rushes outward, there is a temporary depolarization called an **excitatory postsynaptic potential (EPSP)**. Inhibitory neurotransmitters cause K⁺ channels and/or Cl⁻ channels to open. If K⁺ channels open, K⁺ rushes outward; if Cl⁻ channels open, Cl⁻ rushes inward. Either event makes the inside of the membrane even more negative than at the resting potential. This temporary hyperpolarization is called an **inhibitory postsynaptic potential (IPSP)**.
5	After a neurotransmitter binds to its postsynaptic receptors, its action is quickly terminated. Several mechanisms bring this about. Some neurotransmitter molecules are transported back into the synaptic knobs, where they can be repacked into vesicles and used again. Some neurotransmitter molecules are metabolized into inactive compounds by synaptic enzymes. Other neurotransmitter molecules simply diffuse out of the synaptic cleft and are transported into nearby glial cells. The glial cells may release them again for reuptake by the presynaptic neuron, sometimes after breaking them down into another form.

*These steps correspond with the numbered labels in Figure 3-6.

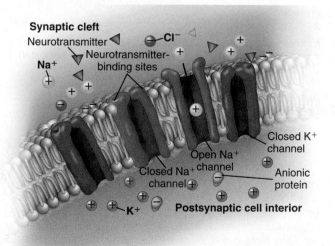

FIGURE 3-7 Direct Stimulation of a Postsynaptic Receptor. Some neurotransmitters, such as *acetylcholine (ACh)*, initiate nerve signals by binding directly to one or both neurotransmitter-binding sites on the stimulus-gated ion channel. Such binding causes the channel to change its shape to an open position. When the neurotransmitter is removed, the channel again closes.

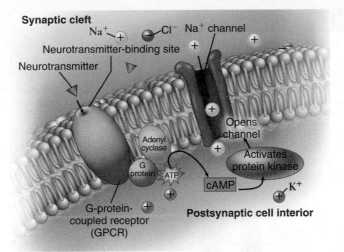

FIGURE 3-8 Second-Messenger Stimulation of a Postsynaptic Receptor. Norepinephrine and many other neurotransmitters initiate nerve signals indirectly by binding to a **G-protein–coupled receptor (GPCR)** that changes shape to activate the enzyme **adenylate cyclase**, which in turn catalyzes the conversion of ATP into **cyclic AMP (cAMP).** cAMP is a "second messenger" that induces a change in the shape of a stimulus-gated channel. (Compare this image with Figure 3-6.)

✧ FIELD NOTES

Sending Messages

As you can imagine, the ability to send messages is critical to the continued stable functioning of the human body. Nerve signals are sent by way of neurotransmitters; endocrine signals are sent by way of hormones; local signals are sent by way of paracrine or autocrine agents. The whole process of a cell's receiving and understanding any of these signals is called *signal transduction.*

Signal transduction is a really big deal. If you really want to understand human physiology—and have any inkling of how most drugs and chemical therapies work—you have to know the basics of signal transduction. It's also a big deal because this is an area of intensely active and important scientific research.

Figures 3-6 and 3-7, which show different methods of signal transduction in postsynaptic cells, give us our first opportunity to learn the basics of this important concept. In either case, you can think of the neurotransmitter as "carrying the message." However, this messenger can't get inside the cell—it's blocked from directly entering the cell. Therefore, it has to send a signal to the inside of the cell—this is the process of signal transduction. It is sort of like when a person needs to deliver a message to someone in a building but can't actually get into the building—that person has to get the message inside some other way.

The direct approach to signal transduction (see Figure 3-7) is to think of a messenger delivering a message such as, "Open the sodium door, please." However, this message can't get inside to the sodium door operator, so the messenger presses the intercom button on the outside of the sodium door and says to the operator inside, "Open the sodium door, please." That's pretty direct: it uses a mechanism that's pretty much built into the doorway itself. Of course, the message could have been, "Close the sodium door, please," or "Open the potassium door, please." It depends on the specific neurotransmitter and the specific receptor/transduction mechanism.

Continued

◈ FIELD NOTES—cont'd

The second-messenger approach (see Figure 3-8) is only one of several such systems, but it is one that serves as a good example. Here, it's like a messenger who gets to the building to deliver the message, "Open the sodium door, please" and can't get in. Therefore, the messenger hands off the message to someone inside the building (maybe through a mail slot). The message is then handed off to a second messenger on the inside who sees that the message is passed along into a system that will eventually get the message to the sodium door operator.

The second-messenger approach seems unnecessarily complex. Such complexity is valuable, however, because its gives more opportunities to the cell (or the outside agents) to modify or adjust the message before it gets to its final destination. In other words, it allows for the operation of "dimmer switches" that increase or decrease certain events that are triggered in the cell.

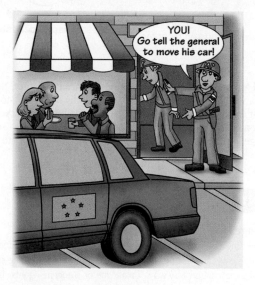

✳ TABLE 3-5   Examples of Neurotransmitters

Neurotransmitter	Location*	Function*
Small-Molecule Transmitters		
Class I		
Acetylcholine (ACh)	Junctions with motor effectors (e.g., muscles, glands); many parts of the brain	Excitatory or inhibitory; involved in memory
Class II: Amines *Monoamines*		
Serotonin (5-HT†)	Several regions of the CNS	Mostly inhibitory; involved in moods, emotions, and sleep
Histamine	Brain	Mostly excitatory; involved in emotions and the regulation of body temperature and water balance

✳ **TABLE 3-5**	**Examples of Neurotransmitters—cont'd**	
Neurotransmitter	**Location***	**Function***
Catecholamines Dopamine (DA)	Brain; autonomic system	Mostly inhibitory; involved in emotions, moods, and the regulation of motor control
Epinephrine	Several areas of the CNS and the sympathetic division of the ANS	Excitatory or inhibitory; acts as a hormone when secreted by sympathetic neurosecretory cells of the adrenal gland
Norepinephrine (NE)	Several areas of the CNS and the sympathetic division of the ANS	Excitatory or inhibitory; regulates sympathetic effectors; in the brain, involved in emotional responses
Class III: Amino Acids		
Glutamate (glutamic acid, Glu)	CNS	Excitatory; most common excitatory neurotransmitter in the CNS
Gamma-aminobutyric acid (GABA)	Brain	Inhibitory; common inhibitory neurotransmitter in the brain
Glycine (Gly)	Spinal cord	Inhibitory; common inhibitory neurotransmitter in the brain
Class IV: Other Small Molecules		
Nitric oxide (NO)	Several regions of the nervous system	May be a signal from a postsynaptic neuron to a presynaptic neuron
Large-Molecule Transmitters		
Neuropeptides		
Vasoactive intestinal peptide (VIP)	Brain; some ANS and sensory fibers; retina; gastrointestinal tract	Function in the nervous system is uncertain
Cholecystokinin (CCK)	Brain; retina	Function in the nervous system is uncertain
Substance P	Brain, spinal cord, sensory pain pathways; gastrointestinal tract	Mostly excitatory; transmits pain information
Enkephalins	Several regions of the CNS; retina; intestinal tract	Mostly inhibitory; act like opiates to block pain
Endorphins	Several regions of the CNS; retina; intestinal tract	Mostly inhibitory; act like opiates to block pain
Neuropeptide Y (NPY)	Brain, some ANS fibers	Variety of functions, including enhancing blood vessel constriction by the ANS, the regulation of energy balance, and learning and memory

*These are examples only; most of these neurotransmitters are also found in other locations, and many have additional functions.
†5-hydroxytryptamine; this is a synonym for *serotonin*.
ANS, Autonomic nervous system; *CNS*, central nervous system.

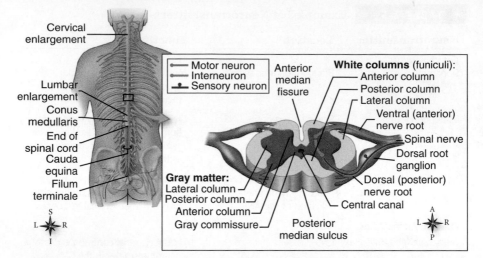

FIGURE 3-9 Spinal Cord. The boxed diagram illustrates a transverse section of the spinal cord shown in the broader view.

✳ TABLE 3-6   Major Ascending Tracts of the Spinal Cord

Name	Function	Location	Origin*	Termination†
Lateral spinothalamic	Pain, temperature, and crude touch on the opposite side	Lateral white columns	Posterior gray column on opposite side	Thalamus
Anterior spinothalamic	Crude touch and pressure	Anterior white columns	Posterior gray column on opposite side	Thalamus
Fasciculi gracilis and cuneatus	Discriminating touch and pressure sensations, including vibration, stereognosis, and two-point discrimination; also conscious kinesthesia	Posterior white columns	Spinal ganglia on same side	Medulla
Anterior and posterior spinocerebellar	Unconscious kinesthesia	Lateral white columns	Anterior or posterior gray column	Cerebellum
Spinotectal	Touch related to visual reflexes	Lateral white columns	Posterior gray columns	Superior colliculus (midbrain)

*The location of the cell bodies of the neurons from which the axons of the tract arise.
†The structure in which the axons of the tract terminate.

| ✳ **TABLE 3-7** | **Major Descending Tracts of the Spinal Cord** |

Name	Function	Location	Origin*	Termination†
Lateral corticospinal (or crossed pyramidal)	Voluntary movement; the contraction of individual or small groups of muscles, particularly those that move the hands, fingers, feet, and toes of the opposite side	Lateral white columns	Motor areas or cerebral cortex of opposite side from tract location in cord	Lateral or anterior gray columns
Anterior corticospinal (direct pyramidal)	Same as lateral corticospinal except mainly muscles of same side	Anterior white columns	Motor cortex but on same side as location in cord	Lateral or anterior gray columns
Reticulospinal	Maintain posture during movement	Anterior white columns	Reticular formation (midbrain, pons, medulla)	Anterior gray columns
Rubrospinal	Coordination of body movement and posture	Lateral white columns	Red nucleus (of midbrain)	Anterior gray columns
Tectospinal	Head and neck movement during visual reflexes	Anterior white columns	Superior colliculus (midbrain)	Medulla and anterior gray columns
Vestibulospinal	Coordination of posture and balance	Anterior white columns	Vestibular nucleus (pons, medulla)	Anterior gray columns

*The location of the cell bodies of the neurons from which the axons of the tract arise.
†The structure in which the axons of the tract terminate.

✴ **TABLE 3-8**   Spinal Nerves and Peripheral Branches

Spinal Nerves	Plexuses Formed from Anterior Rami	Spinal Nerve Branches from Plexuses	Parts Supplied
Cervical 1 2 3 4	Cervical plexus	Lesser occipital Greater auricular Cutaneous nerve of neck Supraclavicular nerves Branches to muscles	Sensory to back of head, front of neck, and upper part of shoulder; motor to numerous neck muscles
		Phrenic nerve	Diaphragm
Cervical 5 6 7 8 Thoracic (or Dorsal) 1	Brachial plexus	Suprascapular and dorsoscapular	Superficial muscles* of scapula
		Thoracic nerves, medial and lateral branches	Pectoralis major and minor
		Long thoracic nerve	Serratus anterior
		Thoracodorsal	Latissimus dorsi
2 3 4 5 6 7 8 9 10 11 12	No plexus formed; branches run directly to intercostal muscles and skin of thorax	Subscapular	Subscapular and teres major muscles
		Axillary (circumflex)	Deltoid and teres minor muscles and skin over deltoid
		Musculocutaneous	Muscles of front of arm (biceps brachii, coracobrachialis, brachialis) and skin on outer side of forearm
		Ulnar	Flexor carpi ulnaris and part of flexor digitorum profundus; some muscles of hand; sensory to medial side of hand and little finger and medial half of fourth finger
		Median	Remaining muscles of front of forearm and hand; sensory to skin of palmar surface of thumb and index and middle fingers
		Radial	Triceps muscle and muscles of back of forearm; sensory to skin of back of forearm and hand
		Medial cutaneous	Sensory to inner surface of arm and forearm

*Although nerves to muscles are considered motor, they do contain some sensory fibers that transmit proprioceptive impulses.
†Sensory fibers from the tibial and peroneal nerves unite to form the medial cutaneous (or sural) nerve that supplies the calf of the leg and the lateral surface of the foot. In the thigh, the tibial and common peroneal nerves are usually enclosed in a single sheath to form the sciatic nerve; this is the largest nerve in the body, with a width of approximately 0.75 inch (2 cm). About two thirds of the way down the posterior part of the thigh, it divides into its component parts. Branches of the sciatic nerve extend into the hamstring muscles.

✳ TABLE 3-8		Spinal Nerves and Peripheral Branches—cont'd	
Spinal Nerves	**Plexuses Formed from Anterior Rami**	**Spinal Nerve Branches from Plexuses**	**Parts Supplied**
Lumbar 1 2 3 4 5	Lumbosacral plexus	Iliohypogastric — Sometimes fused	Sensory to anterior abdominal wall
		Ilioinguinal	Sensory to anterior abdominal wall and external genitalia; motor to muscles of abdominal wall
		Genitofemoral	Sensory to skin of external genitalia and inguinal region
		Lateral femoral cutaneous	Sensory to outer side of thigh
Sacral 1 2 3 4 5		Femoral	Motor to quadriceps, sartorius, and iliacus muscles; sensory to front of thigh and medial side of leg (saphenous nerve)
		Obturator	Motor to adductor muscles of thigh
		Tibial† (medial popliteal)	Motor to muscles of calf of leg; sensory to skin of calf of leg and sole of foot
		Common peroneal (lateral popliteal)	Motor to evertors and dorsiflexors of foot; sensory to lateral surface of leg and dorsal surface of foot
		Nerves to hamstring muscles	Motor to muscles of back of thigh
		Gluteal nerves	Motor to buttock muscles and tensor fasciae latae
		Posterior femoral cutaneous	Sensory to skin of buttocks, posterior surface of thigh, and leg
		Pudendal nerve	Motor to perineal muscles; sensory to skin of perineum
Coccygeal 1	Coccygeal plexus	Anococcygeal nerves	Sensory to skin overlying coccyx

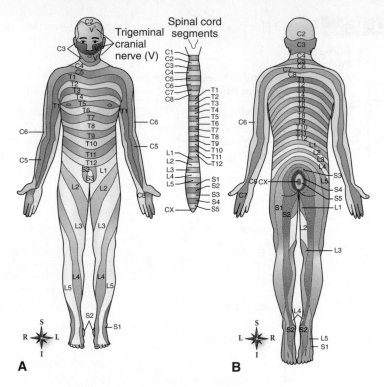

FIGURE 3-10 Dermatome Distribution of the Spinal Nerves.
A, The front of the body's surface.
B, The back of the body's surface.
Cervical segments and spinal nerves *(C)*; thoracic segments and spinal nerves *(T)*; lumbar segments and spinal nerves *(L)*; sacral segments and spinal nerves *(S)*. The inset shows the segments of the spinal cord that are associated with each of the spinal nerves associated with the sensory dermatomes shown.

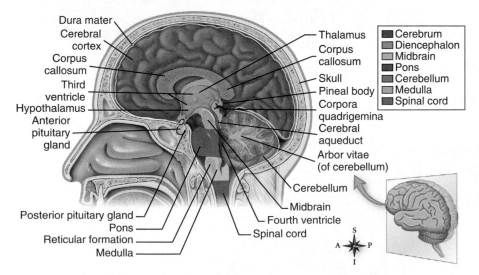

FIGURE 3-11 Divisions of the Brain. A midsagittal section of the brain reveals features of its major divisions.

✳ TABLE 3-9	Summary of Central Nervous System Structures and Functions	

Region	Structure*	Function*
Spinal cord Spinal cord	Elongated cylinder that extends from the brainstem through the foramen magnum of the skull; gray matter interior surrounded by white matter; 31 pairs of spinal nerves attached by dorsal and ventral nerve roots	Integration of simple, subconscious spinal reflexes; conduction of nerve impulses
Gray matter	Numerous synapses and interneurons arranged into anterior, lateral, and posterior gray columns linked by a gray commissure	Integration of spinal reflexes and filtering of information going to higher centers (as in gated pain control)
White matter	Myelinated nerve tracts arranged into anterior, lateral, and posterior white columns (funiculi)	Ascending tracts conduct sensory information to higher CNS centers; descending tracts conduct motor information from higher CNS centers
Brainstem	Extends inferiorly from the diencephalon to the foramen magnum of the skull, where it meets the spinal cord; central gray matter nuclei surrounded and connected by white matter tracts; 10 of the 12 pairs of cranial nerves attached here	Subconscious integration of basic vital functions
Medulla oblongata Medulla oblongata	Inferior region of brainstem between the spinal cord and the pons	Integration of cardiac, vasomotor (vessel muscle), respiratory, digestive, and other reflexes
Pons Pons	Intermediate region of brainstem between the medulla and the midbrain	Integration of numerous autonomic reflexes mediated by cranial nerves V, VI, VII, and VIII (see Chapters 15 and 16); respiration

Continued

✳ **TABLE 3-9**	**Summary of Central Nervous System Structures and Functions—cont'd**

Region	Structure*	Function*
Midbrain Midbrain—	Superior region of the brainstem between the pons and the diencephalon	Integration of numerous cranial nerve reflexes, such as eye movements, pupillary reflex, and ear (sound-muffling) reflexes
Reticular formation Reticular formation—	Roughly cylindrical network of nerve pathways and centers that extend through the brainstem and into the diencephalon	Operates the reticular activating system that regulates the state of consciousness
Cerebellum —Cerebellum	Roughly spherical structure attached at the posterior of the brainstem; wrinkled gray matter cortex, branched network of white fibers inside (arbor vitae), and several small gray nuclei	Coordinates many functions of the cerebrum, including planning and the control of skilled movements, posture, balance, and the coordination of sensory information related to body position and movement
Diencephalon Thalamus —Diencephalon Hypothalamus —Pineal gland	Brain region in the central part of the brain between the cerebrum and the brainstem (midbrain); made up of various gray-matter nuclei	Numerous coordinating and integrating functions
Thalamus	Large ovoid of gray matter that is divided into two large lateral masses connected by an intermediate mass	Crude sensations; coordination of sensory information relayed to the cerebrum; involved in the emotional response to sensory information as well as arousal; general processing of information to and from the cerebrum

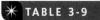 **TABLE 3-9** Summary of Central Nervous System Structures and Functions—cont'd

Region	Structure*	Function*
Hypothalamus	Numerous gray-matter nuclei clustered below the thalamus	Integration and coordination of many autonomic reflexes and hormonal functions; involved in arousal, appetite, and thermoregulation
Pineal gland	Single nucleus of neuroendocrine tissue posterior to the thalamus	Produces melatonin, a timekeeping hormone, as part of the body's biological clock
Cerebrum	Largest and most superior region of brain; divided into right and left hemispheres and connected by the corpus callosum	Complex processing of sensory and motor information; complex integrative functions
Cerebral cortex	Highly wrinkled gray-matter surface of the cerebrum; divided into five major lobes per hemisphere; functionally mapped based on the concept of localization	Higher-level processing of sensory and motor information, including conscious sensation and motor control; complex integrative functions, such as consciousness, language, memory, and emotions
Cerebral tracts	White-matter tracts that connect various regions of the cortex with each other and with inferior CNS structures	Conduction of information between CNS areas to facilitate complex processing and integration
Basal nuclei	Gray-matter nuclei deep in the cerebrum	Integration and regulation of conscious motor control, especially posture, walking, other repetitive movements; possible roles in thinking and learning

*Summary only; see the chapter text and the figures for detailed descriptions of structure and function.
CNS, Central nervous system.

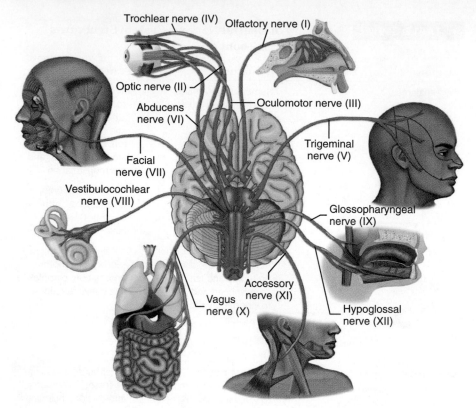

FIGURE 3-12 Cranial Nerves. Ventral surface of the brain showing the attachment of the cranial nerves. Cranial nerves are named by **name** (e.g., *vagus nerve*) and by **number** (e.g., *CN X* or *CN 10*).

✳ TABLE 3-10 Structure and Function of the Cranial Nerves

Nerve	Sensory (Afferent) Fibers			Motor (Efferent) Fibers		
	Receptors	Cell Bodies	Termination	Function	Cell Bodies	Termination	Function

Nerve	Receptors	Cell Bodies	Termination	Cell Bodies	Termination	Function
I Olfactory	Nasal mucosa	Nasal mucosa	Olfactory bulbs (new relay of neurons to olfactory cortex)			Sense of smell
II Optic	Retina (proprioceptive)	Retina	Nucleus in thalamus (lateral geniculate); some fibers terminate in superior colliculus of midbrain			Vision
III Oculomotor	External eye muscles (except superior oblique and lateral rectus)	Trigeminal ganglion	Midbrain (oculomotor nucleus)	Midbrain (oculomotor nucleus)	External eye muscles (except superior oblique and lateral rectus); autonomic fibers terminate in ciliary ganglion and then to ciliary and iris muscles	Eye movements, regulation of size of pupil, accommodation (for near vision), proprioception (muscle sense)

Continued

✳ TABLE 3-10   Structure and Function of the Cranial Nerves—cont'd

Nerve	Sensory (Afferent) Fibers			Motor (Efferent) Fibers		
	Receptors	Cell Bodies	Termination	Cell Bodies	Termination	Function
IV Trochlear	Superior oblique (proprioceptive)	Trigeminal ganglion	Midbrain	Midbrain	Superior oblique muscle of eye	Eye movements, proprioception
V Trigeminal	Skin and mucosa of head; teeth	Trigeminal ganglion	Pons (sensory nucleus)	Pons (motor nucleus)	Muscles of mastication	Sensations of head and face, chewing movements, proprioception
VI Abducens	Lateral rectus (proprioceptive)	Trigeminal ganglion	Pons	Pons	Lateral rectus muscle of eye	Abduction of eye, proprioception

Nerve	Receptors / Structures	Ganglion	CNS Termination / Origin		Motor Structures	Function
VII Facial	Taste buds of anterior two thirds of tongue	Geniculate ganglion	Medulla (nucleus solitarius)	Pons	Superficial muscles of face and scalp; autonomic fibers to salivary and lacrimal glands	Facial expressions, secretion of saliva and tears, taste
VIII Vestibulocochlear						
Vestibular branch	Semicircular canals and vestibule (utricle and saccule)	Vestibular ganglion	Pons and medulla (vestibular nuclei)			Balance or equilibrium sense
Cochlear (auditory) branch	Spiral (Corti) organ in cochlear duct	Spiral ganglion	Pons and medulla (cochlear nuclei)			Hearing
IX Glossopharyngeal	Pharynx; taste buds and other receptors of posterior third of tongue	Jugular and petrous ganglia	Medulla (nucleus solitarius)	Medulla (nucleus ambiguus)	Muscles of pharynx	Sensations of tongue, swallowing movements, secretion of saliva, various reflexes, control of blood pressure and respiration
	Carotid sinus and carotid body	Jugular and petrous ganglia	Medulla (respiratory and vasomotor centers)	Medulla at junction of pons (nucleus salivatorius)	Otic ganglion and then to parotid salivary gland	

Continued

✳ TABLE 3-10 **Structure and Function of the Cranial Nerves—cont'd**

Nerve	Sensory (Afferent) Fibers			Motor (Efferent) Fibers		
	Receptors	Cell Bodies	Termination	Cell Bodies	Termination	Function
X Vagus	Pharynx, larynx, carotid body, thoracic and abdominal viscera	Jugular and nodose ganglia	Medulla (nucleus solitarius) and pons (nucleus of fifth cranial nerve)	Medulla (dorsal motor nucleus)	Ganglia of vagal plexus and then to muscles of pharynx, larynx, and autonomic fibers to thoracic and abdominal viscera	Sensations and movements of organs supplied (e.g., slows heart rate, increases peristalsis, contracts muscles for voice production)
XI Accessory	Trapezius and sternocleidomastoid (proprioceptive)	Upper cervical ganglia	Spinal cord	Anterior gray column of first five or six cervical segments of spinal cord	Trapezius and sternocleidomastoid muscles	Shoulder movements, turning movements of head, proprioception
XII Hypoglossal	Tongue muscles (proprioceptive)	Trigeminal ganglion	Medulla (hypoglossal nucleus)	Medulla (hypoglossal nucleus)	Muscles of tongue and throat	Tongue movements, proprioception

Nervous About Nerves?

Having the names and numbers of the cranial nerves at the tip of your tongue will not only help you learn later topics in A&P, it will also help you in later courses and in clinical situations. So you might as well take some time now to memorize and practice them.

The easiest way to get started is using mnemonics as outlined in the Field Notes on page 160. Although it's best to make up your own mnemonics, here is a set of two sentences that have been used by many students to learn the names, numbers, and general functions of the 12 classic cranial nerves.

Cranial Nerve Mnemonics

Number	Name	Mnemonic	Functional Classification	Mnemonic
I	Olfactory	On	Sensory	Some
II	Optic	Old	Sensory	Say
III	Oculomotor	Olympus'	Motor	"Marry
IV	Trochlear	Tiny	Motor	Money,"
V	Trigeminal	Tops,	Mixed	But
VI	Abducens	A	Motor	My
VII	Facial	Friendly	Mixed	Brothers
VIII	Vestibulocochlear	Viking	Sensory	Say
IX	Glossopharyngeal	Grew	Mixed	"Bad
X	Vagus	Vines	Mixed	Business,
XI	Accessory	And	Motor	Marry
XII	Hypoglossal	Hops.	Motor	Money."

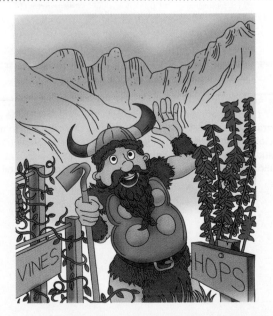

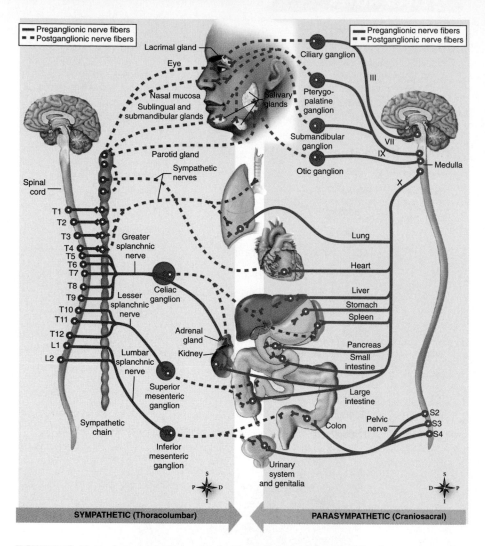

FIGURE 3-13 Major Autonomic Motor Conduction Paths. The left side of the diagram *(orange)* shows the outline of the **sympathetic** motor pathways. The right side of the diagram *(green)* shows the major **parasympathetic** motor pathways. Notice that conduction from the spinal cord to any visceral effector requires a relay of at least two autonomic motor neurons: a preganglionic neuron *(solid line)* and a postganglionic neuron *(broken line)*. Notice also that many of the representative **autonomic effectors** *(center of diagram)* are **dually innervated** by both autonomic motor divisions.

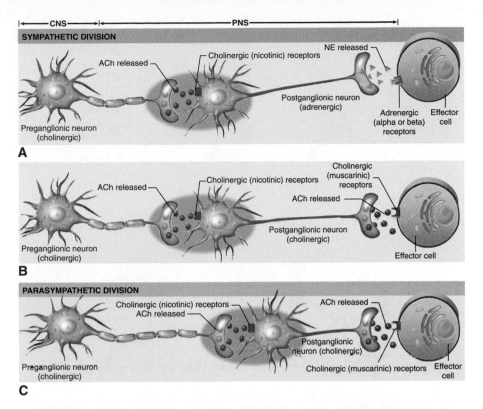

FIGURE 3-14 Locations of Neurotransmitters and Receptors of the Autonomic Nervous System. In all pathways, preganglionic fibers are **cholinergic** and secrete **acetylcholine (Ach),** which stimulates **nicotinic receptors** in the postganglionic neuron.
A, Most sympathetic postganglionic fibers are **adrenergic** and secrete **norepinephrine (NE),** thereby stimulating **alpha-** or **beta-adrenergic receptors**.
B, A few sympathetic postganglionic fibers are **cholinergic**, stimulating **muscarinic receptors** in effector cells.
C, All parasympathetic postganglionic fibers are **cholinergic**, stimulating **muscarinic receptors** in effector cells.

✧ SURVIVAL TIP

☑ Knowing the autonomic nervous system well—including the major *neurotransmitters* and their *receptor types*—is vital to understanding *drug actions*.

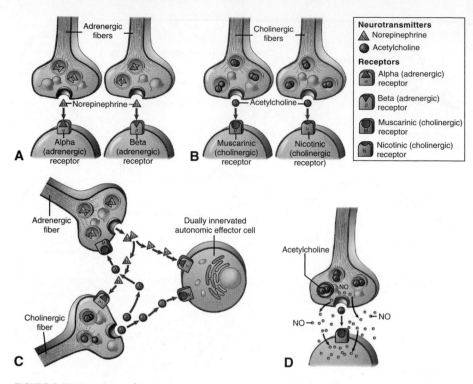

FIGURE 3-15 Functions of Autonomic Neurotransmitters and Receptors.

A, Norepinephrine (NE) released from **adrenergic fibers** binds to **alpha- or beta-adrenergic receptors** according to the lock-and-key model to produce regulatory effects in the postsynaptic cell.

B, Acetylcholine (ACh) released from **cholinergic fibers** similarly binds to **muscarinic or nicotinic cholinergic receptors** to produce postsynaptic regulatory effects.

C, The complex manner in which neurotransmitters and receptors regulate **dually innervated effector** cells shows that a summation of effects on receptors at both presynaptic and postsynaptic locations may occur. For example, norepinephrine released by an adrenergic fiber may bind to postsynaptic alpha (or beta) receptors to influence the effector cell; it may also bind to presynaptic alpha (α_2) receptors in a cholinergic fiber to inhibit the release of acetylcholine, which is a possible antagonist of norepinephrine.

D, Nonadrenergic-noncholinergic (NANC) transmission. In this example, nitric oxide *(NO)* is released from a cholinergic fiber along with acetylcholine *(A)*. A theory of autonomic transmission called **cotransmission** states that all or most postganglionic fibers release either norepinephrine or acetylcholine along with NANC transmitters or modulators and that each substance combines with postsynaptic or presynaptic receptors to produce regulatory effects.

✳ TABLE 3-11	Comparison of Somatic Motor and Autonomic Pathways	

Feature	Somatic Motor Pathways	Autonomic Efferent Pathways
Direction of information flow	Efferent	Efferent
Number of neurons between CNS and effector	One (somatic motor neuron)	Two (preganglionic and postganglionic)
Myelin sheath present	Yes	Preganglionic: yes Postganglionic: no
Location of peripheral fibers	Most cranial nerves and all spinal nerves	Most cranial nerves and all spinal nerves
Effector innervated	Skeletal muscle (voluntary)	Smooth and cardiac muscle, glands, and adipose and other tissues (involuntary)
Neurotransmitter	Acetylcholine	Acetylcholine or norepinephrine

CNS, Central nervous system.

✳ TABLE 3-12	Comparison of Structural Features of the Sympathetic and Parasympathetic Pathways	

Neurons	Sympathetic Pathways	Parasympathetic Pathways
Preganglionic Neurons		
Dendrites and cell bodies	In lateral gray columns of thoracic and first two or three lumbar segments of spinal cord	In nuclei of brainstem and in lateral gray columns of sacral segments of cord
Axons	In anterior roots of spinal nerves to spinal nerves (thoracic and first four lumbar); to and through white rami to terminate in sympathetic ganglia at various levels or to extend through sympathetic ganglia; to and through splanchnic nerves to terminate in collateral ganglia	From brainstem nuclei through cranial nerve III to ciliary ganglion From nuclei in pons through cranial nerve VII to sphenopalatine or submaxillary ganglion From nuclei in medulla through cranial nerve IX to otic ganglion or through cranial nerves X and XI to cardiac and celiac ganglia, respectively
Distribution	Short fibers from CNS to ganglion	Long fibers from CNS to ganglion
Neurotransmitter	Acetylcholine	Acetylcholine

Continued

✳ TABLE 3-12   Comparison of Structural Features of the Sympathetic and Parasympathetic Pathways—cont'd

Neurons	Sympathetic Pathways	Parasympathetic Pathways
Ganglia	Sympathetic chain ganglia (22 pairs); collateral ganglia (celiac, superior, inferior mesenteric)	Terminal ganglia (in or near effector)
Postganglionic Neurons		
Dendrites and cell bodies	In sympathetic and collateral ganglia	In parasympathetic ganglia (e.g., ciliary, sphenopalatine, submaxillary, otic, cardiac, celiac) located in or near visceral effector organs
Receptors	Cholinergic (nicotinic)	Cholinergic (nicotinic)
Axons	In autonomic nerves and plexuses that innervate thoracic and abdominal viscera and blood vessels in these cavities In gray rami to spinal nerves; to smooth muscle of skin, blood vessels, and hair follicles; and to sweat glands	In short nerves to various visceral effector organs
Distribution	Long fibers from ganglion to widespread effectors	Short fibers from ganglion to single effector
Neurotransmitter	Norepinephrine (many); acetylcholine (few)	Acetylcholine

CNS, Central nervous system.

✳ TABLE 3-13   Autonomic Functions

Autonomic Effector	Effect of Sympathetic Stimulation (neurotransmitter: norepinephrine [unless otherwise stated])	Effect of Parasympathetic Stimulation (neurotransmitter: acetylcholine)
Cardiac Muscle	Increased rate and strength of contraction (beta receptors)	Decreased rate and strength of contraction
Smooth Muscle of Blood Vessels		
Skin blood vessels	Constriction (alpha receptors)	No effect
Skeletal muscle blood vessels	Dilation (beta receptors)	No effect
Coronary blood vessels	Constriction (alpha receptors) Dilation (beta receptors)	Dilation

✳ TABLE 3-13   Autonomic Functions—cont'd

Autonomic Effector	Effect of Sympathetic Stimulation (neurotransmitter: norepinephrine [unless otherwise stated])	Effect of Parasympathetic Stimulation (neurotransmitter: acetylcholine)
Abdominal blood vessels	Constriction (alpha receptors)	No effect
Blood vessels of external genitalia	Constriction (alpha receptors)	Dilation of blood vessels that cause erection
Smooth Muscle of Hollow Organs and Sphincters		
Bronchioles	Relaxation (dilation)	Constriction
Digestive tract, except sphincters	Decreased peristalsis	Increased peristalsis
Sphincters of digestive tract	Contraction	Relaxation
Urinary bladder	Relaxation	Contraction
Urinary sphincters	Contraction	Relaxation
Reproductive ducts	Constriction	Relaxation
Eye		
Iris	Contraction of radial muscle; dilated pupil	Contraction of circular muscle; constricted pupil
Ciliary	Relaxation; accommodates for far vision	Contraction; accommodates for near vision
Hairs (arrector pili muscles)	Contraction produces goose pimples or piloerection (alpha receptors)	No effect
Glands		
Sweat	Increased sweat (neurotransmitter: acetylcholine)	No effect
Lacrimal	No effect	Increased secretion of tears
Digestive (e.g., salivary, gastric)	Decreased secretion of saliva; not known for others	Increased secretion of saliva
Pancreas, including islets	Decreased secretion	Increased secretion of pancreatic juice and insulin
Liver	Increased glycogenolysis (beta receptors); increased blood sugar level	No effect
Adrenal medulla*	Increased epinephrine secretion	No effect
Adipose	Increased lipolysis	No effect

Continued

✳ TABLE 3-13   Autonomic Functions—cont'd

Autonomic Effector	Effect of Sympathetic Stimulation (neurotransmitter: norepinephrine [unless otherwise stated])	Effect of Parasympathetic Stimulation (neurotransmitter: acetylcholine)
Skeletal Muscle[†]	During intense exercise, regulates contractility to prevent fatigue (beta receptors)	No effect

*Sympathetic preganglionic axons terminate in contact with secreting cells of the adrenal medulla. Thus, the adrenal medulla functions—to quote a descriptive phrase I once heard—as a "giant sympathetic postganglionic neuron."
[†]Skeletal muscle is primarily a somatic effector. However, during intense exercise, subconscious autonomic stimulation also occurs.

✳ TABLE 3-14   Summary of the Sympathetic "Fight-or-Flight" Reaction

Response	Role in Promoting Energy Use by Skeletal Muscles
Increased heart rate	Increased rate of blood flow, thereby increasing the delivery of oxygen and glucose to the skeletal muscles
Increased strength of cardiac muscle contraction	Increased rate of blood flow, thereby increasing the delivery of oxygen and glucose to the skeletal muscles
Dilation of coronary vessels of the heart	Increased delivery of oxygen and nutrients to the cardiac muscle to sustain increased rate and strength of heart contractions
Dilation of blood vessels in skeletal muscles	Increased delivery of oxygen and nutrients to skeletal muscles
Increased stimulation at neuromuscular junctions and increased ion pump activity in skeletal muscles	Increased availability of ACh at the neuromuscular junction and more efficient restoration of resting ion balance in muscle fibers both reduce fatigue in skeletal muscles
Constriction of blood vessels in digestive and other organs	Shunting of blood to skeletal muscles to increase oxygen and glucose delivery
Contraction of spleen and other blood reservoirs	More blood discharged into the general circulation, thereby increasing the delivery of oxygen and glucose to the skeletal muscles
Dilation of respiratory airways	Increased loading of oxygen into blood
Increased rate and depth of breathing	Increased loading of oxygen into blood (indirect effect)

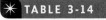 **TABLE 3-14**   Summary of the Sympathetic "Fight-or-Flight" Reaction—cont'd

Response	Role in Promoting Energy Use by Skeletal Muscles
Increased sweating	Increased dissipation of heat generated by skeletal muscle activity
Increased conversion of glycogen into glucose	Increased amount of glucose available to skeletal muscles
Increased breakdown of stored fats	Increased amount of fatty acids and glycerol available to skeletal muscles

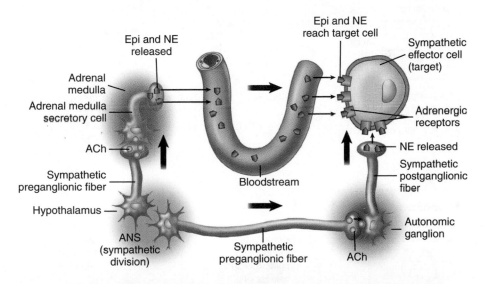

FIGURE 3-16 Combined Nervous and Endocrine Effects During the "Fight-or-Flight" Response.
A sympathetic center in the **hypothalamus** sends efferent impulses through preganglionic fibers. Some preganglionic fibers synapse with postganglionic fibers that deliver **norepinephrine** (NE) across a synapse with the effector cell. Other preganglionic fibers synapse with postganglionic neurosecretory cells in the **adrenal medulla**. These neurosecretory cells secrete **epinephrine** (Epi) and norepinephrine into the bloodstream, where they travel to the target cells (sympathetic effectors) to produce the stress response. Epinephrine in the bloodstream prolongs and enhances the more immediate but short-lived effects of the norepinephrine released at the effector.

✳ TABLE 3-15   Classification of Somatic Sensory Receptors

By Structure	By Location and Type	By Activation Stimulus	By Sensation or Function
Free Nerve Endings			
Nociceptor Dendritic knobs	Either exteroceptor or visceroceptor; found in most body tissues	Almost any noxious stimulus; temperature change; mechanical	Pain; temperature; itch; tickle
Tactile (Merkel) disk (meniscus) Tactile epithelial cell Tactile disk	Exteroceptor	Light pressure; mechanical	Discriminative touch
Root hair plexus	Exteroceptor	Hair movement; mechanical	Sense of "deflection" type of movement of hair
Encapsulated Nerve Endings			
Touch and Pressure Receptors			
Tactile (Meissner) corpuscle	Exteroceptor; found in epidermis and hairless skin	Light pressure; mechanical	Touch; low-frequency vibration
Bulboid (Krause) corpuscle	Exteroceptor; found in mucous membranes	Mechanical	Touch; low-frequency vibration; textural sensation
Bulbous (Ruffini) corpuscle	Exteroceptor; found in dermis of skin	Mechanical	Crude and persistent touch

TABLE 3-15   Classification of Somatic Sensory Receptors—cont'd

By Structure	By Location and Type	By Activation Stimulus	By Sensation or Function
Lamellar (Pacini) corpuscle	Exteroceptor; found in dermis of skin and joint capsules	Deep pressure; mechanical	Deep pressure; high-frequency vibration; stretch
Stretch Receptors Muscle spindles Intrafusal fibers	Interoceptor; found in skeletal muscle	Stretch; mechanical	Sense of muscle length
Golgi tendon receptors	Interoceptor; found in tendons, near muscle tissue	Force of contraction and tendon stretch; mechanical	Sense of muscle tension

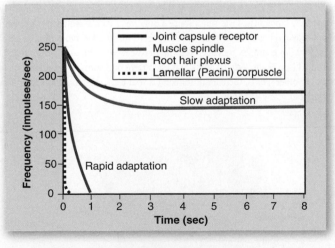

FIGURE 3-17 Adaptation of Sensory Receptors. In the presence of a continuous stimulus, the rate (frequency) of impulses declines quickly in rapidly adapting receptors of the skin. Here the initial stimulus, representing a *change*, is valuable information. However, continued sensation from the skin may be distracting. In slow-adapting joint and muscle receptors, the rate of impulses instead declines gradually and levels off to a constant, moderately high level. Thus, information about body position is continually sent to the central nervous system.

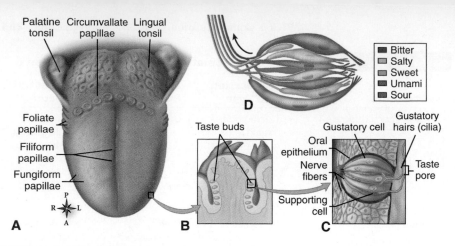

FIGURE 3-18 Lingual Taste Buds.
A, Dorsal surface of the tongue and its adjacent structures.
B, Section through a lingual **papilla** with **taste buds** on the side.
C, Enlarged view of a section through a taste bud.
D, The **labeled-line model** of gustation (taste) holds that each distinct taste has a separate group of taste receptors, with each group sending its impulses along a distinct "line" or neural pathway. (The term *lingual* means "relating to the tongue.")

◇ **FIELD NOTES**

A Taste Map?

For generations, A&P students learned that the location of different taste receptors can be mapped out on the surface of the tongue. However, you won't see many of those maps around anymore. One reason is that they misled us into thinking that taste buds were found only on the tongue. In fact, they are found in many places, including the mouth, the throat, and even the stomach! Another problem is that they limited the taste sensations to only four: sour, sweet, salty, and bitter. More recently umami (savory) has been commonly recognized, many other types of taste sensations are likely to be present (for example, metallic). Yet another issue with the classic taste maps is that the labeled-line model (see Figure 3-18, *D*) holds that each taste bud contains receptors for many different taste sensation. In other words, the current thinking is that taste receptors mix together and are scattered throughout many locations.

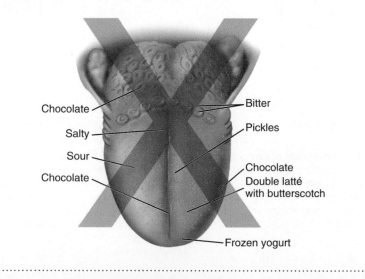

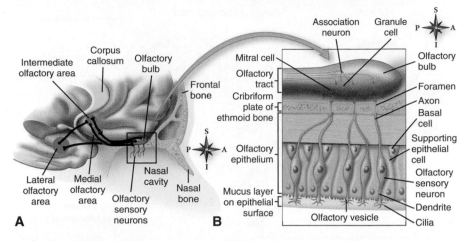

FIGURE 3-19 Olfaction. Olfaction is the sense of smell. The location of the olfactory epithelium, the olfactory bulb, and the neural pathways involved in olfaction are shown here.
A, A midsagittal section of the nasal area shows the locations of major olfactory sensory structures, including the olfactory integration centers of the brain.
B, Details of the olfactory bulb and the olfactory epithelium.

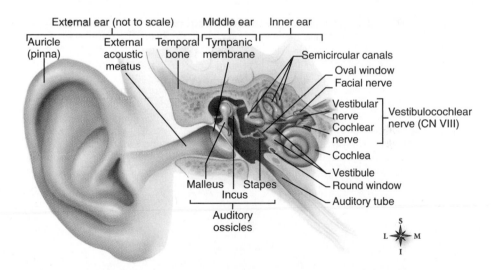

FIGURE 3-20 The Ear. The external, middle, and inner ear. (Anatomic structures are not drawn to scale.) The bony labyrinth is the hard outer wall of the entire inner ear and includes the semicircular canals, the vestibule, and the cochlea. Within the bony labyrinth is the membranous labyrinth (not visible), which is surrounded by perilymph and filled with endolymph. Structures in the vestibule have receptors that detect changes in head position and that send sensory impulses through the vestibular nerve to the brain. Receptors in the cochlea detect sound vibrations in the inner-ear fluids. The vestibular and cochlear nerves join to form the eighth cranial nerve.

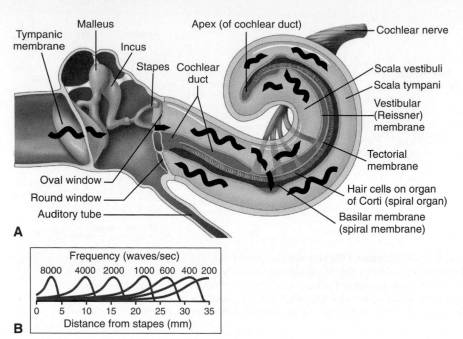

FIGURE 3-21 Effect of Sound Waves on the Cochlear Structures.

A, Sound waves strike the tympanic membrane and cause it to vibrate. This causes the membrane of the oval window to vibrate, which causes the perilymph in the bony labyrinth of the cochlea and the endolymph in the membranous labyrinth of the cochlea (the cochlear duct) to move. This movement of endolymph causes the basilar (spiral) membrane to vibrate, which in turn stimulates hair cells on the organ of Corti (the spiral organ) to transmit nerve impulses along the cochlear nerve. Eventually, nerve impulses reach the auditory cortex and are interpreted as sound.

B, High-frequency (high-pitch) waves stimulate hair cells nearer the stapes (the oval window); low-frequency (low-pitch) waves stimulate hair cells nearer the distal end of the cochlea. The location of peak stimulation of the hair cells allows the brain to interpret the pitch of the sound.

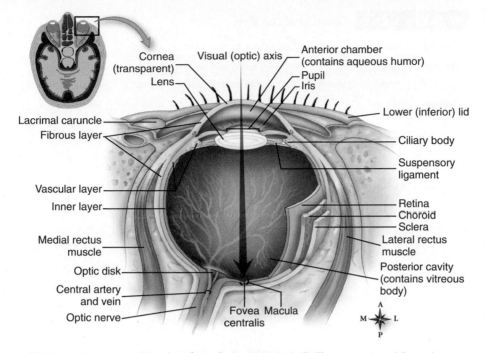

FIGURE 3-22 Horizontal Section Through the Right Eyeball. The eye is viewed from above.

✳ TABLE 3-16		Coats of the Eyeball		
Posterior Location	**Portion**	**Anterior Portion**	**Characteristics**	
Outer coat (sclera)	Sclera proper	Cornea	Protective fibrous coat; the cornea is transparent, and the rest of the coat is white and opaque	
Middle coat (choroid)	Choroid proper	Ciliary body, suspensory ligament, iris (the pupil is a hole in the iris); lens suspended in suspensory ligament	Vascular, pigmented coat	
Inner coat (retina)	Retina	No anterior portion	Nervous tissue; rods and cones (receptors for the second cranial nerve) are located in the retina	

✳ TABLE 3-17	Cavities of the Eye		
Cavity	**Divisions**	**Location**	**Contents**
Anterior	Anterior chamber	Anterior to iris and posterior to cornea	Aqueous humor
	Posterior chamber	Posterior to iris and anterior to lens	Aqueous humor
Posterior	None	Posterior to lens	Vitreous body

B. Endocrine System

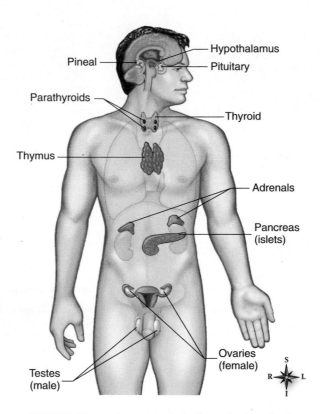

FIGURE 3-23 Locations of Some Major Endocrine Glands.

✳ TABLE 3-18   Names and Locations of Some Major Endocrine Glands

Name	Location
Hypothalamus	Cranial cavity (brain)
Pituitary gland	Cranial cavity
Pineal gland	Cranial cavity (brain)
Thyroid gland	Neck
Parathyroid glands	Neck
Thymus	Mediastinum
Adrenal glands	Abdominal cavity (retroperitoneal)
Pancreatic islets	Abdominal cavity (pancreas)
Ovaries	Pelvic cavity
Testes	Scrotum
Placenta	Pregnant uterus

◆ SURVIVAL TIP

☑ The endocrine system can seem like an overwhelming and unrelated list of hormones and glands. However, it's really more about a *style of regulation*. Before learning the individual glands and their hormones, first get thoroughly familiar with the mechanisms of endocrine regulation and how they relate to nervous regulation—only then will the rest make sense to you.

☑ When learning the names, sources, targets, and actions of hormones, use mnemonics to help you remember them. See **Mnemonics in A&P** (my-ap.us/12WL7BI) for help.

✳ **TABLE 3-19**   Comparison of the Endocrine System and the Nervous System

Feature	Endocrine System	Nervous System
Overall Function	Regulation of effectors to maintain homeostasis	Regulation of effectors to maintain homeostasis
Control by regulatory feedback loops	Yes (endocrine reflexes)	Yes (nervous reflexes)
Effector tissues	Endocrine effectors: virtually all tissues	Nervous effectors: muscle and glandular tissues only
Effector cells	Target cells (throughout the body)	Postsynaptic cells (in muscle and glandular tissues only)
Chemical Messenger	Hormone	Neurotransmitter
Cells that secrete the chemical messenger	Glandular epithelial cells or neurosecretory cells (modified neurons)	Neurons
Distance traveled (and method of travel) by chemical messenger	Long (by way of circulating blood)	Short (across a microscopic synapse)
Location of receptor in effector cell	On the plasma membrane or within the cell	On the plasma membrane
Characteristics of regulatory effects	Slow to appear, long lasting	Appear rapidly, short lived

Cable or Satellite?

Comparing nervous regulation and endocrine regulation as in Table 3-19 is important for understanding the overall regulatory scheme of the body. Often, they are considered together as a single **neuroendocrine** system.

An analogy that can be useful in understanding the difference between these two styles of regulation in the body is based on television signals. As with TV signals, both endocrine and nervous signals are generated in a central location (or several central locations) and then sent out to individuals (individual effector cells, in this case).

How a person gets a TV signal can vary: it may be by cable, a local broadcast, or a satellite. Nervous regulation is more like cable TV, because each effector cell has to be individually "hooked up"—that is, connected to an efferent nerve pathway. Of course, you need a cable decoder box, too. In a nervous effector cell (postsynaptic cell), that takes the form of specific receptors and associated signal transduction mechanisms.

Endocrine regulation is similar to satellite TV: you don't have to have a direct line. Hormones are like satellites, because they are simply sent out everywhere. If you have the right equipment, such as a satellite dish and decoder, then you can receive the signals. If you don't have the equipment, then you're still being bombarded with signals, you just can't receive or interpret them. Similarly, all cells have contact with hormones because hormones move through the entire bloodstream. However, only target cells—that is, those cells with the correct receptors for the specific hormone—actually hear the hormones' messages and respond to them.

We can also consider local regulation here (paracrine regulation). Local regulation is more like local broadcast TV rather than cable or satellite. With a local broadcast, the signals are sent by radio waves to a local community and can travel only a relatively short distance. In other words, you can only receive the signal locally. The TV waves, like local regulatory molecules, can only spread out over the local area. If you have the right equipment (an antenna and a tuner), then you can receive these signals. As with satellite signals, if you don't have the equipment, the signals are still bombarding you, you just can't receive or interpret them. Only those cells with the correct receptors (or some way to respond) for a specific local regulator are affected by the local signal.

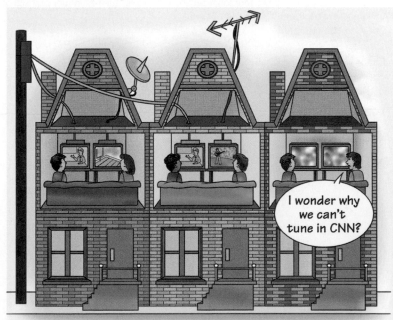

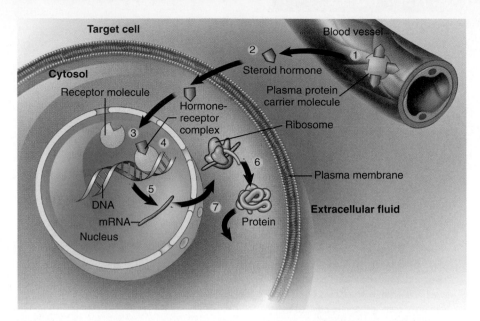

FIGURE 3-24 Steroid Hormone Mechanism. According to the **mobile-receptor model,** lipid-soluble steroid hormone molecules detach from a carrier protein (1) and pass through the plasma membrane (2). The hormone molecules then pass into the nucleus, where they bind with a mobile receptor to form a hormone-receptor complex (3). This complex then binds to a specific site on a DNA molecule (4), thereby triggering the transcription of the genetic information encoded there (5). The resulting mRNA molecule moves to the cytosol, where it associates with a ribosome and initiates the synthesis of a new protein (6). This new protein, which is usually an enzyme or a channel protein, produces specific effects in the target cell (7). Some steroid hormones also have additional secondary effects, such as influencing signal transduction pathways at the plasma membrane.

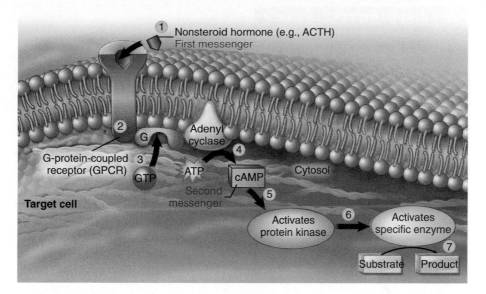

FIGURE 3-25 Example of a Second-Messenger Mechanism. A nonsteroid hormone (the **first messenger**) binds to a fixed *G-protein-coupled receptor (GPCR)* in the plasma membrane of the target cell *(1)*. The hormone-receptor complex activates the *G protein (2)*. The activated G protein reacts with GTP, which in turn activates the membrane-bound enzyme *adenyl cyclase (3)*. Adenyl cyclase removes phosphates from ATP, converting it to *cAMP* (the **second messenger**) *(4)*. cAMP activates or inactivates protein *kinases (5)*. Protein kinases activate specific intracellular enzymes *(6)*. These activated enzymes then influence specific cellular reactions, thereby producing the target cell's response to the hormone *(7)*.
ATP, Adenosine triphosphate; *cAMP*, cyclic adenosine monophosphate; *GTP*, guanosine triphosphate.

✧ FIELD NOTES

Hormone Styles

As you can see in the table on the next page, steroid and nonsteroid hormones don't just work differently at the cellular and molecular levels—they have different styles of action. Nonsteroid hormones are like your "first responders." They work quickly to trigger their effects in the body. However, their effects don't last very long. Steroid hormones, on the other hand, take a while to produce their effects, but their effects last quite a while. The availability of both types of responses allows the body more options when it comes to carefully regulating the internal environment.

The conventional view of the steroid hormone regulation of gene activity states that one or more hours pass before the effects of the hormone reach their peak, as you can see in the table. However, steroid hormones can also produce some rapid effects in target cells, sometimes within just seconds or minutes. How is this possible? We now know that additional steroid hormone receptors at the plasma membrane enable many steroid hormones to regulate signal transduction in target cells. In other words, steroid hormones have a secondary effect that can change the messages sent by other regulatory molecules, such as other hormones or neurotransmitters.

Continued

✧ FIELD NOTES—cont'd

The emerging view is that steroid hormones produce both slow and rapid effects in target cells. Slow effects result from stimulating the transcription of specific genes in the target cell's nucleus, thereby producing new proteins. Rapid effects result from altering signal transduction mechanisms in the plasma membrane of the target cell.

Comparison of Steroid and Nonsteroid Hormones

Characteristic	Steroid Hormones	Nonsteroid Hormones*
Chemical structure	Lipid	One or more amino acids, sometimes with added sugar groups
Stored in secretory cell	No	Yes; stored in secretory vesicles before release
Interaction with plasma membrane	No; simple diffusion through plasma membrane and into target cell	Yes; binds to specific plasma membrane receptor
Receptor	Mobile receptor in cytoplasm or nucleus	Embedded in plasma membrane
Action	Regulates gene activity (transcription of new proteins that eventually produce effects in the cell)	Triggers signal transduction cascade, producing internal "second messengers" that trigger rapid effects in the target cell
Response time	1 hour to several days	Several seconds to a few minutes

*Some nonsteroid hormones derived from amino acids (e.g., the thyroid hormones T_3 and T_4) have gene-activating actions that are similar to those of steroid hormones.

✷ TABLE 3-20		Chemical Classification of Selected Hormones*
Category	**Subcategory**	**Hormone**
Steroid		Cortisol
		Aldosterone
		Estrogen
		Progesterone
		Testosterone
Nonsteroid	Protein	Growth hormone (GH)
		Prolactin (PRL)
		Parathyroid hormone (PTH)
		Calcitonin (CT)
		Adrenocorticotropic hormone (ACTH)
		Insulin
		Glucagon
	Glycoprotein	Follicle-stimulating hormone (FSH)
		Luteinizing hormone (LH)
		Thyroid-stimulating hormone (TSH)
		Human chorionic gonadotropin (hCG)
	Peptide	Antidiuretic hormone (ADH) Arginine vasopressin (AVP)
		Oxytocin (OT)
		Somatostatin (SS)
		Thyrotropin-releasing hormone (TRH)
		Gonadotropin-releasing hormone (GnRH)
		Atrial natriuretic hormone (ANH) Atrial natriuretic peptide (ANP)
	Amino acid derivative	Norepinephrine (NE)
	Amine	Noradrenaline (NA)
		Epinephrine Adrenaline
		Melatonin
	Iodinated amino	Tetraiodothyronine (T_4) Thyroxine
		Triiodothyronine (T_3)

*Does not include prostaglandins and related compounds.

✳ TABLE 3-21   Prostaglandins and Related Hormones

Hormone	Source	Target	Principal Action
Prostaglandins (PGs)	Many diverse tissues of the body	Local cells within the source tissue	Diverse local (paracrine/autocrine) effects, such as the regulation of inflammation and muscle contraction in the blood vessels
Thromboxanes (TXs)	Platelets	Other platelets; muscles in the blood vessel walls	Increase the stickiness of platelets; promote blood clotting; cause constriction of the blood vessels
Leukotrienes	Several types of white blood cells (leukocytes)	Local cells of various types	Regulate local inflammation triggered by allergens, including the constriction of airways (as in asthma) and other inflammatory responses

✳ TABLE 3-22   Hormones of the Hypothalamus

Hormone	Source	Target	Principal Action
Growth-hormone–releasing hormone (GHRH)	Hypothalamus	Adenohypophysis (somatotrophs)	Stimulates secretion (release) of growth hormone
Growth-hormone–inhibiting hormone (GHIH) or somatostatin	Hypothalamus	Adenohypophysis (somatotrophs)	Inhibits secretion of growth hormone
Corticotropin-releasing hormone (CRH)	Hypothalamus	Adenohypophysis (corticotrophs)	Stimulates release of adrenocorticotropic hormone (ACTH)
Thyrotropin-releasing hormone (TRH)	Hypothalamus	Adenohypophysis (thyrotrophs)	Stimulates release of thyroid-stimulating hormone (TSH)
Gonadotropin-releasing hormone (GnRH)	Hypothalamus	Adenohypophysis (gonadotrophs)	Stimulates release of gonadotropins (FSH and LH)
Prolactin-releasing hormone (PRH)	Hypothalamus	Adenohypophysis (corticotrophs)	Stimulates secretion of prolactin
Prolactin-inhibiting hormone (PIH)	Hypothalamus	Adenohypophysis (corticotrophs)	Inhibits secretion of prolactin

✳ **TABLE 3-23**   **Hormones of the Pituitary Gland**

Hormone	Source	Target	Principal Action
Growth hormone (GH) (somatotropin [STH])	Adenohypophysis (somatotrophs)	General	Promotes growth by stimulating protein anabolism and fat mobilization
Prolactin (PRL) (lactogenic hormone)	Adenohypophysis (lactotrophs)	Mammary glands (alveolar secretory cells)	Promotes milk secretion
Thyroid-stimulating hormone (TSH)*	Adenohypophysis (thyrotrophs)	Thyroid gland	Stimulates development and secretion in the thyroid gland
Adrenocorticotropic hormone (ACTH)*	Adenohypophysis (corticotrophs)	Adrenal cortex	Promotes development and secretion in the adrenal cortex
Follicle-stimulating hormone (FSH)*	Adenohypophysis (gonadotrophs)	Gonads (primary sex organs)	*Female:* promotes development of ovarian follicle; stimulates estrogen secretion *Male:* promotes development of testes; stimulates sperm production
Luteinizing hormone (LH)*	Adenohypophysis (gonadotrophs)	Gonads	*Female:* triggers ovulation; promotes development of corpus luteum *Male:* stimulates production of testosterone
Antidiuretic hormone (ADH) or arginine vasopressin (AVP)	Neurohypophysis	Kidney	Promotes water retention by kidney tubules; raises blood pressure by stimulating muscles in walls of small arteries
Oxytocin (OT)	Neurohypophysis	Uterus and mammary glands	Stimulates uterine contractions; stimulates ejection of milk into ducts of mammary glands; involved in social bonding

*Tropic hormones.

✳ **TABLE 3-24**	**Hormones of the Thyroid and Parathyroid Glands**		
Hormone	**Source**	**Target**	**Principal Action**
Triiodothyronine (T₃)	Thyroid gland (follicular cells)	General	Increases rate of metabolism
Tetraiodothyronine (T₄) or thyroxine	Thyroid gland (follicular cells)	General	Increases rate of metabolism (usually converted to T₃ first)
Calcitonin (CT)	Thyroid gland (parafollicular cells)	Bone tissue	Increases calcium storage in bone; lowers blood Ca⁺⁺ levels
Parathyroid hormone (PTH) or parathormone	Parathyroid glands	Bone tissue and kidney	Increases calcium removal from storage in bone; produces the active form of vitamin D in the kidneys; increases absorption of calcium by intestines; increases blood Ca⁺⁺ levels

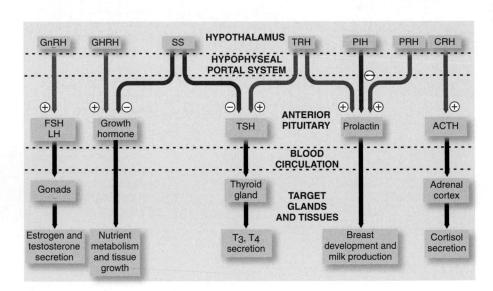

FIGURE 3-26 Actions of Hypothalamic Hormones. Hypothalamic hormones have releasing or inhibiting effects on the various cells of the anterior pituitary, thereby regulating anterior pituitary secretion and ultimately regulating the effects of anterior pituitary hormones throughout the body.

ACTH, Adrenocorticotropic hormone; *CRH,* corticotropin-releasing hormone; *FSH,* follicle-stimulating hormone; *GHRH,* growth hormone-releasing hormone; *GnRH,* gonadotropin-releasing hormone; *LH,* luteinizing hormone; *PIH,* prolactin-inhibiting hormone; *PRH,* prolactin-releasing hormone; *SS,* somatostatin; *T₃,* triiodothyronine; *T₄,* thyroxine; *TRH,* thyroid-releasing hormone; *TSH,* thyroid-stimulating hormone.

Endocrine Feedback Loops

As in most types of regulation in the body, endocrine regulation relies on both **negative feedback loops** (see Figure 1-22 on pages 128 and 129) and **positive feedback loops** (see Figure 1-23 on page 130) to maintain the balance of function in the body that is known as **homeostasis**.

Because some glands regulate the secretion of hormones by other glands, sometimes in multiple levels, we talk about long feedback loops or **long-loop feedback** and short feedback loops or **short-loop feedback**. This simply refers to how many "levels" up in the hierarchy of glands the regulatory response occurs. It's sort of like what occurs in a business, when the quality of service is regulated by the CEO, the district manager, the store manager, and the clerk. The clerk may respond to a problem to satisfy a customer—this is short-loop feedback. However, the store manager or the district manager may be the one to recognize a problem and fix it—this is long-loop feedback. An even longer loop would involve a response from the CEO.

To get used to the idea of a feedback loop in endocrine regulation, look at the illustration of a short feedback loop.

Here, each parathyroid gland is sensitive to changes in the physiological variable that its hormone (parathyroid hormone [PTH]) controls: blood calcium (Ca^{++}) concentration. When lactation (milk production) in a breastfeeding woman consumes Ca^{++} and thus lowers blood Ca^{++} concentration, the parathyroids sense the change and respond by increasing their secretion of PTH. PTH stimulates osteoclasts in bone to release more Ca^{++} from storage in bone tissue (among other effects), which increases maternal blood Ca^{++} concentration to the set point level.

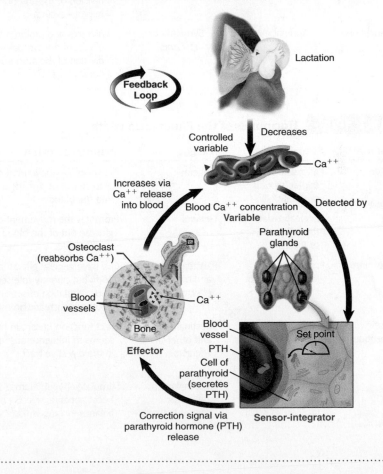

✳ TABLE 3-25   Hormones of the Adrenal Glands

Hormone	Source	Target	Principal Action
Aldosterone	Adrenal cortex (zona glomerulosa)	Kidney	Stimulates kidney tubules to conserve sodium, which in turn triggers the release of ADH and the resulting conservation of water by the kidney
Cortisol (hydrocortisone)	Adrenal cortex (zona fasciculata)	General	Influences metabolism of food molecules; in large amounts, it has an anti-inflammatory effect
Adrenal androgens	Adrenal cortex (zona reticularis)	Sex organs and other effectors	Exact role uncertain but may support sexual function
Adrenal estrogens	Adrenal cortex (zona reticularis)	Sex organs	Thought to be physiologically insignificant
Epinephrine (Epi) or adrenaline	Adrenal medulla	Sympathetic effectors	Enhances and prolongs the effects of the sympathetic division of the autonomic nervous system
Norepinephrine (NE)	Adrenal medulla	Sympathetic effectors	Enhances and prolongs the effects of the sympathetic division of the autonomic nervous system

✳ TABLE 3-26   Hormones of the Pancreatic Islets

Hormone	Source	Target	Principal Action
Glucagon	Pancreatic islets (alpha [α] cells or A cells)	General	Promotes the movement of glucose out of storage and into the blood
Insulin	Pancreatic islets (beta [β] cells, or B cells)	General	Promotes the movement of glucose out of the blood and into the cells
Somatostatin (SS)	Pancreatic islets (delta [δ] cells or D cells)	Pancreatic cells and other effectors	Can have general effects in the body but primary role seems to be regulation of secretion of other pancreatic hormones
Pancreatic polypeptide (PP)	Pancreatic islets (pancreatic polypeptide [PP] or F cells)	Intestinal cells and other effectors	Exact function uncertain but seems to influence absorption in the digestive tract
Ghrelin (GHRL)	Stomach mucosa, pancreatic islets (epsilon [ε] cells)	Hypothalamus and other diverse tissues	Stimulates hypothalamus to boost appetite; affects energy balance in various tissues

✳ **TABLE 3-27**   **Examples of Additional Hormones of the Body**

Hormone	Source	Target	Principal Action
Cholecalciferol (vitamin D₃)	Skin, liver, and kidney (in progressive steps)	Intestines, bones, and most other tissues	Promotes calcium absorption from food; regulates mineral balance in bones; regulates growth and differentiation of many cell types
Dehydroepiandrosterone (DHEA)	Adrenal gland, testis, ovary, and other tissues	Converted to other hormones	Eventually converted to estrogens, testosterone, or both
Melatonin	Pineal gland	Timekeeping tissues of the nervous system	Helps "set" the biological clock mechanisms of the body by signaling light changes during the day, month, and seasons; may help to induce sleep
Testosterone	Testis (small amounts in adrenal gland and ovary)	Sperm-producing tissues of testis, muscles, and other tissues	Stimulates sperm production; stimulates growth and maintenance of male sexual characteristics; promotes muscle growth
Estrogen, including estradiol (E₂) and estrone	Ovary and placenta (small amounts in adrenal gland and testis)	Uterus, breasts, and other tissues	Stimulates development of female sexual characteristics and breast development; maintains bone and nervous system
Progesterone	Ovary and placenta	Uterus, mammary glands, and other tissues	Helps maintain proper conditions for pregnancy
Human chorionic gonadotropin (hCG)	Placenta	Ovary	Stimulates secretion of estrogen and progesterone during pregnancy
Human placental lactogens (hPLs)	Placenta	Mammary glands, pancreas, and other tissues	Promote development of mammary glands during pregnancy; help regulate energy balance in fetus
Relaxin	Placenta	Uterus and joints	Inhibits uterine contractions during pregnancy; softens pelvic joints to facilitate childbirth

Continued

✳ **TABLE 3-27**   **Examples of Additional Hormones of the Body—cont'd**

Hormone	Source	Target	Principal Action
Thymosins and thymopoietins	Thymus gland	Certain lymphocytes (type of white blood cell)	Stimulate development of T lymphocytes, which are involved in immunity
Gastrin	Stomach mucosa	Exocrine glands of the stomach	Triggers increased secretion of gastric juice
Secretin	Intestinal mucosa	Stomach and pancreas	Increases alkaline secretions of the pancreas and slows emptying of stomach; helps regulate water homeostasis
Cholecystokinin (CCK)	Intestinal mucosa	Gallbladder and pancreas	Triggers release of bile from gallbladder and enzymes from the pancreas
Atrial natriuretic hormone (ANH) and other atrial natriuretic peptides (ANPs)	Heart muscle	Kidney	Promote loss of sodium from body into urine, thereby promoting water loss from body and a resulting decrease in blood volume and pressure
Inhibins	Ovary and testis	Hypothalamus and adenohypophysis (anterior pituitary)	Inhibit secretion of GnRH by hypothalamus and FSH by anterior pituitary, thereby helping to regulate the female reproductive cycle
Leptin	Adipose tissue	Hypothalamus and other diverse tissues	Affects energy balance, perhaps as a signal of how much fat is stored; affects various immune, neuroendocrine, and developmental functions throughout the body
Resistin	Adipose tissue and macrophages	Liver and other tissues	Reduces sensitivity to insulin (a pancreatic islet hormone), thereby increasing blood glucose levels
Insulin-like growth factor 1 (IGF-1)	Liver, kidney, and other tissues	Bone, muscle, and other tissues	Secreted in response to growth hormone (GH); carries out many of the functions attributed to GH

CHAPTER FOUR

Transportation and Defense

Navigation Guide

A. Cardiovascular System

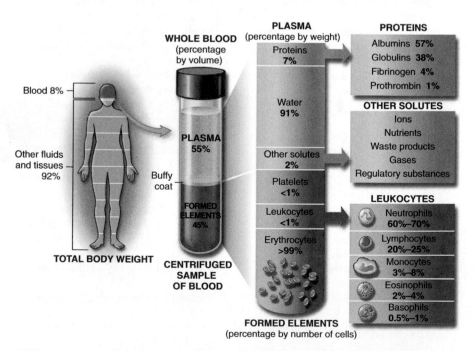

FIGURE 4-1 Composition of Whole Blood. Approximate values for the components of blood in a normal adult.

✳ TABLE 4-1 Classes of Blood Cells

Cell Type	Description	Function	Life Span
Erythrocyte	7 μm in diameter; concave disk shape; entire cell stains pale pink; no nucleus	Transportation of respiratory gases (O_2 and CO_2)	105 to 120 days
Neutrophil	12 to 15 μm in diameter; spherical shape; multilobed nucleus; small, pink-purple–staining cytoplasmic granules	Cellular defense—phagocytosis of small pathogenic microorganisms	Hours to 3 days
Basophil	11 to 14 μm in diameter; spherical shape; generally two-lobed nucleus; large purple-staining cytoplasmic granules	Secretes heparin (anticoagulant) and histamine (important in inflammatory response)	Hours to 3 days
Eosinophil	10 to 12 μm in diameter; spherical shape; generally two-lobed nucleus; large, orange-red–staining cytoplasmic granule	Cellular defense—some phagocytosis; chemical attack of large pathogenic microorganisms (such as protozoa) and parasitic worms; helps regulate allergic reactions and other inflammatory responses	10 to 12 days
Lymphocyte	6 to 9 μm in diameter; spherical shape; round, single-lobed nucleus; small lymphocytes have scant cytoplasm	Humoral defense—secretes antibodies; involved in immune system response and regulation	Days to years
Monocyte	12 to 17 μm in diameter; spherical shape; nucleus generally kidney-bean or horseshoe shaped with a convoluted surface; ample cytoplasm often steel blue in color	Capable of migrating out of the blood to enter tissue spaces as a macrophage—an aggressive phagocytic cell capable of ingesting bacteria, cellular debris, and cancerous cells	Months
Platelet	2 to 5 μm in diameter; irregularly shaped fragments; cytoplasm contains very small, pink-staining granules	Releases clot-activating substances and helps in the formation of actual blood clots by forming platelet plugs	7 to 10 days

✦ FIELD NOTES

Field Marks

Recall from *Special Survival Skills: The Student Laboratory* course (see page 58) that **field marks** are used by naturalists to quickly distinguish between two similar species of plant or animal (or whatever) while out on a field trip. *Field guides* often highlight these distinguishing characteristics with arrows or some other way to tell you what to look for. For many animals, such as birds, you may only have a moment to look at them. If all you remember is that *it was big and gray*, then you probably won't be able to accurately identify it. However, if your field guide shows that the several kinds of big gray birds can be distinguished by the color of their beaks, you can figure that out quickly and accurately.

This method works wonderfully for many structures of the body, too, as we have seen. Tissues, bones and bone features, muscles, and so on can all be easily distinguished once you've discovered their one or two unique characteristics: their field marks.

This *field mark method* is especially helpful when trying to distinguish between different types of white blood cells (WBCs, leukocytes) when doing a differential WBC count—that is, a count of how many of each type of WBC you have in your sample (see Table 4-2).

Use Table 4-1 to make your own field guide to the WBCs. Enlarge the table on a color photocopier or snap a photo with your phone and then print it, and cut out the blood cell images. Even better, draw your own color sketches of them. Put arrows on the figures where each cell type differs from other similar cell types. Then write a brief notation, such as "two-lobed nucleus" to tell what the field mark arrow points to or how to distinguish it.

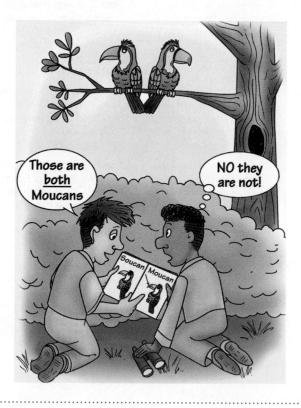

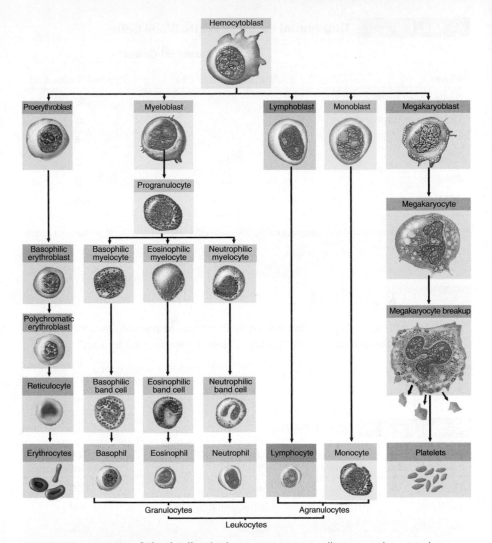

FIGURE 4-2 Formation of Blood Cells. The *hematopoietic stem cell* serves as the original stem cell from which all formed elements of the blood are derived. Note that all five precursor cells, which ultimately produce the different components of the formed elements, are derived from the hematopoietic stem cell called a **hemocytoblast.**

TABLE 4-2   Differential Count of White Blood Cells

Class	Differential Count*	
	Normal Range (%)	Typical Value (%)
Neutrophils	65-75	65
Lymphocytes (large and small)	20-25	25
Monocytes	3-8	6
Eosinophils	2-5	3
Basophils	½-1	1
TOTAL	100	100

*In any differential count, the sum of the percentages of the different kinds of white blood cells must, of course, total 100%.

◈ SURVIVAL TIP

☑ When you look at Table 4-2, this mnemonic phrase may help you to remember percent values in decreasing order by class of WBC: "**N**ever **L**et **M**onkeys **E**at **B**ananas."

TABLE 4-3   Blood Typing

Blood Type (ABO and RH)	Antigens Present*	Antibodies Present*	Percent of General Population
O+	Rh	Anti-A, anti-B	35%
O– †	None	Anti-A, anti-B, anti-Rh?	7%
A+	A, Rh	Anti-B	35%
A–	A	Anti-B, anti-Rh?	7%
B+	B, Rh	Anti-A	8%
B–	B	Anti-A, anti-Rh?	2%
AB+ ‡	A, B, Rh	None	4%
AB–	A, B	Anti-Rh?	2%

*Anti-Rh antibodies may be present, depending on the individual's exposure to Rh antigens.
†Universal donor.
‡Universal recipient.
Adapted from Pagana KD, Pagana TJ: *Mosby's manual of diagnostic and laboratory tests*, ed 4, St. Louis, 2010, Mosby.

Recipient's blood		Reactions with donor's blood			
RBC antigens	Plasma antibodies	Donor type O	Donor type A	Donor type B	Donor type AB
None (Type O)	Anti-A Anti-B				
A (Type A)	Anti-B				
B (Type B)	Anti-A				
AB (Type AB)	(None)				

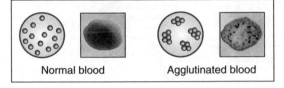

Normal blood	Agglutinated blood

FIGURE 4-3 ABO Blood Types. Results of different combinations of donor and recipient blood. The left columns show the recipient's blood characteristics, and the top row shows the donor's blood type.

✳ TABLE 4-4   Hemostasis (Stopping Blood Loss)

Step	Name	Time Frame*	Description
1	Platelet plug	Seconds	Damage to the endothelial lining of the vessel promotes the sticking of platelets to form a temporary plug at the injury site; platelets release chemicals that promote more platelet adhesion (positive feedback) and that trigger the clotting mechanism (see Step 2)
2	Clot formation (coagulation)	Minutes	Chemicals from injured tissue cells and from platelets trigger a cascade of chemical reactions that result in the formation of a fibrin mesh that traps blood cells to form a clot (see Figure 4-4)
3	Clot dissolution	Days or weeks	Chemicals that trigger clot formation also trigger clot dissolution (fibrinolysis); the clot slowly dissolves as the underlying tissue is repaired

*Time frames can vary with the extent of the injury and the location in the body.

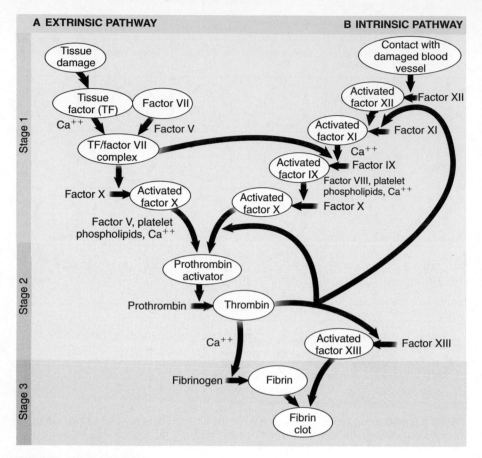

FIGURE 4-4 Clot Formation.

A, Extrinsic clotting pathway.

Stage 1: Damaged tissue releases tissue factor, which with factor VII and calcium ions activates factor X. Activated factor X, factor V, phospholipids, and calcium ions form prothrombin activator (prothrombinase).

Stage 2: Prothrombin is converted to thrombin by prothrombin activator.

Stage 3: Fibrinogen is converted to fibrin by thrombin. Fibrin forms a clot.

B, Intrinsic clotting pathway.

Stage 1: Damaged vessels cause the activation of factor XII. Activated factor XII activates factor XI, which activates factor IX. Factor IX, along with factor VIII and platelet phospholipids, activates factor X. Activated factor X, factor V, phospholipids, and calcium ions form prothrombin activator.

Stages 2 and 3: These follow the same course as the extrinsic clotting pathway.

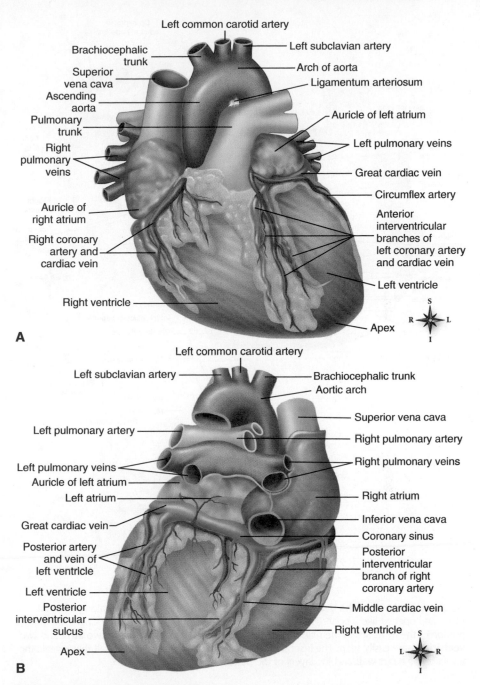

Left common carotid artery

Brachiocephalic trunk

Superior vena cava

Ascending aorta

Pulmonary trunk

Right pulmonary veins

Auricle of right atrium

Right coronary artery and cardiac vein

Right ventricle

Left subclavian artery

Arch of aorta

Ligamentum arteriosum

Auricle of left atrium

Left pulmonary veins

Great cardiac vein

Circumflex artery

Anterior interventricular branches of left coronary artery and cardiac vein

Left ventricle

Apex

A

Left common carotid artery

Left subclavian artery

Left pulmonary artery

Left pulmonary veins

Auricle of left atrium

Left atrium

Great cardiac vein

Posterior artery and vein of left ventricle

Left ventricle

Posterior interventricular sulcus

Apex

Brachiocephalic trunk

Aortic arch

Superior vena cava

Right pulmonary artery

Right pulmonary veins

Right atrium

Inferior vena cava

Coronary sinus

Posterior interventricular branch of right coronary artery

Middle cardiac vein

Right ventricle

B

FIGURE 4-5 The Heart and the Central Vessels.
A, Anterior view of the heart and the great vessels.
B, Posterior view of the heart and the great vessels.

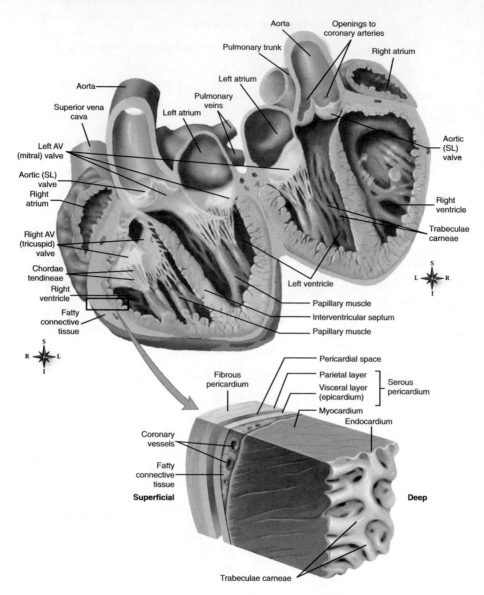

FIGURE 4-6 Interior of the Heart. The heart as it would appear if it were cut along a frontal plane and opened like a book. The front portion of the heart lies to the reader's right; the back portion of the heart lies to the reader's left. The four chambers of the heart—two **atria** and two **ventricles**—are easily seen. The inset shows a small slice of the ventricular wall that reveals the layers of the **heart wall** and the layers of the **pericardium**.

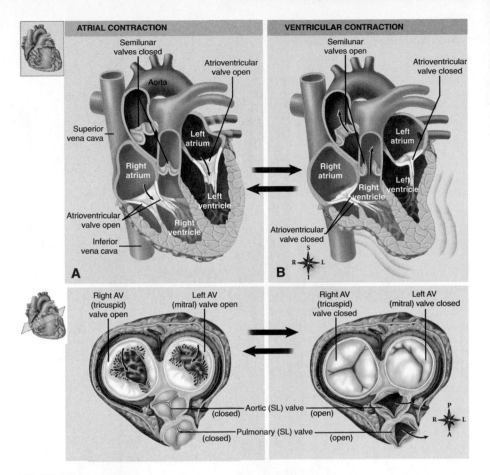

FIGURE 4-7 Heart Action.
A, During **atrial systole** (contraction), cardiac muscle in the atrial wall contracts, forcing blood through the **atrioventricular (AV) valves** and into the ventricles. The bottom illustration shows a superior view of all four valves (with the atria removed), with the **semilunar (SL) valves** closed and the AV valves open.
B, During **ventricular systole** that follows, the AV valves close, and blood is forced out of the ventricles through the SL valves and into the arteries. The bottom illustration shows a superior view with the SL valves open and the AV valves closed.

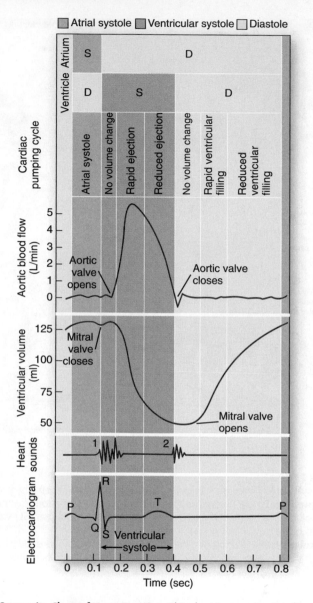

FIGURE 4-8 Composite Chart of Heart Function. This chart is a composite of several diagrams of heart function—cardiac pumping cycle, blood flow and volume, heart sounds, and electrocardiogram (ECG)—all adjusted to the same time scale. Although daunting at first glance, it is a good summary to use as a reference, and it will help you "put it all together" when applying principles of heart function.

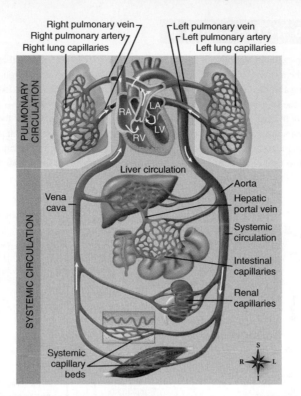

FIGURE 4-9 Blood Flow Through the Circulatory System. In the **pulmonary circulation**, blood is pumped from the right side of the heart to the gas-exchange tissues of the lungs. In the **systemic circulation**, blood is pumped from the left side of the heart to all other tissues of the body.

◇ FIELD NOTES

Tracing the Flow of Blood
An important skill for A&P as well as for later courses and clinical experiences is to be able to trace the flow of blood through the circulatory system. To list the vessels through which blood flows to reach a designated part of the body or when returning to the heart from another part, you should remember the following tips:

☑ Blood always flows in this direction: left ventricle of heart → arteries → arterioles → capillaries of each body part → venules → veins → right atrium → right ventricle → pulmonary artery → lung capillaries → pulmonary veins → left atrium → back to left ventricle of heart (see Figure 4-9).

☑ When blood is in the capillaries of the abdominal digestive organs, it must flow through the hepatic portal system (see Figure 4-9) before returning to the heart.

☑ Be familiar with the names of the main arteries and veins of body (see Figure 4-11 on page 300 and Figure 4-12 on page 301). Although many of the small arteries and veins have names, many can be referred to simply by the organ that they supply or drain. They can also be looked up on a case-by-case basis.

Continued

✦ FIELD NOTES—cont'd

Let's try an example. We can use the figure shown here to help us. Suppose that glucose were instilled into the rectum. To reach the cells of the right little finger, the vessels through which it would pass after being absorbed from the intestinal mucosa into capillaries would be as follows: capillaries → venules of the large intestine into the inferior mesenteric vein → splenic vein → portal vein → capillaries of the liver → hepatic veins → inferior vena cava → right atrium of the heart → right ventricle → pulmonary artery → pulmonary capillaries → pulmonary veins → left atrium → left ventricle → ascending aorta → aortic arch → innominate artery → right subclavian artery → right axillary artery → right brachial artery → right ulnar artery → arteries of the palmar arch → arterioles → capillaries of the right little finger.

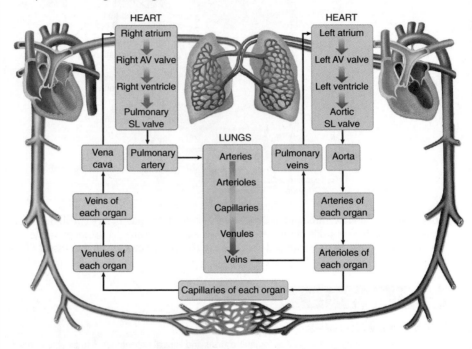

Diagram of blood flow in the circulatory system.

In this illustration, blood passes through a single capillary bed in the systemic circulation—this is the most typical route. After leaving the heart and entering the major arteries of the body, blood travels through the arterioles to a capillary bed and then to the venules and veins before returning to the opposite side of the heart.

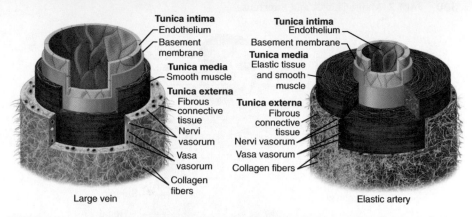

Tunica intima
— Endothelium
— Basement
   membrane
Tunica media
— Smooth muscle
Tunica externa
Fibrous
connective
tissue
Nervi
vasorum
Vasa
vasorum
Collagen
fibers

Large vein

Tunica intima
Endothelium —
Basement membrane —
Tunica media
Elastic tissue
and smooth —
muscle
Tunica externa
Fibrous
connective
tissue
Nervi vasorum —
Vasa vasorum —
Collagen fibers —

Elastic artery

FIGURE 4-10 Artery and Vein Structure. Schematic drawings of a large and medium vein *(left)* and a large and medium artery *(right)* show the comparative thicknesses of the three main layers: the outer layer (or **tunica externa**), the muscle layer (or **tunica media**), and the inner **tunica intima,** which is made of **endothelium.** Note that the middle and outer layers are much thinner in veins than in arteries and that veins have valves.

✳ **TABLE 4-5**   **Structure of Blood Vessels**

Typical Histology	Typical Diameter	Typical Wall Thickness (Endothelium)	Tunica Intima (Smooth muscle; elastic fibers)	Tunica Media (Collagen fibers)	Tunica Externa
Arteries	Aorta: 25 mm Small artery: 4 mm Arteriole: 30 μm	Aorta: 2 mm Small artery: 1 mm Arteriole: 8 μm	Smooth lining	Allows for the constriction and dilation of vessels; thicker than in the veins; muscle innervated by autonomic fibers	Provides flexible support that resists collapse or injury; thicker than in the veins; thinner than in the tunica media
Veins	Vena cava: 30 mm Vein: 5 mm Venule: 20 μm	Vena cava: 1.5 mm Vein: 0.5 mm Venule: 1 μm	Smooth lining with valves to ensure one-way flow	Allows for the constriction and dilation of vessels; thinner than in the arteries; muscle innervated by autonomic fibers	Provides flexible support that resists collapse or injury; thinner than in the arteries; thicker than in the tunica media
Capillaries	5 μm	0.5 μm	Makes up entire wall of capillary; thinness permits ease of transport across vessel wall	(Absent)	(Absent)

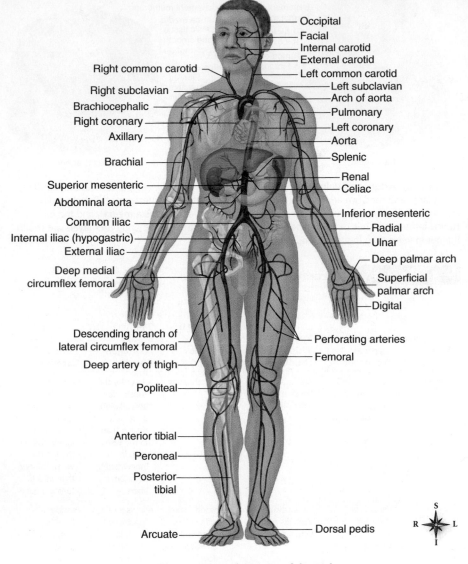

FIGURE 4-11 Principal Arteries of the Body.

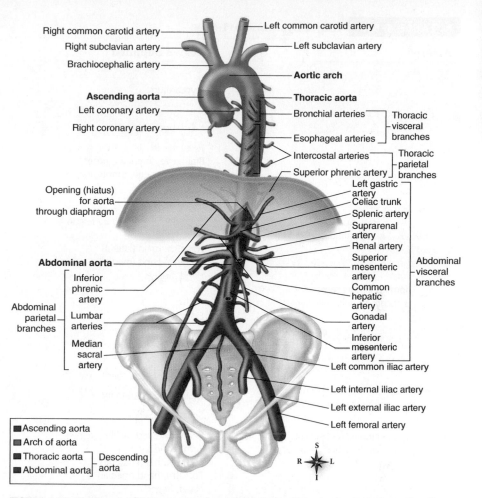

Right common carotid artery
Right subclavian artery
Brachiocephalic artery

Left common carotid artery
Left subclavian artery

Aortic arch

Ascending aorta
Left coronary artery
Right coronary artery

Thoracic aorta
Bronchial arteries ⎤ Thoracic
 ⎱ visceral
Esophageal arteries ⎦ branches

Intercostal arteries ⎤ Thoracic
 ⎱ parietal
Superior phrenic artery ⎦ branches

Opening (hiatus)
for aorta
through diaphragm

Left gastric
artery
Celiac trunk
Splenic artery
Suprarenal
artery
Renal artery
Superior
mesenteric
artery
Common
hepatic
artery
Gonadal
artery
Inferior
mesenteric
artery

Abdominal
visceral
branches

Abdominal aorta

Abdominal
parietal
branches

Inferior
phrenic
artery
Lumbar
arteries
Median
sacral
artery

Left common iliac artery
Left internal iliac artery
Left external iliac artery
Left femoral artery

■ Ascending aorta
■ Arch of aorta
■ Thoracic aorta ⎤ Descending
■ Abdominal aorta ⎦ aorta

S
R ✦ L
I

FIGURE 4-12 Divisions and Primary Branches of the Aorta. This anterior view shows that the aorta is the main systemic artery, serving as a trunk from which other arteries branch. Blood is conducted from the heart first through the ascending aorta, then through the arch of the aorta, and then through the thoracic and abdominal segments of the descending aorta. Note the designations of the visceral and parietal branches in the thoracic and abdominal aortic divisions. Compare this with the tables and charts of arterial blood flow that follow.

✳ TABLE 4-6   **Major Systemic Arteries**

Artery*	Region Supplied
Ascending Aorta	
Coronary arteries	Myocardium
Arch of Aorta	
Brachiocephalic (Innominate)	Head, upper extremity
Right common carotid	Head, neck
Right internal carotid[†]	Brain, eye, forehead, nose
Right external carotid[†]	Thyroid, tongue, tonsils, ear, etc.
Right subclavian	Head, upper extremity
Right vertebral[†]	Spinal cord, brain
Right axillary (continuation of subclavian)	Shoulder, chest, axillary region
Right brachial (continuation of axillary)	Arm, hand
Right radial	Forearm, hand (lateral)
Right ulnar	Forearm, hand (medial)
Superficial and deep palmar arches (formed by anastomosis of branches of radial and ulnar)	Hand, fingers
Digital	Fingers
Left Common Carotid	Head, neck
Left internal carotid[†]	Brain, eye, forehead, nose
Left external carotid[†]	Thyroid, tongue, tonsils, ear, etc.
Left Subclavian	Head, upper extremity
Left vertebral[†]	Spinal cord, brain
Left axillary (continuation of subclavian)	Shoulder, chest, axillary region
Left brachial (continuation of axillary)	Arm, hand
Left radial	Forearm, hand (lateral)
Left ulnar	Forearm, hand (medial)
Superficial and deep palmar arches (formed by the anastomosis of branches of the radial and ulnar)	Hand, fingers
Digital	Fingers
Descending Thoracic Aorta	
Visceral Branches	Thoracic viscera
Bronchial	Lungs, bronchi
Esophageal	Esophagus
Parietal Branches	Thoracic walls
Intercostal	Lateral thoracic walls (ribcage)
Superior phrenic	Superior surface of diaphragm

*The branches of each artery are indented below the artery name.
†See the flowcharts that follow or your text or anatomy atlas for branches of this artery.

✳ **TABLE 4-6**   Major Systemic Arteries—cont'd

Artery*	Region Supplied
Descending Abdominal Aorta	
Visceral Branches	Abdominal viscera
Celiac artery (trunk)	Abdominal viscera
Left gastric	Stomach, esophagus
Common hepatic	Liver
Splenic	Spleen, pancreas, stomach
Superior mesenteric	Pancreas, small intestine, colon
Inferior mesenteric	Descending colon, rectum
Suprarenal	Adrenal (suprarenal) gland
Renal	Kidney
Ovarian	Ovary, uterine tube, ureter
Testicular	Testis, ureter
Parietal Branches	Walls of abdomen
Inferior phrenic	Inferior surface of diaphragm, adrenal gland
Lumbar	Lumbar vertebrae, muscles of back
Median sacral	Lower vertebrae
Common Iliac (formed by terminal branches of aorta)	Pelvis, lower extremity
External Iliac	Thigh, leg, foot
Femoral (continuation of external iliac)	Thigh, leg, foot
Popliteal (continuation of femoral)	Leg, foot
Anterior tibial	Leg, foot
Posterior tibial	Leg, foot
Plantar arch (formed by the anastomosis of branches of the anterior and posterior tibial arteries)	Foot, toes
Digital	Toes
Internal Iliac	Pelvis
Visceral branches	Pelvic viscera
Middle rectal	Rectum
Vaginal	Vagina, uterus
Uterine	Uterus, vagina, uterine tube, ovary
Parietal branches	Pelvic wall, external regions
Lateral sacral	Sacrum
Superior gluteal	Gluteal muscles
Obturator	Pubic region, hip joint, groin
Internal pudendal	Rectum, external genitals, floor of pelvis
Inferior gluteal	Lower gluteal region, coccyx, upper thigh

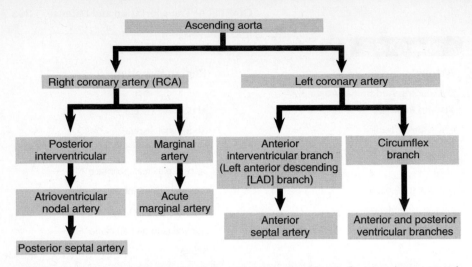

FIGURE 4-13 Blood Flow Through the Coronary Arteries. Blood leaves the ascending aorta and flows through the myocardium of the heart.

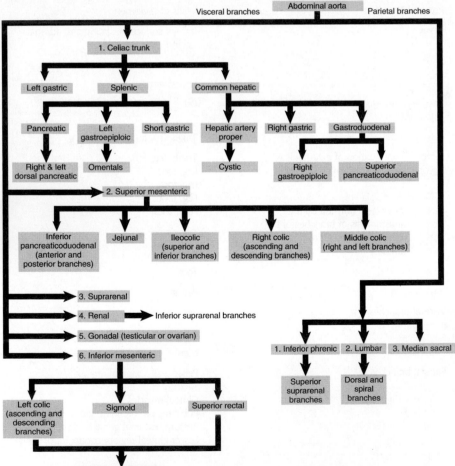

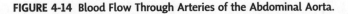

FIGURE 4-14 Blood Flow Through Arteries of the Abdominal Aorta.

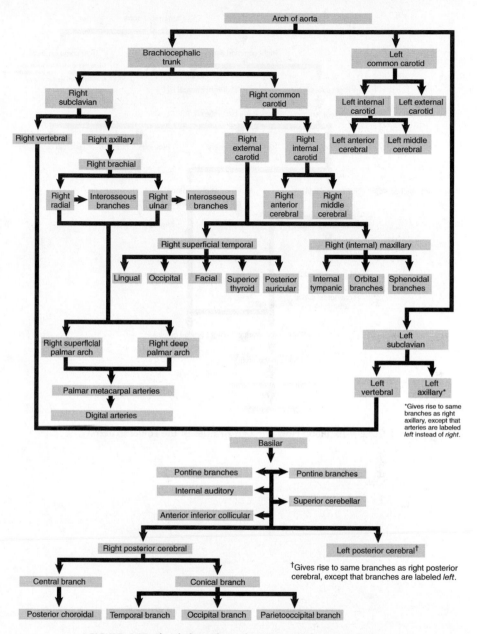

FIGURE 4-15 Blood Flow Through Arteries of the Aortic Arch.

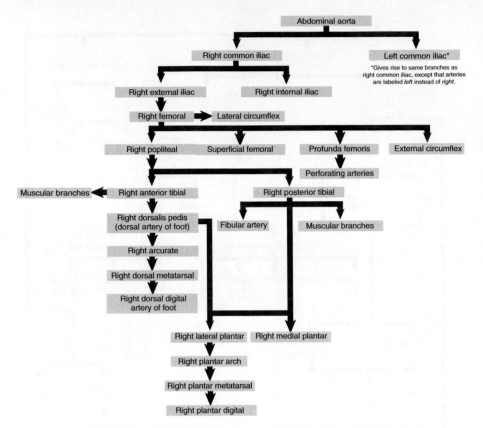

FIGURE 4-16 Blood Flow Through Arteries of the Lower Extremity.

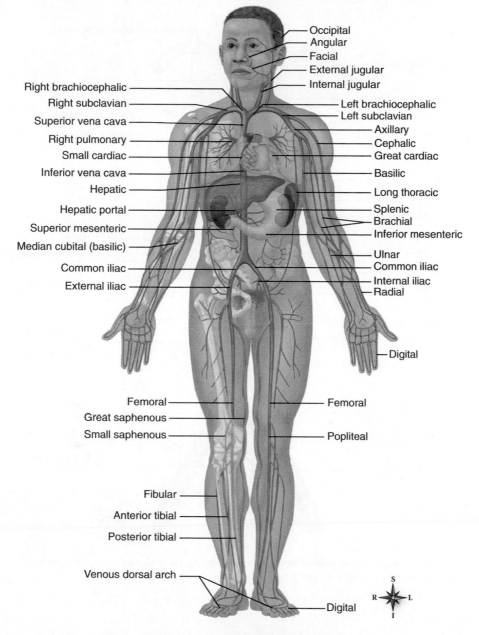

Occipital
Angular
Facial
External jugular
Internal jugular

Right brachiocephalic
Right subclavian
Superior vena cava
Right pulmonary
Small cardiac
Inferior vena cava
Hepatic
Hepatic portal
Superior mesenteric
Median cubital (basilic)
Common iliac
External iliac

Left brachiocephalic
Left subclavian
Axillary
Cephalic
Great cardiac
Basilic
Long thoracic
Splenic
Brachial
Inferior mesenteric
Ulnar
Common iliac
Internal iliac
Radial

Digital

Femoral
Great saphenous
Small saphenous

Femoral

Popliteal

Fibular
Anterior tibial
Posterior tibial

Venous dorsal arch

Digital

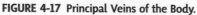

FIGURE 4-17 Principal Veins of the Body.

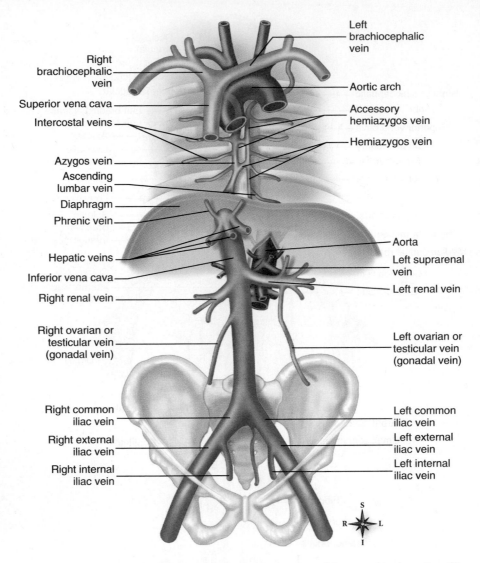

FIGURE 4-18 Superior and Inferior Venae Cavae. Anterior view of the ventral body cavity with many of the viscera removed. Note the close anatomical relationship between the venae cavae and the aorta.

✳ **TABLE 4-7**	Major Systemic Veins

Vein*	Region Drained
SUPERIOR VENA CAVA	Head, neck, thorax, upper extremity
Brachiocephalic (Innominate)	Head, neck, upper extremity
Internal jugular (continuation of sigmoid sinus)	Brain
Lingual	Tongue, mouth
Superior thyroid	Thyroid, deep face
Facial	Superficial face
Sigmoid sinus (continuation of transverse sinus; direct tributary of the internal jugular)	Brain, meninges, skull
Superior and inferior petrosal sinuses	Anterior brain, skull
Cavernous sinus	Anterior brain, skull
Ophthalmic veins	Eye, orbit
Transverse sinus (direct tributary of the sigmoid sinus)	Brain, meninges, skull
Occipital sinus	Inferior, central region of the cranial cavity
Straight sinus	Central region of the brain, meninges
Inferior sagittal sinus	Central region of the brain, meninges
Superior sagittal (longitudinal) sinus	Superior region of the cranial cavity
External jugular	Superficial, posterior head, neck
Subclavian (continuation of axillary; direct tributary of the brachiocephalic)	Axilla, lower extremity
Cephalic	Lateral arm and forearm, hand
Axillary (continuation of basilic; direct tributary of the subclavian)	Axilla, lower extremity
Brachial	Deep arm
Radial	Deep lateral forearm
Ulnar	Deep medial forearm
Basilic (direct tributary of the axillary)	Medial arm and forearm, hand
Median cubital (formed by the anastomosis of the cephalic and basilic)	Forearm, hand
Deep and superficial palmar venous arches (formed by the anastomosis of the cephalic and basilic)	Hand
Digital	Fingers
Azygos (anastomoses with right ascending lumbar)	Right posterior wall of the thorax and the abdomen, esophagus, bronchi, pericardium, mediastinum
Hemiazygos (anastomoses with left renal)	Left inferior posterior wall of the thorax and the abdomen, esophagus, mediastinum
Accessory hemiazygos	Left superior posterior wall of the thorax
INFERIOR VENA CAVA	Lower trunk and extremity
Phrenic	Diaphragm
Hepatic portal system	Upper abdominal viscera
Hepatic veins (continuations of liver venules and the sinusoids and ultimately the hepatic portal vein)	Liver

Continued

✳ TABLE 4-7   Major Systemic Veins—cont'd

Vein*	Region Drained
Hepatic portal vein	Gastrointestinal organs, pancreas, spleen, gallbladder
Cystic	Gallbladder
Gastric	Stomach
Splenic	Spleen
Inferior mesenteric	Descending colon, rectum
Pancreatic	Pancreas
Superior mesenteric	Small intestine, most of colon
Gastroepiploic	Stomach
Renal	Kidneys
Suprarenal	Adrenal (suprarenal) gland
Left ovarian	Left ovary
Left testicular	Left testis
Left ascending lumbar (anastomoses with the hemiazygos)	Left lumbar region
Right ovarian (gonadal)	Right ovary
Right testicular (gonadal)	Right testis
Right ascending lumbar (anastomoses with the azygos)	Right lumbar region
Common iliac (continuation of the external iliac; common iliacs unite to form the inferior vena cava)	Lower extremity
External iliac (continuation of the femoral direct tributary of the common iliac)	Thigh, leg, foot
Femoral (continuation of the popliteal direct tributary of the external iliac)	Thigh, leg, foot
Popliteal	Leg, foot
Small (external, short) saphenous	Superficial posterior leg, lateral foot
Dorsal veins of foot (also drain into the great saphenous)	Anterior (dorsal) foot, toes
Medial and lateral plantar	Sole of foot
Anterior tibial	Anterior leg, foot
Fibular (peroneal)	Lateral and anterior leg, foot
Posterior tibial	Deep posterior leg
Great (internal, long) saphenous	Superficial medial and anterior thigh, leg, foot
Dorsal veins of the foot	Anterior (dorsal) foot, toes
Dorsal venous arch	Anterior (dorsal) foot, toes
Digital	Toes
Internal iliac (unites with the external iliac to form the common iliac)	Pelvic region

*Tributaries of each vein are identified below each vein's name; deep veins are printed in dark blue, and superficial veins are printed in light blue.

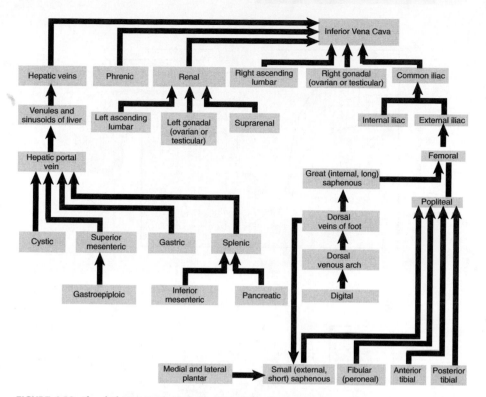

FIGURE 4-19 Blood Flow into the Inferior Vena Cava from Its Major Tributaries. Keep in mind that venous pathways show great variability among individuals.

✦ FIELD NOTES

What Makes Blood Flow?

There are many factors that affect blood flow—so many, in fact, that it can easily get confusing. However, there is a basic principle that explains the effects of all these factors. It's sometimes called the **primary principle of circulation** and it states that *blood flows down a pressure gradient*. A pressure gradient is a difference in pressure between two points. Anything that flows from one place to another does so because of a difference in pressure.

If you squeeze a bottle of ketchup, it will flow out of the bottle because you've increased the pressure inside the bottle to be above that outside of the bottle. Thus, the ketchup moves from an area of higher pressure to an area of lower pressure. That's all there is to it!

The inset of the diagram shows that blood (or ketchup) in a tank flows from the area of high pressure in the tank toward the area of low pressure above the bucket. The graph below shows that, when we map out blood pressures (which are measured in **mm Hg** or *millimeters of mercury*), we can easily see the pressure gradient that exists in the bloodstream as the blood exits the heart (the left side of diagram) to the point at which it returns back to the heart (the right side of the diagram). All of the factors that influence blood flow (see Figure 4-21 on p. 313) somehow maintain this gradient by keeping the left side of the graph higher than the right side of the graph.

If you keep this simple principle in mind, any further explanations will make more sense to you!

Continued

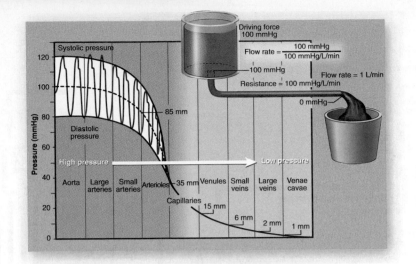

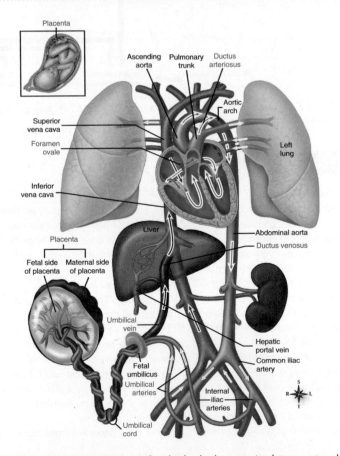

FIGURE 4-20 Plan of Fetal Circulation. Before birth, the human circulatory system has several special features that adapt the body to life in the womb. These features (labeled in red type) include two umbilical arteries, one **umbilical vein, ductus venosus, foramen ovale, ductus arteriosus, placenta,** and **umbilical cord.**

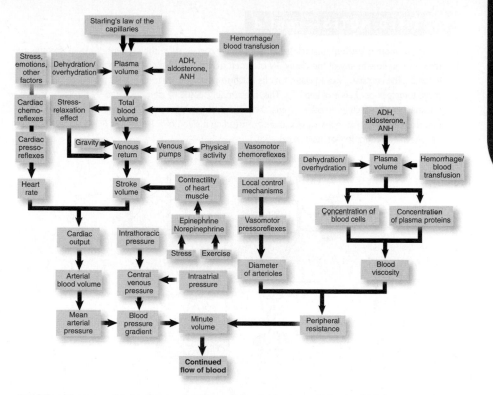

FIGURE 4-21 Factors That Influence the Flow of Blood. The flow of blood, which is expressed as volume of blood flowing per minute (or **minute volume**), is determined by various factors. This chart shows only some of the major factors that influence blood flow. Notice that some factors appear more than once in the chart, which indicates that they can influence blood flow in several ways.

✦ FIELD NOTES

Blood and Ketchup

Learning about all of the factors that affect blood flow can be daunting. One of the tough things about it is trying to visualize *how* all of the factors influence blood flow.

One factor that affects blood flow is **peripheral resistance.** This is the resistance to blood flow in the peripheral vessels ... the arterioles.

What kinds of things can cause blood to "resist" flowing as freely as possible? Well, one factor is the **viscosity** of blood. One way to think of viscosity is "thickness" of a fluid. What makes blood thick? One factor is the viscous nature of blood plasma, which is made more viscous than plain water by the presence of **plasma proteins** such as *albumin.* A bigger factor in blood viscosity is how concentrated the red blood cells (RBCs) are in each drop of blood. It is often expressed as the **PCV** (packed cell volume) or the **hematocrit level** of the blood. *The more blood cells that there are in a drop of blood, the thicker—or more viscous—the blood is and the more it resists flow.*

Continued

Using another ketchup analogy (see page 311), we can visualize the concept of blood viscosity and resistance to flow in any of the classic TV commercials once used by a major brand to promote their ketchup. The company would claim that its ketchup was better than the other brands because it had more tomatoes per bottle of ketchup. This, presumably, could be demonstrated by the comparative thickness of the ketchup. In other words, their brand of ketchup was more viscous than some other brands of ketchup. For more on this analogy, including a video of a TV ad, see *Blood Viscosity and Peripheral Resistance* (my-ap.us/XiJCc7).

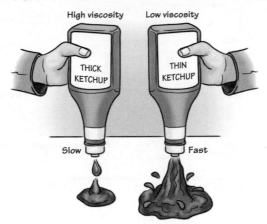

So, to summarize this analogy:

☑ More tomatoes per bottle of ketchup make the ketchup thicker or more viscous. *The higher the viscosity of ketchup, the more it resists flow* and thus the slower it will flow out the narrow neck of a tipped bottle.

☑ Likewise, more RBCs per drop of blood make the blood thicker or more viscous. *The higher the viscosity of blood, the more it resists flow.* This resistance can be significant where the blood vessels narrow at the peripheral vessels called arterioles.

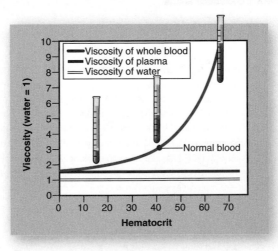

B. Lymphatic System

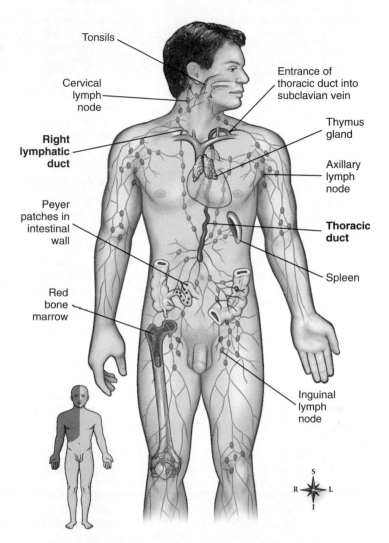

FIGURE 4-22 Principal Organs of the Lymphatic System. The inset shows the areas that are drained by the **right lymphatic duct(s)** in green and the areas that are drained by the **thoracic duct** in blue.

✳ **TABLE 4-8**   **Major Lymphatic Organs**

Organ	Structure	Function
Lymphatic vessels	Thin-walled vessels with numerous valves that ensure the one-way flow of lymphatic fluid (lymph); larger vessels have three layers (similar to veins)	Collect fluid that drains from the tissues of the body (lymph) and return it to the blood circulation
Lymphatic capillaries	Microscopic, blind-end vessels made up of a single endothelial layer with many gaps	Collect tissue fluid (forming lymph) Transport lymph to larger lymphatic vessels
Lymphatic ducts	Large lymphatic vessels formed by many tributaries throughout the body; connect to the subclavian veins	Collect lymph from the network of lymphatic vessels and drain it into the blood circulation
Lymphoid organs	Have a significant component of lymphoid tissue (developing white blood cells)	Hematopoiesis (WBCs) Immunity Filter body fluids
Lymph nodes	Fibrous capsule that surrounds a maze of sinuses, each with a lymphoid tissue nodule suspended by reticular fibers	Filtration of lymph before it enters the bloodstream Mechanical filtration: removing particles Biological filtration: cells destroy and remove particles
Aggregated lymph nodules (tonsils, Peyer patches)	Groupings of nodules (lumps of lymphoid tissue) embedded in mucous membranes	Provide immunity at common points of entry for pathogenic microbes
Thymus	Two pyramid-shaped lobes subdivided into smaller lobules that contain lymphoid tissue	Hematopoiesis: the site of T-lymphocyte (T-cell) development Hormone production: thymosin regulates T-cell development
Spleen	Ovoid fibrous capsule with internal maze of sinuses that contain dense lymphoid tissue (white pulp) surrounded by blood sinusoids with cords of lymphoid tissue (red pulp)	Hematopoiesis (WBCs) Immunity Filtration of blood Tissue repair Destruction of old RBCs and platelets Blood reservoir

RBC, Red blood cell; *WBC*, white blood cell.

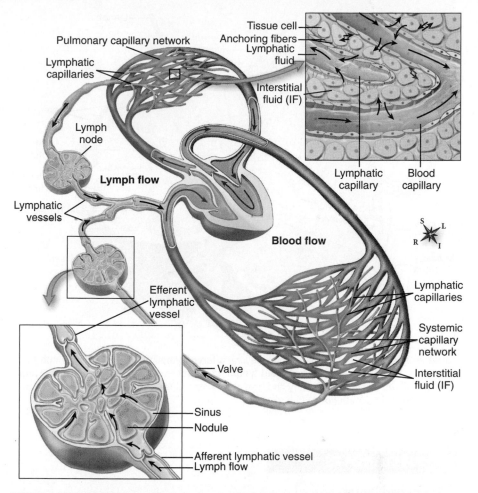

FIGURE 4-23 Role of the Lymphatic System in Fluid Balance. Fluid from plasma flowing through the capillaries moves into the interstitial spaces. Although *most* of this **interstitial fluid (IF)** is either absorbed by tissue cells or reabsorbed by capillaries, *some* of the fluid tends to accumulate in the interstitial spaces. As this fluid builds up, it tends to drain into the **lymphatic vessels**, where it is called **lymph** or *lymphatic fluid*. Lymph is "cleaned up" by **lymph nodes** and eventually returns to the venous blood.

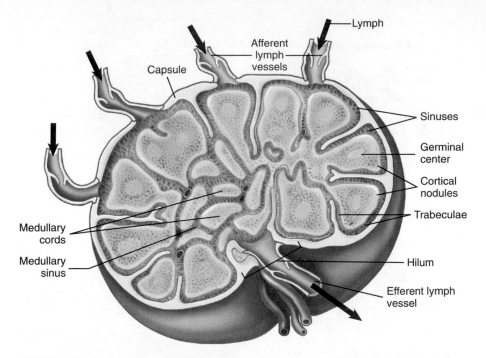

FIGURE 4-24 Structure of a Lymph Node. Several **afferent lymphatic vessels** bring lymph to the node. In this example, a single **efferent lymphatic vessel** leaves the node at a concave area called the **hilum.** Note that the artery and vein also enter and leave at the hilum. Arrows show the direction of the lymph flow.

✦ FIELD NOTES

Sewers and Drains

The overall role of the lymphatic system in the body is always a little confusing for beginning students. Perhaps because we don't hear much about this system in our culture, the way we do with nearly all of the other parts of the body.

It really is pretty easy to understand, however. The best way to look at the role of the lymphatic system is to use the analogy of the system of storm drains and sewage treatment in a city.

Let's start with the city. It rains, and the rain soaks into the ground, evaporates, or runs off into the local rivers and streams. Then the water proceeds through the water cycle. Remember the water cycle from middle school science class? It's the idea that water all eventually gets back into the clouds and returns as rain.

However, some of the rain falls on the streets, roofs, and parking lots and doesn't soak into the ground, and it doesn't all evaporate. Instead, it runs off into drains and sewers scattered around the city. If we didn't have such drainage networks, any good rain would flood streets and homes and make a big mess all around.

Where does all that drained water go? It goes through a network of drainpipes that conduct the wastewater off toward the sewage treatment plants. Some cities don't send all wastewater to a treatment plant, but they should. At the wastewater treatment plant, the chunks of stuff that have been carried along by the storm runoff are filtered out (**mechanical filtration** or *primary filtration*),

◆ FIELD NOTES—cont'd

and bacteria convert chemical wastes into something harmless (**biological filtration** or *secondary filtration*).

Next, the cleaned-up wastewater goes out of the treatment plant and into the local river or lake. Now it's back in the water cycle, and it will someday return as rain.

Likewise, the tissues of the body are constantly being rained on by fluids that are leaving the blood capillaries. That water becomes **interstitial fluid (IF).** Some of it is used by cells, and some of it diffuses or filters back into the bloodstream. However, some of it collects in drains—these are the **lymphatic capillaries.** This prevents "flooding" or swelling (edema) of tissues. Once it is in the lymphatic system, the runoff IF is called **lymphatic fluid** or simply *lymph.*

The lymph collects within larger lymphatic vessels (like larger drainpipes) and goes to small little wastewater treatment plants called **lymph nodes.** As it passes through a lymph node, the lymph is *mechanically filtered* and *biologically filtered.* Thus, the lymph that leaves the lymph node is relatively free of damaged cells or cell parts, bacteria, cancer cells, and so on. The cleaned-up lymph then moves into larger and larger **lymphatic vessels** until it is eventually dumped into the bloodstream (via a *subclavian vein*).

Thus, the fluid that started out as blood plasma became IF, became lymph, and is now returned to the bloodstream again. The lymphatic system completes the body's form of the "water cycle" in a way that not only constantly recycles water but that also prevents the swelling or **edema** of tissues.

C. Immunity

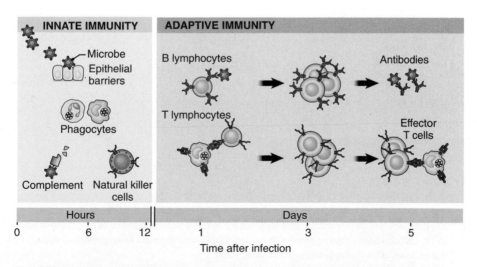

FIGURE 4-25 Innate and Adaptive Immunity. Innate *(nonspecific)* **immune mechanisms** are "built in" and ready for action, thereby providing the initial defense against infections and other assaults on the body. **Adaptive** *(specific)* **immune mechanisms** develop later, as lymphocytes are activated to work against specific foreign or abnormal cells and particles. The time frames are generalizations.

✳ TABLE 4-9 Innate and Adaptive Immunity

		Innate Immunity	Adaptive Immunity
Synonyms	Frequently used alternate terminology	Nonspecific immunity, native immunity, genetic immunity	Specific immunity, acquired immunity
Characteristics			
Specificity	Unique antigens produce unique responses of the immune system	Not specific; recognizes a variety of different groups of foreign cells or particles	Specific; recognizes specific antigens on specific cells or particles
Speed of reaction	Reaction time of the immune responses	Rapid: immediate or up to several hours	Slower: several hours to several days
Memory	Enhanced responses to repeated exposures to the same antigen	None	Yes
Does not react to self	Prevents injury to the individual's own cells*	Yes	Yes
Components			
Barriers	Prevent the entry of harmful particles	Skin, mucosa, antimicrobial chemicals	Lymphocytes in the epithelia; antibodies released at epithelial surfaces
Blood proteins	Circulate throughout the body to provide a wide area of protection	Complement, interferon (IFN), others	Antibodies
Cells	Types of leukocytes involved in immunity	Phagocytes (macrophages, neutrophils), natural killer (NK) cells	Lymphocytes (B cells and T cells)

*Assumes healthy function. Anti-self immunity (autoimmunity) is a characteristic of many disorders.

◈ FIELD NOTES

Patton's Army

I have an army inside of me—and so do you! It's the immune system. All immunologists use the "military model" when thinking about how our immune defenses work. If you think very broadly about military function—including defending against invaders from outside as well as troublemakers inside, restoring balance during times of injury and disaster, and generally keeping order—*military science serves as an excellent model of immune function.*

Agents of the immune system are not just ready on a moment's notice; they are *continually* patrolling the body for foreign or internal enemies and shoring up the various lines of defense to fend off a possible attack. Before you begin studying the specifics of immunity, let's spend a moment mapping out the overall defensive strategy of the immune system.

◆ FIELD NOTES—cont'd

First, it is important to recognize that cells, viruses, and other particles have unique molecules and groups of molecules on their surfaces that can be used to identify them. These molecular markers visible to the immune system are called **antigens.** This is similar to military operations in which enemy aircraft, vehicles, or soldiers can be identified by their distinctive insignia that are different from the insignia seen on "our side." Likewise, our own cells have unique cell markers embedded in our plasma membranes that identify each of our cells as **self**—that is, belonging to us as an individual. And foreign cells or particles have **nonself** molecules that serve as recognition markers for our immune system. The ability of our immune system to attack abnormal or foreign cells but spare our own normal cells is called **self-tolerance.**

In human society, any good security force employs numerous and varied strategies to guard its territory and take action if necessary. So, too, does the body's "society of cells" employ a system that uses many different kinds of mechanisms to ensure the integrity and survival of the internal environment. All of these defense mechanisms can be categorized into one of two major categories of immune mechanisms: **innate immunity** and **adaptive immunity.**

Innate immunity is called such because it is "in place" before a person is exposed to a particular harmful particle or condition. The word *innate* refers to something that is already present naturally at birth. Because it includes mechanisms that resist a wide variety of threatening agents or conditions, innate immunity is also called **nonspecific immunity.** The term *nonspecific* implies that these immune mechanisms do not act on only one or two specific invaders but rather provide a more general defense by simply acting against a wide variety of particles recognized as *nonself.*

Going back to the military analogy, innate immune strategies are like the "general purpose" strategies a soldier may learn during basic training: sounding alarms and responding to alarms, communications and codes, rescue techniques, use of basic weapons, and other strategies commonly used in a variety of combat conditions.

Adaptive immunity, on the other hand, involves mechanisms that recognize *specific* threatening agents and then *adapt,* or respond, by targeting their activity against these agents—and these agents only. Because it targets only specific harmful particles, adaptive immunity is also called **specific immunity.** Adaptive immune strategies can be compared with specialized military strategies that have been developed to combat specific enemies.

Adaptive immune mechanisms often take some time to recognize their targets and react with sufficient force to overcome the threat, at least on their first exposure to a specific kind of threatening agent. Innate mechanisms, because they are already in place, have the advantage of being able to meet an enemy as soon as it presents itself. In **antibody-mediated immunity,** lymphocytes called **B cells** "shoot guided missiles" at specific enemy particles—plasma proteins called **antibodies** or *immunoglobulins.* In *cell-mediated immunity,* lymphocytes called *T cells* engage in "hand-to-hand combat" by latching onto abnormal cells and killing them. T cells often use chemical "knives" to puncture a cell as well as "poisons" to do further damage.

As you study the immune system, you will come to appreciate the value in having many complementary "military" strategies for defending the body.

✳ TABLE 4-10   Mechanisms of Innate Defense

Mechanism	Description
Species Resistance	Genetic characteristics of the human species protect the body from certain pathogens
Mechanical and Chemical Barriers	Physical impediments to the entry of foreign cells or substances
Skin and mucosa	Form a continuous wall that separates the internal environment from the external environment, thereby preventing the entry of pathogens
Secretions	Secretions such as sebum, mucus, acids, and enzymes chemically inhibit the activity of pathogens
Inflammation	The inflammatory response isolates the pathogens and stimulates the speedy arrival of large numbers of immune cells
Fever	Fever may enhance immune reactions and inhibit pathogens
Phagocytosis	Ingestion and destruction of pathogens by phagocytic cells
Neutrophils	Granular leukocytes that are usually the first phagocytic cell to arrive at the scene of an inflammatory response
Macrophages	Monocytes that have enlarged to become giant phagocytic cells capable of consuming many pathogens; often called by other, more specific names when found in specific tissues of the body
Natural Killer (NK) Cells	Group of lymphocytes that kill many different types of cancer cells and virus-infected cells
Interferon	Protein produced by cells after they become infected by a virus; inhibits the spread or further development of a viral infection
Complement	Group of plasma proteins (inactive enzymes) that produce a cascade of chemical reactions that ultimately causes the lysis (rupture) of a foreign cell; the complement cascade can be triggered by adaptive or innate immune mechanisms
Toll-like Receptors (TLRs)	Membrane receptors that recognize nonspecific patterns in microbial molecules (not human molecules) and that trigger a variety of innate immune responses (many of those listed in this table)

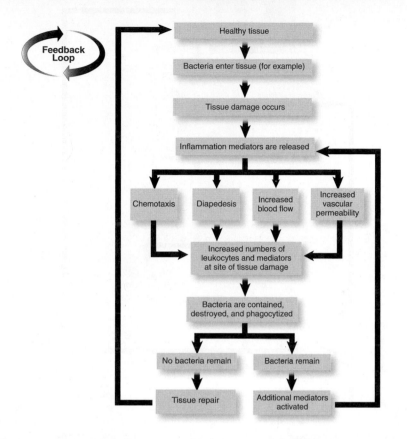

FIGURE 4-26 Example of the Inflammatory Response. Tissue damage caused by bacteria triggers a series of events that produces the inflammatory response and that promotes phagocytosis at the site of injury. These responses tend to inhibit or destroy the bacteria, eventually bringing the tissue back to its healthy state. Similar reactions will occur in the presence of other abnormal or injurious particles or conditions.

✳ TABLE 4-11   Four Classic Signs of Inflammation

English	Latin*	Mechanisms†
Redness	*Rubor*	Increased blood flow to the site of injury; pooling of blood at the site of injury
Heat	*Calor*	Increased blood flow to the injury site from deeper, warmer tissues; body-wide fever may also occur when chemical mediators (**pyrogens**) reset the body's set point temperature
Swelling	*Tumor*	Increased permeability of vessels at the site of injury causes the buildup of interstitial fluid (**edema**); increased blood flow around the injury site contributes to swelling; fibrin clot formation occurs in affected tissues
Pain	*Dolor*	Chemical mediators such as **kinins** (especially bradykinin) can trigger pain; swelling can trigger pain

*The Latin terms are sometimes used in clinical practice.
†Some of these mechanisms can also be seen in Figure 4-26.

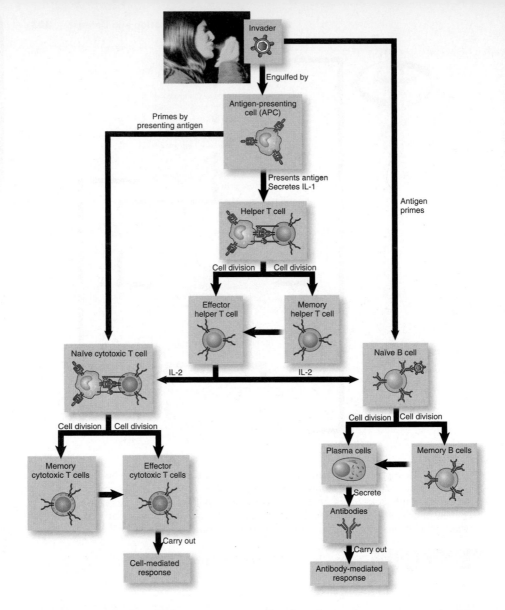

FIGURE 4-27 Summary of Adaptive Immunity. A flowchart that summarizes an example of the adaptive immune response when an individual is exposed to a microbial pathogen.

✳ TABLE 4-12	Types of Adaptive Immunity
Type	**Description or Example**
Natural Immunity	Exposure to the causative agent is not deliberate
Active (exposure)	A child develops measles and acquires an immunity to a subsequent infection
Passive (exposure)	A fetus receives protection from the mother through the placenta, or an infant receives protection through the mother's milk

✴ **TABLE 4-12**	**Types of Adaptive Immunity—cont'd**

Type	Description or Example
Artificial Immunity	Exposure to the causative agent is deliberate
Active (exposure)	Injection of the causative agent, such as a vaccination against polio, confers immunity
Passive (exposure)	Injection of protective material (antibodies) that was developed by another individual's immune system confers immunity

D. Stress

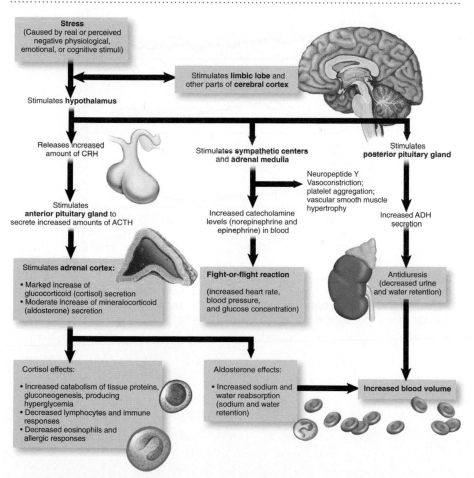

FIGURE 4-28 Summary of the Stress Syndrome. Some effects are immediate, such as the sympathetic **fight-or-flight reaction,** and some effects are longer term, such as the hormonal effects.
ACTH, Adrenocorticotropic hormone; *ADH,* antidiuretic hormone; *CRH,* corticotropin-releasing hormone.

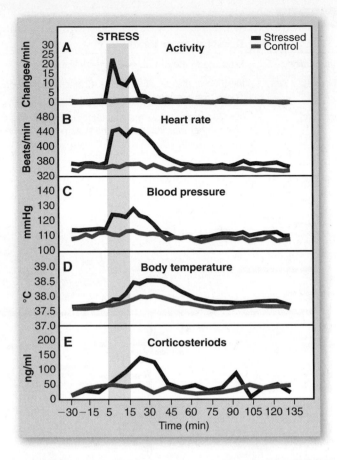

FIGURE 4-29 Stress Indicators. Graphs showing a variety of physiological changes in mice when presented with the following stressors: **A,** increased movements; **B,** elevated heart rate; **C,** elevated blood pressure; **D,** elevated body temperature; and **E,** increased plasma corticosteroids. Similar stress responses occur in all mammals.

◈ FIELD NOTES

The Load of Stress

Stress, in a physiological sense, is anything that is perceived as a threat to the homeostatic balance of the body. According to a current operational definition, stress can include any stimulus that directly or indirectly stimulates neurons of the *hypothalamus* to release *corticotropin-releasing hormone (CRH).* CRH acts as a trigger that initiates many diverse changes in the body (see Figure 4-28). Together, these changes constitute a collection of signs and symptoms commonly called the **stress syndrome.**

The term **allostasis** is sometimes used to refer to the body's attempts to reestablish homeostatic balance while under stress. The word part *allo-* means "different." One can think of allostasis as the body's coping mechanisms when things are different. **Allostatic load** refers to the broad effects of allostasis on the body, such as increased energy expenditure, alterations of neural and endocrine mechanisms, and changes in behavior. One can think of allostatic load as the physiological load placed on the body as one copes with stress.

As the cartoon implies, one may be able to bear a large allostatic load—or stress load—but it will take a lot of effort by the body, and it may put one at risk of a serious health threat.

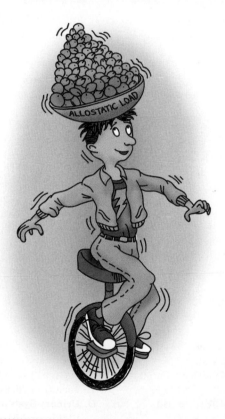

5 Respiration, Nutrition, and Excretion

Navigation Guide

A. Respiratory System

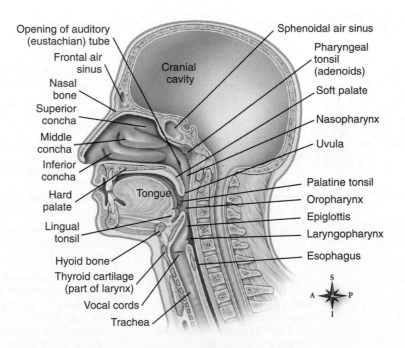

FIGURE 5-1 Sagittal Section of the Head and Neck. The upper respiratory structures are clearly visible. In the section through the nose and the nasal cavity, the nasal septum has been removed to reveal the turbinates (nasal conchae) of the lateral wall of the nasal cavity.

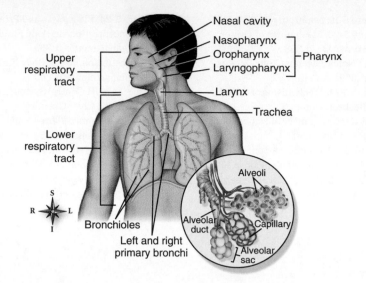

FIGURE 5-2 Structural Plan of the Respiratory System. The inset shows the alveolar sacs, where the interchange of oxygen (O_2) and **carbon dioxide (CO_2)** takes place through the walls of the grape-like **alveoli.**

✳ **TABLE 5-1**   **Summary of Respiratory Tract Structures***

Structure	Description	Functions
Upper respiratory tract	Portion of the respiratory tract outside of the thoracic cavity	Processing of incoming air Conducting of air to and from the lungs Vocalization and phonation Olfaction
Nasal cavity	Lumen of the nose, which is separated into left and right portions by the nasal septum Supported by cartilage, the vomer, the perpendicular plate of ethmoid, and the nasal conchae	Conducts air between the atmosphere (external environment) and the pharynx Warms, humidifies, and cleans inspired air
Anterior nares (external nares)	Nostrils (external openings of nasal cavity)	Boundary between the external environment and the nasal cavity
Vestibule	Extends from the anterior nares to the inferior meatus Supported by the cartilage of the septum and the ala Lined with skin epidermis (keratinized stratified squamous epithelium) that has vibrissae (hairs)	Conducts air between the external environment and the respiratory portion of the nasal cavity Vibrissae prevent the entry of large contaminants

✳ TABLE 5-1	Summary of Respiratory Tract Structures—cont'd	
Structure	**Description**	**Functions**
Respiratory portion	Extends from the vestibule to the posterior nares Supported by the bones of the septum and the nasal conchae, which curve to form meatuses Lined with highly vascular respiratory mucosa (pseudostratified ciliated columnar epithelium) Olfactory epithelium in the superior lining contains numerous sensory receptors	Conducts air between the vestibule and the pharynx Meatuses create turbulence to assist with the processing of inspired air Mucosa warms, humidifies, and cleans inspired air Olfaction
Paranasal sinuses	Four pairs of air-filled spaces within the frontal, maxillary, ethmoid, and sphenoid bones of the skull Lined with pseudostratified ciliated columnar epithelium Drain into the nasal cavity	Reduce weight of skull Help warm and humidify air
Posterior nares (internal nares)	Openings from the nasal cavity into the pharynx	Boundary between the nasal cavity and the pharynx
Pharynx	Throat Extends from the posterior nares to the esophagus Supported by the occipital bone and the skeletal muscle Lined with mucous membrane (nonkeratinized stratified squamous epithelium)	Conducts air between the nasal cavity and the larynx
Nasopharynx	Segment of the pharynx posterior to the nasal cavity Includes the pharyngeal tonsils in the posterior wall	Conducts air between the posterior nares and the oropharynx
Oropharynx	Segment of the pharynx posterior to the oral cavity Includes a pair of palatine tonsils in the lateral walls and the lingual tonsils in the anterior wall at the base of the tongue	Conducts air between the nasopharynx or oral cavity and the laryngopharynx
Laryngopharynx	Segment of the pharynx posterior to the opening of the larynx and superior to the opening of the esophagus	Conducts air between the oropharynx and the larynx
Tonsils	Ring of individual aggregations of lymphoid nodules	Immune protection of the respiratory and digestive mucosa

Continued

✳ TABLE 5-1	Summary of Respiratory Tract Structures—cont'd	
Structure	**Description**	**Functions**
Larynx	Voice box Extends from the laryngopharynx to the trachea Supported by nine cartilages that are connected by muscle and ligaments Lined with mucosa (pseudostratified ciliated columnar epithelium, except the epiglottis and the vocal folds)	Conducts air between the pharynx and the trachea Prevents food from entering the lower airways Vocalization Ciliary escalator removes contaminants
Epiglottis	Flexible "lid" of the larynx Covered and lined with nonkeratinized stratified squamous epithelium that transitions through simple columnar epithelium to pseudostratified ciliated columnar epithelium at the border with the vestibule	Flexes during swallowing to cover the larynx and to prevent food from entering the lower airways
Vestibule	Extends from the base of the epiglottis to the vestibular folds	Conducts air between the pharynx and the vestibular folds
Vestibular folds (false vocal folds)	Superior pair of lateral mucosal folds	Slow contaminants that are dripping toward the lower airways
Ventricle (laryngeal ventricle)	Space between the vestibular folds and the vocal folds	Conducts air among the mucosal folds of the larynx
Vocal folds (true vocal folds or vocal cords)	Inferior pair of lateral mucosal folds Each fold is supported by skeletal muscle and strong vocal ligaments at the medial edge Covered with nonkeratinized stratified squamous epithelium Glottis includes vocal folds and the spaces between them (rima glottidis)	Prevent contaminants from entering the lower airways Produce vibrations when pulled together during expiration (vocalization)
Infraglottic cavity	Segment below the glottis, between the vocal folds and the trachea	Conducts air between the vocal folds and the trachea

✳ TABLE 5-1	Summary of Respiratory Tract Structures—cont'd	
Structure	**Description**	**Functions**
Lower respiratory tract	Portion of respiratory tract within the thoracic cavity Also called the *bronchial tree*	Conducts air to and from the gas-exchange tissues of the lungs
Trachea	Windpipe Extends from the larynx to the primary bronchi Supported by C-shaped cartilage rings Lined with respiratory mucosa (pseudostratified ciliated columnar epithelium)	Conducts air between the larynx and the bronchi Ciliary escalator removes contaminants
Bronchi	Tree-like branching of airways 23 levels of branching that produce a huge number of individual airways Supported by cartilage rings (incomplete outside of the lungs, complete inside of the lungs) Lined with respiratory mucosa (pseudostratified ciliated columnar epithelium)	Conduct air between the trachea and the lungs Ciliary escalator removes contaminants
Primary bronchi	Left and right branches from trachea, with one going to each lung	Conduct air to and from the lungs
Secondary bronchi (lobar bronchi)	Branches of the primary bronchi: three from the right, two from the left	Conduct air to and from the lobes of the lungs
Tertiary bronchi (segmental bronchi)	Branches of the secondary bronchi	Conduct air to and from the various bronchopulmonary segments of the lungs
Bronchioles	Smallest branches (20 levels of branching)	Conduct air to and from the alveoli
Alveoli	Microscopic air spaces at the terminals of the bronchial tree Lined with simple squamous epithelium that joins with pulmonary capillary endothelium to form the respiratory membrane	Exchange of gases (CO_2, O_2) between the air and the pulmonary blood Surfactant that lines the alveoli prevents the collapse of air spaces

*Listed in order of air flow during inspiration.

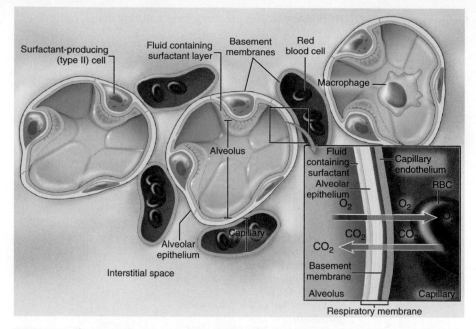

FIGURE 5-3 The Gas-Exchange Structures of the Lung. Each **alveolus** is continually ventilated with fresh air. The inset shows a magnified view of the **respiratory membrane,** which is composed of the alveolar wall (fluid coating, epithelial cells, and basement membrane), the interstitial fluid, and the wall of a pulmonary capillary (basement membrane and endothelial cells). The gases—CO_2 (carbon dioxide) and O_2 (oxygen)—diffuse across the respiratory membrane.

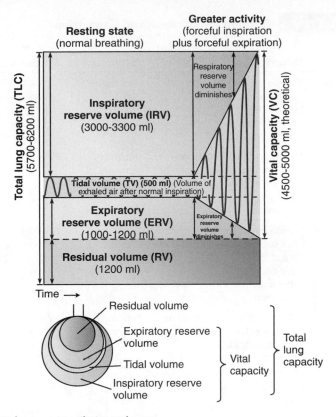

FIGURE 5-4 Pulmonary Ventilation Volumes.
A, Graph produced by a spirometer.
B, Figure showing the **pulmonary volumes** at rest as relative proportions of an inflated balloon. During normal, quiet respirations, the atmosphere and lungs exchange about 500 ml of air (**tidal volume [TV]**). With a forcible inspiration, about 3300 ml more air can be inhaled (**inspiratory reserve volume [IRV]**). After a normal inspiration and a normal expiration, approximately 1000 ml more air can be forcibly expired (**expiratory reserve volume [ERV]**). **Vital capacity (VC)** is the amount of air that can be forcibly expired after a maximal inspiration and therefore indicates the largest amount of air that can enter and leave the lungs during respiration. **Residual volume (RV)** is the air that remains trapped in the alveoli.

✳ TABLE 5-2   Pulmonary Volumes and Capacities

Volume	Description	Typical Value	Capacity	Formula	Typical Value
Tidal volume (TV)	Volume moved into or out of the respiratory tract during a normal respiratory cycle	500 ml	Vital capacity (VC)	TV + IRV + ERV	4500 to 5000 ml
Inspiratory reserve volume (IRV)	Maximum volume that can be moved into the respiratory tract after a normal inspiration	3000 to 3300 ml	Inspiratory capacity (IC)	TV + IRV	3500 to 3800 ml
Expiratory reserve volume (ERV)	Maximum volume that can be moved out of the respiratory tract after a normal expiration	1000 to 1200 ml	Functional residual capacity (FRC)	ERV + RV	2200 to 2400 ml
Residual volume (RV)	Volume that remains in the respiratory tract after maximum expiration	1200 ml	Total lung capacity (TLC)	TV + IRV + ERV + RV	5700 to 6200 ml

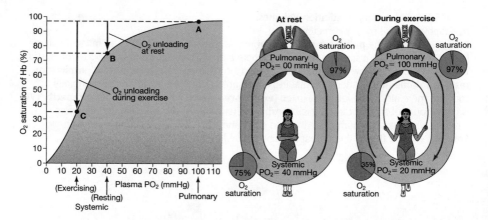

FIGURE 5-5 Oxyhemoglobin Dissociation Curve. This graph shows **oxygen (O_2)** unloading at rest and during exercise. At rest, fully saturated **hemoglobin (Hb)** unloads almost 25% of its O_2 load when it reaches the low **O_2 partial pressure (PO_2)** (40 mm Hg) environment in systemic tissues *(left)*. During exercise, the tissue PO_2 is even lower (20 mm Hg), thereby causing fully saturated Hb to unload about 70% of its O_2 load *(right)*. As you can see in the graph, a slight drop in tissue PO_2—from point B to point C—causes a large increase in O_2 unloading *(top)*.

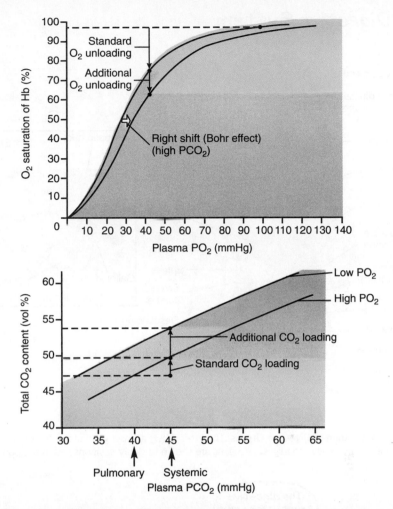

FIGURE 5-6 Interaction of Oxygen Partial Pressure and Carbon Dioxide Partial Pressure During Gas Transport by the Blood.
A, The increased **carbon dioxide partial pressure (PCO$_2$)** in systemic tissues decreases the affinity between **hemoglobin (Hb)** and **oxygen (O$_2$)**, which is shown as a right shift of the oxyhemoglobin dissociation curve. This phenomenon is known as the **Bohr effect.** A right shift can also be caused by a decrease in plasma pH or an increase in temperature.
B, At the same time, the decreased **oxygen partial pressure (PO$_2$)** commonly observed in systemic tissues increases the carbon dioxide (CO$_2$) content of the blood, shown as a left shift of the CO$_2$ dissociation curve. This phenomenon is known as the **Haldane effect.**

B. Digestive System

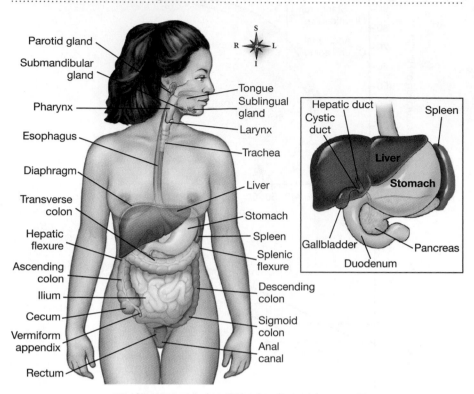

FIGURE 5-7 Location of Digestive Organs. The inset shows a closer view of the upper abdominal organs. A few nondigestive organs are shown to clarify positions within the body.

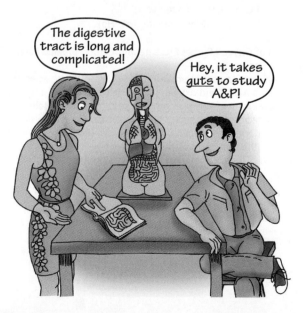

✳ TABLE 5-3	Modifications of Layers of the Digestive Tract Wall		
Organ	**Mucosa**	**Muscularis**	**Serosa**
Esophagus	Stratified squamous epithelium that resists abrasion	Has two layers: an inner one made of circular fibers and an outer one made of longitudinal fibers; includes striated muscle in the upper part and smooth muscle in the lower part of the esophagus and in the rest of the tract	Outer layer is fibrous (adventitia); serous serosa is found around the part of the esophagus in the thoracic cavity
Stomach	Arranged in flexible longitudinal folds called *rugae;* allows for distention; contains gastric pits with microscopic gastric glands	Has three layers instead of the usual two: circular, longitudinal, and oblique fibers; also includes two sphincters: the lower esophageal sphincter at the entrance of the stomach and the pyloric sphincter at its exit, both of which are formed by circular fibers	Outer layer is the visceral peritoneum; it hangs in a double fold from the lower edge of the stomach over the intestines and forms an apron-like structure (greater omentum); the lesser omentum connects the stomach to the liver
Small intestine	Contains permanent circular folds (plicae circulares), microscopic finger-like projections, villi with a brush border, crypts of Lieberkühn, microscopic duodenal (Brunner) mucous glands, aggregated lymphoid nodules (Peyer patches), and numerous single lymphoid nodules called *solitary nodules*	Has two layers: an inner one made of circular fibers and an outer one made of longitudinal fibers	Outer layer is the visceral peritoneum, which is continuous with the mesentery
Large intestine (colon)	Solitary lymph nodes and intestinal mucous glands; anal columns form in the anal region	The outer longitudinal layer is condensed to form three tape-like strips (taeniae coli); the inner circular layer is condensed to form small sacs (haustra) that give the rest of the wall a puckered appearance; internal anal sphincters are formed by circular smooth fibers; and external anal sphincters are formed by striated fibers	Outer layer is the visceral peritoneum, which is continuous with the mesocolon

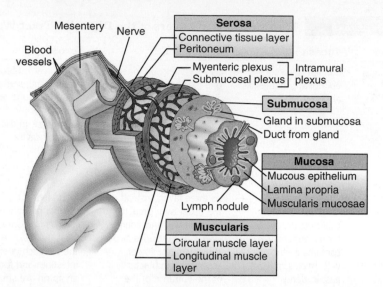

FIGURE 5-8 Wall of the Gastrointestinal Tract. The wall of the **gastrointestinal (GI) tract** is made up of four layers, which are shown here in a generalized diagram of a segment of the GI tract. Notice that the **serosa** is continuous, with a fold of serous membrane called a **mesentery.** Notice also that the digestive glands may empty their products into the lumen of the GI tract by way of ducts.

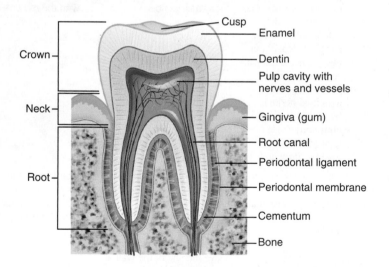

FIGURE 5-9 Typical Tooth. A molar tooth that has been sectioned to show its bony socket and details of its three main parts: the **crown**, the **neck**, and the **root. Enamel** *(over the crown)* and **cementum** *(over the neck and root)* surround the **dentin** layer. The **pulp** contains nerves and blood vessels.

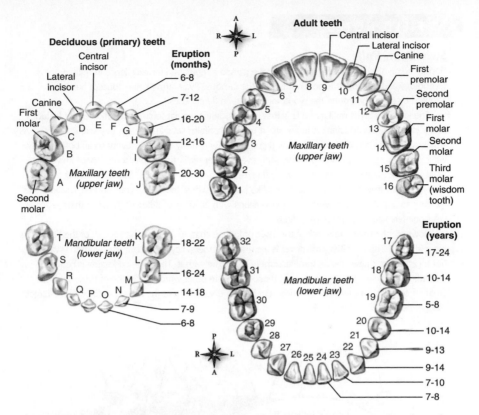

FIGURE 5-10 Dentition. In the **deciduous** (baby teeth) set, where letters are used in place of numbers, there are no premolars and only two pairs of molars in each jaw. Generally, the lower teeth erupt before the corresponding upper teeth.

✳ **TABLE 5-4**	**Dentition**	
	Number per Jaw	
Name of Tooth	**Deciduous Set**	**Permanent Set**
Central incisors	2	2
Lateral incisors	2	2
Canines (cuspids)	2	2
Premolars (bicuspids)	0	4
First molars (tricuspids)	2	2
Second molars	2	2
Third molars (wisdom teeth)	0	2
Total (per jaw)	10	16
Total (per set)	20	32

◆ FIELD NOTES

Swiss Army Knife

Despite being officially neutral, the Swiss have gained a reputation for excellence in military technology and training. It is no wonder that the famous "Swiss army knife" concept has been adopted by so many around the world for so many different uses.

The idea of a Swiss military knife is that it is basically a regular folding pocketknife that includes many extra gadgets. In addition to a knife, it usually contains several different tiny screwdrivers, a very small can opener, a miniature corkscrew (I guess the Swiss army is rationed very small bottles of Swiss wine with tiny corks), a tiny saw blade, and several other really tiny implements. These knives are great because they are easy to carry around (except into secure buildings) but have the capabilities of a wide assortment of different tools. It's like having a whole tool set in your pocket! This idea has become so popular that now you can get versions with all kinds of different things in them, such as laser pointers and other modern gadgets.

However, the main drawback of this style of knife is that, to make it "handy," all of the little tools are really tiny. The itty-bitty screwdriver is great for an emergency repair, but you wouldn't want to put together your new "needs some assembly" furniture with it. That little corkscrew is cool, but would a wine steward really use one of those? Nope. In other words, each one of those tools is great for occasional use while "traveling light," but it does not have the full capabilities of the larger, independent version of the tool.

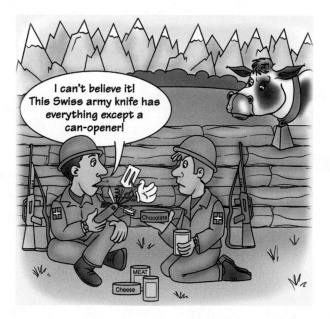

This is analogous to the dentition of the human mouth. The dentition is the type and number of teeth that are found in an organism.

Human dentition is outlined in Figure 5-10 and listed in Table 5-4. Humans are classified as omnivores, which means that we have the ability to eat and digest a wide variety of different organisms: plants, animals, fungi, and more. Herbivores have a different sort of dentition, because they mainly eat plants. Therefore, herbivores like horses and rabbits have really big incisors for biting off plants and really broad, flat molars for grinding them up. Carnivores have the sort of dentition that is needed for eating mainly animals. Carnivores like cats and dogs have really small incisors but really big, pointed canines for killing animals and tearing meat. Their premolars and molars are like saw blades for cutting through meat and bone.

Humans, being omnivores, have a sort of *Swiss-army-knife dentition*. In other words, we have one of everything that both the herbivores and the carnivores have, but none of our teeth are very capable in comparison. For example, our incisors can bite off a carrot but not a tree limb. Our canines can help rip the meat from barbeque ribs but not the thigh muscles of an antelope. Our molars can grind up some salad but not raw whole oats (at least not very effectively). Basically, our mouth holds a variety of moderately useful tools. This analogy also helps us to understand the role of teeth: they are tools. Think about how you use the different types of teeth in your mouth for biting and chewing.

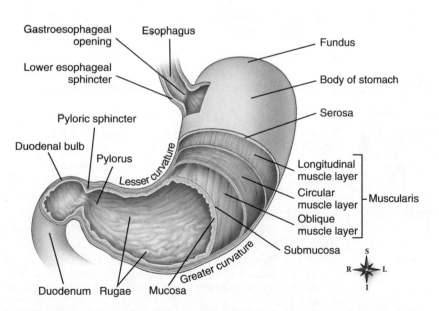

FIGURE 5-11 Stomach. A portion of the anterior wall has been cut away to reveal the muscle layers of the stomach wall. Notice that the mucosa lining the stomach forms folds called **rugae.**

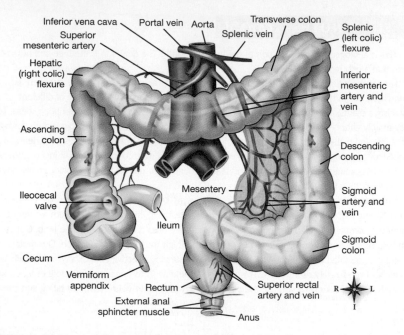

FIGURE 5-12 Divisions of the Large Intestine. An illustration that shows the divisions of the large intestine and the adjacent vascular structures.

✳ TABLE 5-5	Primary Mechanisms of the Digestive System
Mechanism	**Description**
Ingestion	The process of taking food into the mouth and starting it on its journey through the digestive tract
Digestion	A group of processes that break complex nutrients into simpler ones, thereby facilitating their absorption; mechanical digestion physically breaks large chunks into small bits; chemical digestion breaks molecules apart
Motility	Movement by the muscular components of the digestive tube, including processes of mechanical digestion; examples include peristalsis and segmentation
Secretion	The release of digestive juices that contain enzymes, acids, bases, mucus, bile, or other products that facilitate digestion; some digestive organs also secrete endocrine hormones that regulate digestion or the metabolism of nutrients
Absorption	The movement of digested nutrients through the gastrointestinal (GI) mucosa and into the internal environment
Elimination	The excretion of the residues of the digestive process (feces) from the rectum, through the anus; defecation
Regulation	The coordination of digestive activity (e.g., motility, secretion)

✳ **TABLE 5-6** Processes of Mechanical Digestion

Organ	Mechanical Process	Nature of Process
Mouth (teeth and tongue)	Mastication	Chewing movements that reduce the size of food particles and mix them with saliva
	Deglutition	Swallowing; the movement of food from the mouth to the stomach
Pharynx	Deglutition	See above
Esophagus	Deglutition	See above
	Peristalsis	Rippling movements that squeeze food downward in the digestive tract; a constricted ring forms first in one section, then the next, and so on, thereby causing waves of contraction that spread along the entire canal
Stomach	Churning	Forward and backward movements (propulsion and retropulsion) of the gastric contents that mix food with gastric juices to form chyme
	Peristalsis	Wave that starts in the body of the stomach that occurs about three times per minute and that sweeps toward the closed pyloric sphincter; at intervals, strong peristaltic waves press chyme past the sphincter and into the duodenum
Small intestine	Segmentation (mixing contractions)	Forward and backward movement within segment of the intestine; the purpose is to mix food and digestive juices thoroughly and to bring all digested food into contact with intestinal mucosa to facilitate absorption; the purpose of peristalsis, on the other hand, is to propel the intestinal contents along the digestive tract
	Peristalsis	
Large intestine		
Colon	Segmentation	Churning movements within the haustral sacs
	Peristalsis	See above
Descending colon	Mass peristalsis	The entire contents are moved into the sigmoid colon and the rectum; this occurs three or four times a day, usually after a meal
Rectum	Defecation	Emptying of rectum; "bowel movement"

TABLE 5-7   Chemical Digestion

Digestive Juices and Enzymes	Substance Digested or Hydrolyzed	Resulting Product*
Saliva		
Amylase (ptyalin)	Starch (polysaccharide)	Maltose (disaccharide)
Gastric Juice		
Protease (pepsin)† plus hydrochloric acid	Proteins	Partially digested proteins
Pancreatic Juice		
Proteases (e.g., trypsin)‡	Proteins (intact or partially digested)	Peptides and **amino acids**
Lipases	Fats emulsified by bile	**Fatty acids, monoglycerides,** and **glycerol**
Amylase	Starch	Maltose
Nucleases	Nucleic acids (DNA, RNA)	Nucleotides
Intestinal Enzymes§		
Peptidases	Peptides	**Amino acids**
Sucrase	Sucrose (cane sugar)	**Glucose** and **fructose**¶ (monosaccharides)
Lactase	Lactose (milk sugar)	**Glucose** and **galactose** (monosaccharides)
Maltase	Maltose (malt sugar)	**Glucose**
Nucleotidases and phosphatases	Nucleotides	Nucleosides

*Substances in **boldface type** are end products of digestion (i.e., completely digested nutrients that are ready for absorption).
†Secreted in an inactive form (pepsinogen); activated by low pH (hydrochloric acid).
‡Secreted in an inactive form (trypsinogen); activated by enterokinase, an enzyme that is found in the intestinal brush border.
§Brush-border enzymes.
¶Glucose is also called *dextrose*; fructose is also called *levulose*.

✳ TABLE 5-8   Digestive Secretions

Digestive Juice	Source	Substance	Functional Role*
Saliva	Salivary glands	Mucus	*Lubricates bolus of food; facilitates mixing of food*
		Amylase (ptyalin)	**Enzyme; begins digestion of starches**
		Sodium bicarbonate	Increases pH (for optimum amylase function)
		Water	*Dilutes food and other substances; facilitates mixing*
Gastric juice	Gastric glands	Pepsin	**Enzyme; digests proteins**
		Hydrochloric acid	Denatures proteins; decreases pH (for optimum pepsin function)
		Intrinsic factor	**Protects and allows later absorption of vitamin B$_{12}$**
		Mucus	*Lubricates chyme; protects stomach lining*
		Water	*Dilutes food and other substances; facilitates mixing*
Pancreatic juice	Pancreas (exocrine portion)	Proteases (e.g., trypsin, chymotrypsin, collagenase, elastase)	**Enzymes; digest proteins and polypeptides**
		Lipases (e.g., lipase, phospholipase)	**Enzymes; digest lipids**
		Colipase	**Coenzyme; helps lipase digest fats**
		Nucleases	**Enzymes; digest nucleic acids (RNA and DNA)**
		Amylase	**Enzyme; digests starches**
		Water	*Dilutes food and other substances; facilitates mixing*
		Mucus	*Lubricates*
		Sodium bicarbonate	**Increases pH** (for optimum enzyme function)

Continued

✳ **TABLE 5-8**   **Digestive Secretions—cont'd**

Digestive Juice	Source	Substance	Functional Role*
Bile	Liver (stored and concentrated in gallbladder)	Lecithin and bile salts	*Emulsify lipids*
		Sodium bicarbonate	**Increases pH** (for optimum enzyme function)
		Cholesterol	Excess cholesterol from body cells; excreted with feces
		Products of detoxification	From detoxification of harmful substances by hepatic cells; excreted with feces
		Bile pigments (mainly bilirubin)	Products of breakdown of heme groups during hemolysis; excreted with feces
		Mucus	*Lubrication*
		Water	Dilutes food and other substances; facilitates mixing
Intestinal juice	Mucosa of small and large intestine	Mucus	*Lubrication*
		Sodium bicarbonate	**Increases pH** (for optimum enzyme function)
		Water	Small amount to carry mucus and sodium bicarbonate

*__Boldface type__ indicates a chemical digestive process; *italic type* indicates a mechanical process.

✳ **TABLE 5-9**   **Actions of Some Digestive Hormones Summarized**

Hormone	Source	Action
Gastrin	Secreted by the gastric mucosa in the presence of partially digested proteins when stimulated by the vagus nerve or when the stomach is stretched	Stimulates the secretion of gastric juice that is rich in pepsin and hydrochloric acid
Gastric inhibitory peptide (GIP)	Secreted by the intestinal mucosa in the presence of glucose, fats, and perhaps other nutrients	Inhibits gastric secretion and motility; enhances insulin secretion by the pancreas
Secretin	Secreted by the intestinal mucosa in the presence of acid, partially digested proteins, and fats	Inhibits gastric secretion; stimulates the secretion of pancreatic juice that is low in enzymes and high in alkalinity (bicarbonate); enhances the effects of CCK
Cholecystokinin (CCK)	Secreted by the intestinal mucosa in the presence of fats, partially digested proteins, and acids	Stimulates the ejection of bile from the gallbladder and the secretion of pancreatic juice that is high in enzymes; relaxes the sphincters that regulate flow from the common bile duct; opposes the action of gastrin, thereby raising the pH of gastric juice

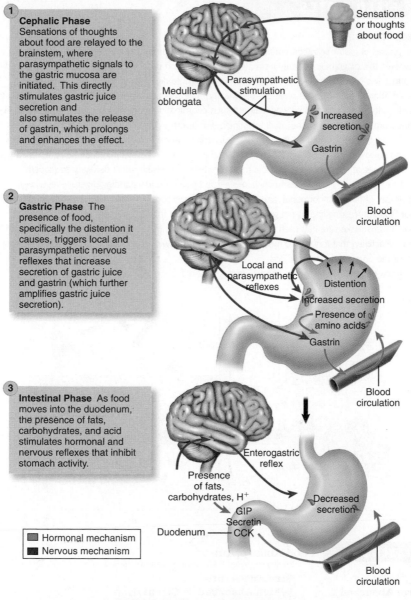

1

Cephalic Phase Sensations of thoughts about food are relayed to the brainstem, where parasympathetic signals to the gastric mucosa are initiated. This directly stimulates gastric juice secretion and also stimulates the release of gastrin, which prolongs and enhances the effect.

Sensations or thoughts about food

Parasympathetic stimulation

Medulla oblongata

Increased secretion

Gastrin

Blood circulation

2

Gastric Phase The presence of food, specifically the distention it causes, triggers local and parasympathetic nervous reflexes that increase secretion of gastric juice and gastrin (which further amplifies gastric juice secretion).

Local and parasympathetic reflexes

Distention

Increased secretion

Presence of amino acids

Gastrin

Blood circulation

3

Intestinal Phase As food moves into the duodenum, the presence of fats, carbohydrates, and acid stimulates hormonal and nervous reflexes that inhibit stomach activity.

Enterogastric reflex

Presence of fats, carbohydrates, H$^+$

GIP
Secretin
CCK

Duodenum

Decreased secretion

Blood circulation

☐ Hormonal mechanism
■ Nervous mechanism

FIGURE 5-13 Phases of Gastric Secretion.

◇ **FIELD NOTES**

Keep It Moving

The phases of gastric secretion outlined in Figure 5-13 seem pretty complicated at first glance. However, this diagram is not only a simplification of a much more complex process than shown but also just one of many examples of regulation in the whole digestive tract.

What are the advantages of all this complexity? The short answer is that it helps us to keep things moving along in a coordinated way. Without such coordination, your midday meal might be whisked along from the stomach to the small intestine before room exists to receive it. In addition, when the meal does begin moving from the stomach, you don't want it to all move at once—the intestines are too narrow to handle it. You also need to make sure that digestive juices are being released into the intestines at the same time that the meal is entering, or else it won't be digested properly.

The analogy of a factory assembly line is a good one for understanding digestive regulation. A number of nervous, hormonal, and local regulatory mechanisms make sure that one part of your "food-processing line" is not going faster than the part that comes next. In addition, these mechanisms make sure that each process has the secretions that it needs to be effective, the motility (muscle activity) that it needs to move things along (or to swish them around a little), and the proper pH for the enzymes to do their jobs.

Think of this analogy as you review Figure 5-13 and Table 5-9.

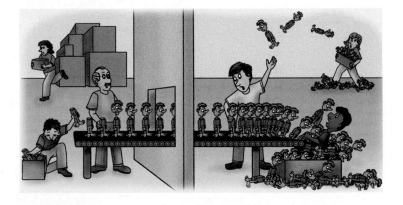

✳ **TABLE 5-10**   Food Absorption

Form Absorbed	Structures into Which Absorbed	Circulation
Protein, as amino acids Perhaps minute quantities of some short-chain polypeptides and whole proteins are absorbed (e.g., some antibodies)	Blood in the intestinal capillaries	Portal vein, liver, hepatic vein, inferior vena cava to heart, and so on
Carbohydrates, as simple sugars	Same as amino acids	Same as amino acids

✳ **TABLE 5-10**	Food Absorption—cont'd	
Form Absorbed	**Structures into Which Absorbed**	**Circulation**
Fats		
Glycerol and monoglycerides	Lymph in the intestinal lacteals	During absorption (i.e., while in epithelial cells of the intestinal mucosa), glycerol and fatty acids recombine to form microscopic packages of fats (chylomicrons); lymphatics carry them by way of the thoracic duct to the left subclavian vein, the superior vena cava, the heart, and so on; some fats are transported by blood in the form of phospholipids or cholesterol esters
Fatty acids combine with bile salts to form water-soluble substances	Lymph in the intestinal lacteals	
Some finely emulsified, undigested fats are absorbed	A small fraction enters the intestinal blood capillaries	

Mouth
Breaks up food particles
Assists in producing spoken language

Salivary glands
Saliva moistens and lubricates food
Amylase digests polysaccharides

Pharynx
Swallows

Esophagus
Transports food

Liver
Breaks down and builds up many biological molecules
Stores vitamins and iron
Destroys old blood cells
Destroys poisons
Bile aids in digestion

Stomach
Stores and churns food
Pepsin digests protein
HCl activates enzymes, breaks up food, kills germs
Mucus protects stomach wall
Limited absorption

Gallbladder
Stores and concentrates bile

Pancreas
Hormones regulate blood glucose levels
Bicarbonates neutralize stomach acid
Trypsin and chymotrypsin digest proteins
Amylase digests polysaccharides
Lipase digests lipids
Nucleases digest RNA and DNA

Small intestine
Completes digestion
Mucus protects gut wall
Absorbs nutrients, most water
Peptidase digests proteins
Sucrases digest sugars
Nucleotidases and phosphatases digest nucleotides

Large intestine
Reabsorbs some water and ions
Forms and stores feces

Rectum
Stores and expels feces

Anus
Opening for elimination of feces

FIGURE 5-14 Summary of Digestive Function.

C. Nutrition and Metabolism

✳ TABLE 5-11   Amino Acids

Essential (Indispensable)	Nonessential (Dispensable)	Essential (Indispensable)	Nonessential (Dispensable)
Histidine (His)*	Alanine (Ala)	Threonine (Thr)	Glutamine (Gln)
Isoleucine (Ile)	Arginine (Arg)	Tryptophan (Trp)	Glycine (Gly)
Leucine (Leu)	Asparagine (Asn)	Valine (Val)	Proline (Pro)
Lysine (Lys)	Aspartic acid (Asp)		Selenocysteine (Sec)
Methionine (Met)	Cysteine (Cys)		Serine (Ser)
Phenylalanine (Phe)	Glutamic acid (Glu)		Tyrosine (Tyr)†

*Essential in infants and perhaps in adult males.
†Can be synthesized from phenylalanine; therefore, this is considered nonessential as long as there is phenylalanine in the diet.

✳ TABLE 5-12   Metabolism

Nutrient	Anabolism	Catabolism	
Carbohydrates	Temporary excess changed into glycogen by liver cells in the presence of insulin; stored in the liver and skeletal muscles until needed and then changed back to glucose; true excess beyond the body's energy requirements is converted into adipose tissue and stored in various fat depots of the body	Oxidized, in the presence of insulin, to yield energy (4.1 kcal per g) and wastes (carbon dioxide and water): $C_6H_{12}O_6 + 6\ O_2 \rightarrow$ Energy $+ 6\ CO_2 + 6\ H_2O$	
Fats	Built into the adipose tissue; stored in fat depots of the body	Fatty acids ↓ (beta-oxidation) Acetyl CoA ⇌ Ketones ↓ (tissues; citric acid cycle) Energy (9.3 kcal/g) + $CO_2 + H_2O$	Glycerol ↓ (glycolysis) Acetyl CoA
Proteins	Synthesized into tissue proteins, blood proteins, enzymes, hormones, and so on	Deaminated by liver, thereby forming ammonia (which is converted to urea) and keto acids (which are either oxidized or changed into glucose or fat)	

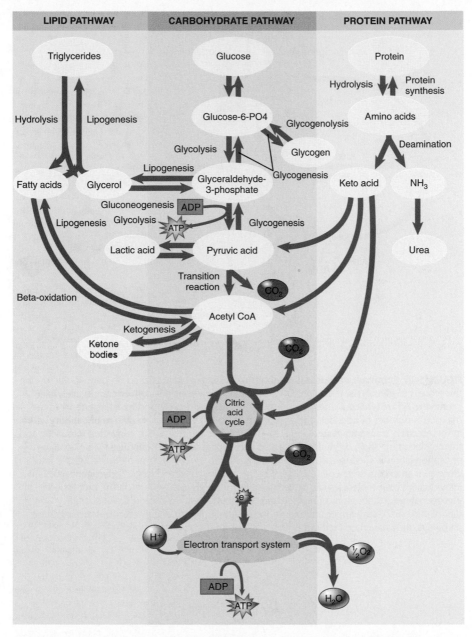

FIGURE 5-15 Summary of Metabolism. Notice the central role played by the **citric acid cycle** *(Krebs cycle)* and the **electron transport system.** Notice also how different nutrient molecules can be converted into forms that may enter other pathways.

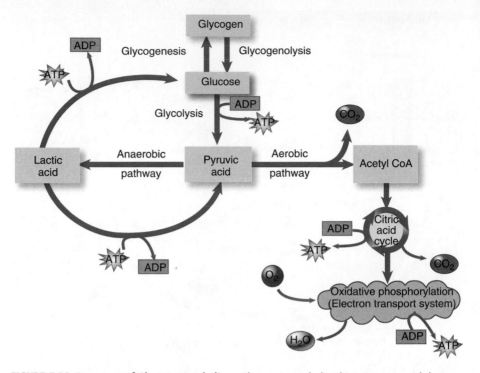

FIGURE 5-16 Summary of Glucose Metabolism. Glucose is catabolized into pyruvic acid during the process of **glycolysis.** If oxygen (O_2) is available, pyruvic acid is converted into acetyl **coenzyme A (acetyl-CoA)**, and it then enters the **citric acid cycle** and transfers energy to the maximum number of **adenosine triphosphate (ATP)** molecules via **oxidative phosphorylation** in the **electron transport system.** If O_2 is not available, pyruvic acid is converted into lactic acid, thereby incurring an **O_2 debt.** The O_2 debt is later repaid when ATP produced via oxidative phosphorylation is used to convert lactic acid back into pyruvic acid or all the way back into glucose. If an excess of glucose exists, the cell may convert it to glycogen (**glycogenesis**). Later, individual glucose molecules can be removed from the glycogen chain via the process of **glycogenolysis.** Although *nicotinamide adenine dinucleotide (NAD)* and *flavin adenine dinucleotide (FAD)* play important roles in the shuttling of high-energy electrons among these pathways, they have been left out of this diagram for the sake of simplicity.

✳ TABLE 5-13   Major Vitamins

Vitamin	Dietary Sources	Functions	Symptoms of Deficiency
Vitamin A	Green and yellow vegetables, dairy products, and liver	Maintains epithelial tissue and produces visual pigments	Night blindness and flaking skin
B-complex vitamins			
B₁ (thiamine)	Grains, meat, and legumes	Helps enzymes during the citric acid cycle	Nerve problems (beriberi), heart muscle weakness, and edema
B₂ (riboflavin)	Green vegetables, organ meats, eggs, and dairy products	Helps enzymes during the citric acid cycle	Inflammation of the skin and eyes
B₃ (niacin)	Meat and grains	Helps enzymes during the citric acid cycle	Pellagra (scaly dermatitis and mental disturbances) and nervous disorders
B₅ (pantothenic acid)	Organ meat, eggs, and liver	Helps enzymes that connect fat and carbohydrate metabolism	Loss of coordination (rare) and decreased gut motility
B₆ (pyridoxine)	Vegetables, meats, and grains	Helps enzymes that catabolize amino acids	Convulsions, irritability, and anemia
B₉ (folic acid)	Vegetables	Helps enzymes with amino acid catabolism and blood production	Digestive disorders and anemia
B₁₂ (cyanocobalamin)	Meat and dairy products	Involved in blood production and other processes	Pernicious anemia
Biotin (vitamin H)	Vegetables, meat, and eggs	Helps enzymes with amino acid catabolism and fat and glycogen synthesis	Mental and muscle problems (rare)
Vitamin C (ascorbic acid)	Fruits and green vegetables	Helps with the manufacture of collagen fibers; antioxidant	Scurvy and degeneration of skin, bone, and blood vessels
Vitamin D (calciferol)	Dairy products and fish liver oil	Helps with calcium absorption	Rickets and skeletal deformities
Vitamin E (tocopherol)	Green vegetables and seeds	Protects cell membranes from being destroyed; antioxidant	Muscle and reproductive disorders (rare)

✳ TABLE 5-14   Major Minerals

Mineral	Dietary Sources	Functions	Symptoms of Deficiency
Calcium (Ca)	Dairy products, legumes, and vegetables	Helps with blood clotting, bone formation, and nerve and muscle function	Bone degeneration and nerve and muscle malfunction
Chlorine (Cl)	Salty foods	Helps with stomach acid production and acid–base balance	Acid–base imbalance
Cobalt (Co)	Meat	Helps vitamin B_{12} with blood cell production	Pernicious anemia
Copper (Cu)	Seafood, organ meats, and legumes	Involved in the extraction of energy from the citric acid cycle and in blood production	Fatigue and anemia
Iodine (I)	Seafood and iodized salt	Required for thyroid hormone synthesis	Goiter (thyroid enlargement) and decrease in metabolic rate
Iron (Fe)	Meat, eggs, vegetables, and legumes	Involved in the extraction of energy from the citric acid cycle and in blood production	Fatigue and anemia
Magnesium (Mg)	Vegetables and grains	Helps many enzymes	Nerve disorders, blood vessel dilation, and heart rhythm problems
Manganese (Mn)	Vegetables, legumes, and grains	Helps many enzymes	Muscle and nerve disorders
Phosphorus (P)	Dairy products and meat	Helps with bone formation and used to make ATP, DNA, RNA, and phospholipids	Bone degeneration and metabolic problems
Potassium (K)	Seafood, milk, fruit, and meats	Helps with muscle and nerve function	Muscle weakness, heart problems, and nerve problems
Selenium (Se)	Nuts, grains, meat, fish, mushrooms, and eggs	Needed to make some amino acids and serves as a cofactor for certain enzymes	Heart muscle damage, cartilage degeneration, and hypothyroidism
Sodium (Na)	Salty foods	Helps with muscle and nerve function and fluid balance	Weakness and digestive upset
Zinc (Zn)	Many foods	Helps many enzymes	Inadequate growth

D. Urinary System and Balance of pH, Fluids, and Electrolytes

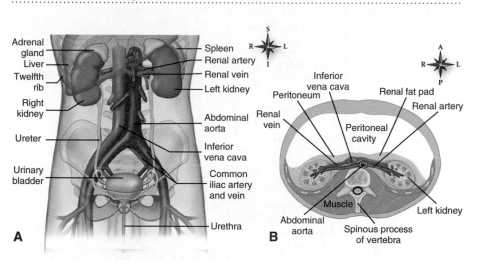

FIGURE 5-17 Location of Urinary System Organs.
A, Anterior view of the urinary organs, with the peritoneum and the visceral organs removed.
B, Horizontal (transverse) section of the abdomen showing the retroperitoneal position of the kidneys.

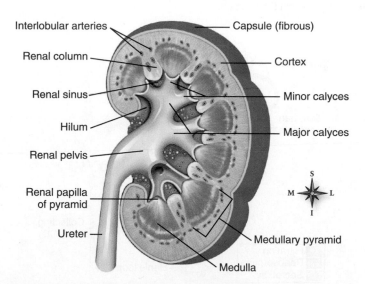

FIGURE 5-18 Gross Structure of the Kidney. A coronal section of a kidney showing the structures of the inner **renal medulla** and the outer **renal cortex.**

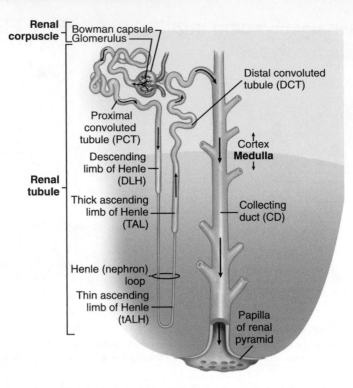

FIGURE 5-19 Nephron. The nephron is the basic functional unit of the kidney. The arrows show the direction of flow within the nephron.

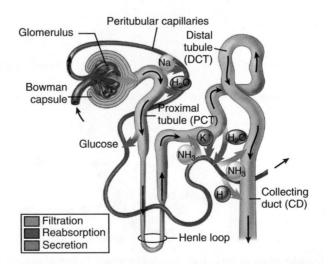

FIGURE 5-20 Mechanism of Urine Formation. This diagram shows the primary mechanisms of urine formation—**filtration, reabsorption,** and **secretion**—and where they occur in the nephron (see Figure 5-19).

Cleaning Your Drawers

Kidney function—especially the processes that occur within the nephrons—is often troublesome for beginning students. It needn't be, because the basic concepts are fairly simple and straightforward when you know the overall plan. However, that's the tricky part. If you just dive right into this area of study without considering the overall plan, then it doesn't seem to add up.

One way to think about the kidney's function is that it balances or cleans up the blood that passes through it. Each nephron has the job of doing its small share of the cleanup duties. The three basic methods that the nephron uses to do its job are **filtration**, **reabsorption**, and **secretion**. These are outlined in Figure 5-20. However, the figure makes it looks like things are coming into and out of the blood and doesn't show anything being cleaned or balanced.

Here's an analogy that may help: You are going to clean out your junk drawer. (You must be really bored, or maybe you are really trying to avoid studying.) You realize that your drawer contains a lot of junk and not much that is very useful. Besides, it's so packed that you probably won't be able to close it up again.

You decide that the best method for attacking this project would be to just dump the entire contents of the drawer out onto a clear spot on the floor. Now you can see all of the stuff that was in the drawer, all spread out. This is like *filtration*. When the bloodstream first hits the nephron at the glomerulus, a huge amount of fluid and solutes (around 50 gallons a day!) moves into the Bowman capsule. Obviously, you don't want to get rid of all of it, so you dump everything into the nephron so that the nephron can decide what to keep (put back into the blood) and what not to keep (release as urine).

The next step is to pick up those things that you want to keep and put them back into your junk drawer. This is like *reabsorption*. The cells in the wall of the nephron are constructed in a way that promotes the movement of most of the water, sodium, chloride, and glucose (and a few other needed molecules) back into the blood. Recall that the bloodstream has returned again to the nephron (in the peritubular blood supply) before leaving the kidney.

Before you're done cleaning your junk drawer, you decide that some last-minute adjustments are needed. You probably should get rid of those licorice candies that are stuck to the side of the drawer and that old chocolate, too. You pull those off of the inside of the drawer, one by one, and then put them into your trash pile on the floor. This is like *secretion*, the process by which the nephron cells push molecules from the peritubular blood into the lumen of the nephron, where they'll be lost with the urine.

The final step, of course, is taking the trash out of your home. This is like moving the fluid in the nephron into the emptying system of the kidney: the calyces, the renal pelvis, the ureter, the bladder, the urethra, and then out. After it leaves the microscopic kidney tubules, the fluid, which is now entirely waste, is called *urine*.

Continued

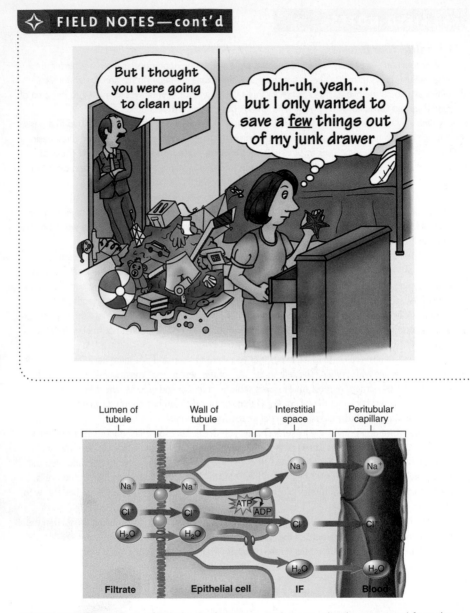

FIGURE 5-21 Mechanisms of Tubular Reabsorption. Sodium ions (Na⁺) are pumped from the tubule cell to the interstitial fluid (IF), thereby increasing the interstitial Na⁺ concentration to a level that drives the diffusion of Na⁺ into the blood. As Na⁺ is pumped out of the cell, more Na⁺ passively diffuses in from the filtrate to maintain an equilibrium of concentration. Enough Na⁺ moves out of the tubule and into the blood that an electrical gradient is established (i.e., blood is positive relative to the filtrate). Electrical attraction between oppositely charged particles drives the diffusion of negative ions in the filtrate, such as chloride (Cl⁻), into the blood. As the ion concentration of the blood increases, osmosis of water from the tubule occurs. Thus, the active transport of sodium creates a situation that promotes the passive transport of negative ions and water. Such a mechanism is often called *secondary active transport*.

✳ TABLE 5-15   Summary of Nephron Function

Part of Nephron	Function	Substance Moved
Renal corpuscle	Filtration (passive)	Water Smaller solute particles (e.g., ions, glucose)
Proximal convoluted tubule (PCT)	Reabsorption (active)	Active transport: Na^+ Cotransport: glucose and amino acids
	Reabsorption (passive)	Diffusion: Cl^-, $PO_4^{\equiv}$, urea, and other solutes Osmosis: water
Henle loop		
Descending limb (DLH) and thin ascending limb (tALH)	Reabsorption (passive)	Osmosis: water
	Secretion (passive)	Diffusion: urea
Thick ascending limb (TALH)	Reabsorption (active)	Active transport: Na^+
	Reabsorption (passive)	Diffusion: Cl^-
Distal convoluted tubule (DCT)	Reabsorption (active)	Active transport: Na^+
	Reabsorption (passive)	Diffusion: Cl^- and other anions Osmosis: water (only in the presence of antidiuretic hormone)
	Secretion (passive)	Diffusion: ammonia
	Secretion (active)	Active transport: K^+, H^+, and some drugs
Collecting duct (CD)	Reabsorption (active)	Active transport: Na^+
	Reabsorption (passive)	Diffusion: urea Osmosis: water (only in the presence of antidiuretic hormone)
	Secretion (passive)	Diffusion: ammonia
	Secretion (active)	Active transport: K^+, H^+, and some drugs

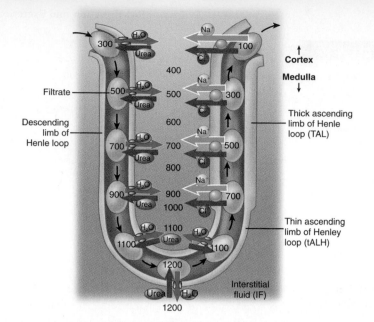

FIGURE 5-22 Countercurrent Multiplier System in the Henle Loop. Na^+ and Cl^- are pumped from the ascending limb and moved into the interstitial fluid (IF) to maintain high osmolality there. Because the salt content of the medullary IF increases, this is called a *multiplier mechanism*. Ion pumping also lowers the tubule fluid's osmolality by 200 mOsm, so fluid leaving the Henle loop is only 100 mOsm (hypotonic); it was 300 mOsm (isotonic) when it entered the loop. Values in this diagram are expressed in milliosmoles (mOsm).

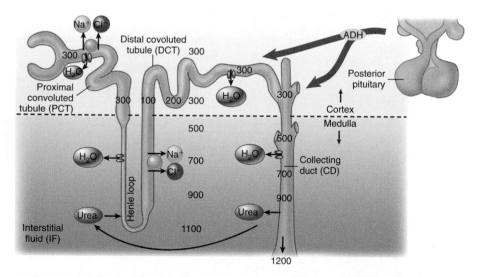

FIGURE 5-23 Production of Hypertonic Urine. Hypertonic urine can be formed when **antidiuretic hormone (ADH)** is present. ADH, which is a posterior pituitary hormone, increases the water permeability of the distal tubule and the collecting duct. Thus, hypotonic (100 mOsm) tubule fluid leaving the Henle loop can equilibrate first with the isotonic (300 mOsm) interstitial fluid (IF) of the cortex and then with the increasingly hypertonic (400 to 1200 mOsm) IF of the medulla. As H_2O leaves the collecting duct by osmosis, the filtrate becomes more concentrated with the solutes that are left behind. The concentration gradient causes urea to diffuse into the IF, where some of it is eventually picked up by tubule fluid in the descending limb of the Henle loop *(long arrow)*. This countercurrent movement of urea helps to maintain a high solute concentration in the medulla. Values in this diagram are expressed in milliosmoles.

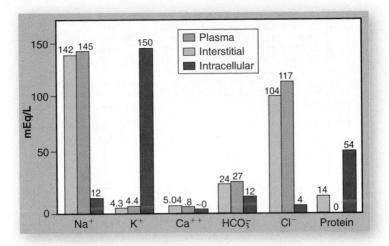

FIGURE 5-24 Electrolyte and Protein Concentrations in Body Fluid Compartments. This graph compares the individual electrolyte and anionic (negatively charged) protein concentrations of the three fluid compartments.

✱ **TABLE 5-16**   Volumes of Body Fluid Compartments*

Body Fluid	Infant	Adult Male	Adult Female
Extracellular Fluid			
Plasma	4%	4%	4%
Interstitial fluid	26%	16%	11%
Intracellular fluid	45%	40%	35%
Total	75%	60%	50%

*Percentage of body weight.

✱ **TABLE 5-17**   pH Control Systems

Type	Response Time	Example
Chemical buffer systems	Immediate	Bicarbonate buffer system Phosphate buffer system Protein buffer system
Physiological buffer systems	Minutes Hours	Respiratory response system Renal response system

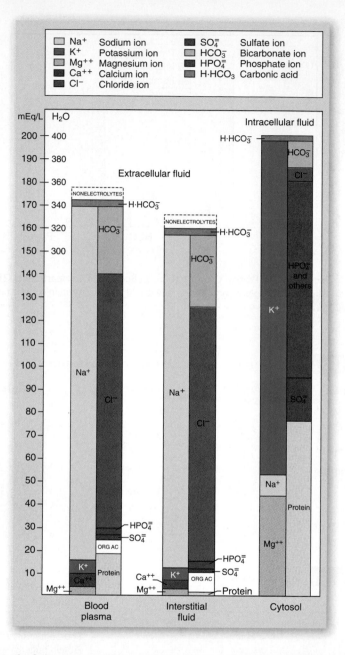

FIGURE 5-25 Chief Chemical Constituents of Three Fluid Compartments. The left component of each bar in the graph shows the amounts of **cation** (positive ion) or **anion** (negative ion), whereas the right component of each bar shows the combined sum of all of the cations and anions.

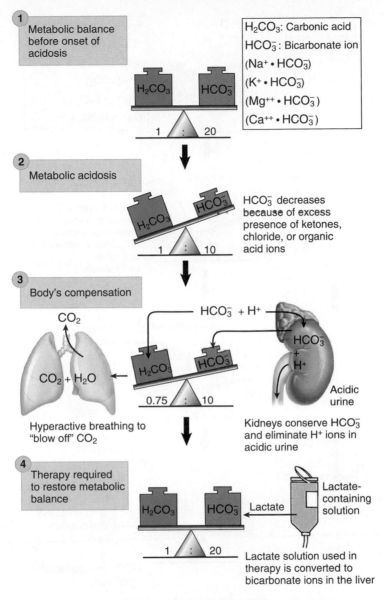

1 Metabolic balance before onset of acidosis

H_2CO_3: Carbonic acid
HCO_3^-: Bicarbonate ion
$(Na^+ \cdot HCO_3^-)$
$(K^+ \cdot HCO_3^-)$
$(Mg^{++} \cdot HCO_3^-)$
$(Ca^{++} \cdot HCO_3^-)$

H_2CO_3 HCO_3^-

1 : 20

2 Metabolic acidosis

HCO_3^- H_2CO_3

1 : 10

HCO_3^- decreases because of excess presence of ketones, chloride, or organic acid ions

3 Body's compensation

CO_2

$HCO_3^- + H^+$

$CO_2 + H_2O$

H_2CO_3 HCO_3^-

0.75 : 10

HCO_3^- + H^+

Acidic urine

Hyperactive breathing to "blow off" CO_2

Kidneys conserve HCO_3^- and eliminate H^+ ions in acidic urine

4 Therapy required to restore metabolic balance

H_2CO_3 HCO_3^-

Lactate

Lactate-containing solution

1 : 20

Lactate solution used in therapy is converted to bicarbonate ions in the liver

FIGURE 5-26 Metabolic Acidosis.

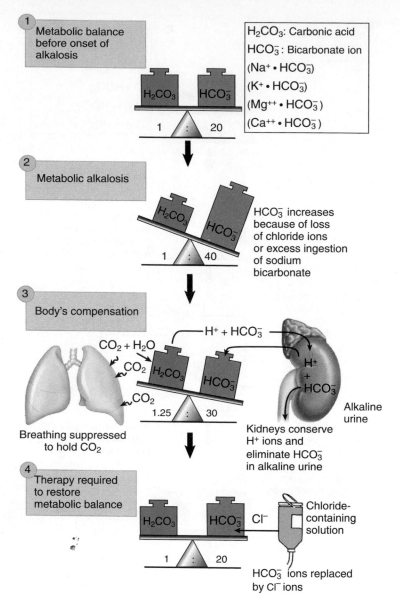

FIGURE 5-27 Metabolic Alkalosis.

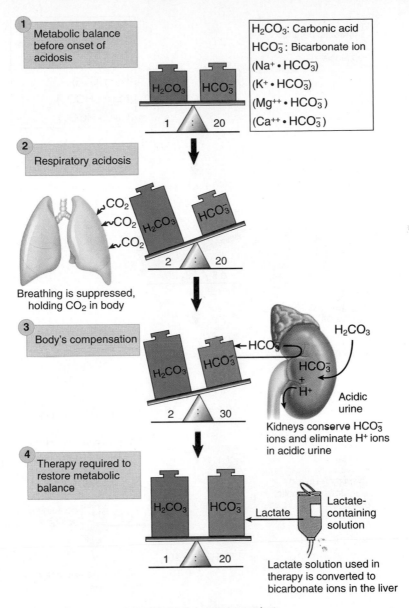

FIGURE 5-28 Respiratory Acidosis.

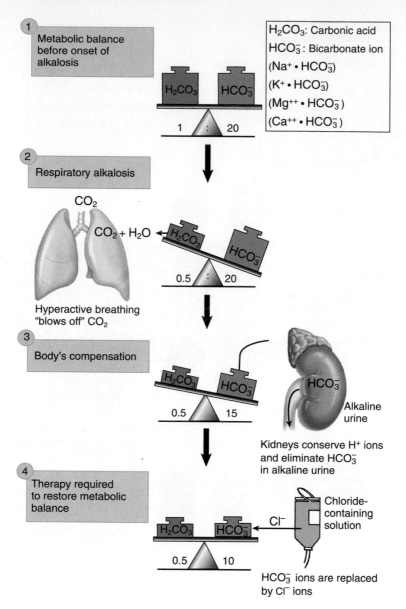

1. Metabolic balance before onset of alkalosis

H_2CO_3: Carbonic acid
HCO_3^-: Bicarbonate ion
$(Na^+ \cdot HCO_3^-)$
$(K^+ \cdot HCO_3^-)$
$(Mg^{++} \cdot HCO_3^-)$
$(Ca^{++} \cdot HCO_3^-)$

H_2CO_3 HCO_3^-

1 : 20

2. Respiratory alkalosis

CO_2
$CO_2 + H_2O$ ← H_2CO_3 HCO_3^-

0.5 : 20

Hyperactive breathing "blows off" CO_2

3. Body's compensation

H_2CO_3 HCO_3^- HCO_3^-

0.5   15

Alkaline urine

Kidneys conserve H^+ ions and eliminate HCO_3^- in alkaline urine

4. Therapy required to restore metabolic balance

Cl^- Chloride-containing solution

H_2CO_3 HCO_3^-

0.5   10

HCO_3^- ions are replaced by Cl^- ions

FIGURE 5-29 Respiratory Alkalosis.

6

Reproduction and Development

Navigation Guide

A. Reproductive Systems

✦ FIELD NOTES

Nudity

Before we move further through the reproductive system, I should tell you something about nudity. You have to look at naked bodies—fully naked breasts and genitals—to study human anatomy. Even more importantly, most A&P students will move along into professions that require them to look at naked bodies—this means breasts and genitals, too. You simply can't completely and practically know the body or treat the body without such exposure.

Continued

✦ FIELD NOTES—cont'd

The problem with this is that our culture often tells us that looking at nakedness—especially the external reproductive organs and the breasts—is not nice and perhaps even wrong. We can't avoid feeling this way simply by changing our minds; this idea is ingrained in our culture, which is a very powerful force that affects the development of our attitudes and beliefs. Because of this, nudity can also be very distracting.

It's good to be aware of this cultural view as you begin your study of the reproductive system. You're going to have to look at genitals and breasts (or at least at pictures of them). It's also good to be aware of this as you prepare for a profession in which you'll probably see far more breasts and genitals than you may realize. Keep in mind that we all experience this built-in attitude (some more than others, of course); however, we learn through time and experience to put it aside. Fortunately, cultural beliefs that involve nakedness generally don't apply to anatomy classes or healing professions. However, nudity does take some getting used to for most people.

It's also good to be aware of this attitude when we do eventually deal with clients and colleagues so that we can be sensitive to their possible attitudes and beliefs.

The same goes for terminology, too. If you can't say "penis" or "vagina" without giggling, then you had better find some way to overcome that before your A&P lab class and certainly before your first clinical assignment. In addition, when you do get comfortable with the terms, you should cultivate sensitivity for the times when you are dealing with others who haven't reached the same comfort level.

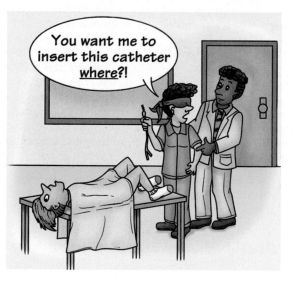

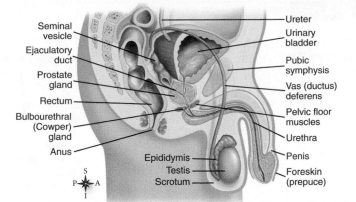

FIGURE 6-1 Male Reproductive Organs. Sagittal section of the pelvis showing the placement of the male reproductive organs.

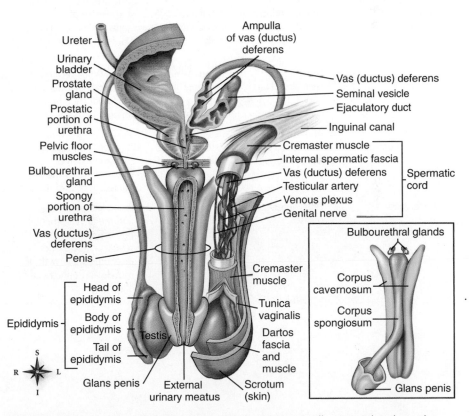

FIGURE 6-2 Anterior View of the Male Reproductive System. An illustration that shows the **testes**, the **epididymis**, the **ductus deferens**, and the glands of the male reproductive system in an isolation/dissection format.

✳ TABLE 6-1   Male Reproductive Hormones

Hormone	Source	Target	Action
Dehydroepiandrosterone (DHEA)	Adrenal gland, testis, other tissues	Converted into other hormones	Eventually converted into estrogens, testosterone, or both
Estrogen	Testis (interstitial cells), liver, other tissues	Testis (spermatogenic tissue), other tissues	Role of estrogen in men is still uncertain; may play a role in spermatogenesis, the inhibition of gonadotropins, male sexual behavior, and partner preference
Follicle-stimulating hormone (FSH)	Anterior pituitary (gonadotroph cells)	Testis (spermatogenic tissue)	Gonadotropin; promotes the development of the testes and stimulates spermatogenesis
Gonadotropin-releasing hormone (GnRH)	Hypothalamus (neuroendocrine cells)	Anterior pituitary (gonadotroph cells)	Stimulates the production and release of gonadotropins (FSH and LH) from the anterior pituitary
Inhibin	Testis (sustentacular cells)	Hypothalamus, anterior pituitary (gonadotroph cells)	Inhibits GnRH secretion by the hypothalamus and FSH production in the anterior pituitary
Luteinizing hormone (LH)	Anterior pituitary (gonadotroph cells)	Testis (interstitial cells)	Gonadotropin; stimulates the production of testosterone by the interstitial cells of the testis
Testosterone	Testis (interstitial cells)	Spermatogenic cells, skeletal muscle, bone, other tissues	Stimulates spermatogenesis and the development of primary and secondary sexual characteristics; promotes the growth of muscle and bone (anabolic effect)

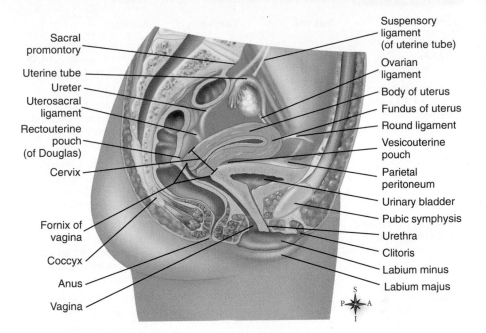

FIGURE 6-3 Female Reproductive Organs. Sagittal section of the pelvis showing the location of the female reproductive organs.

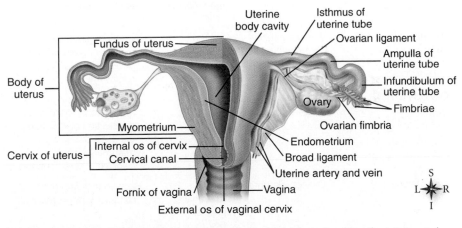

FIGURE 6-4 Female Pelvic Organs. An illustration of a partial frontal section; the interior and exterior features of the female reproductive organs of the pelvis are visible.

Hormone	Source	Target	Action
Dehydroepiandrosterone (DHEA)	Adrenal gland, ovary, other tissues	Converted into other hormones	Eventually converted into estrogens, testosterone, or both
Estrogens (including estradiol [E_2] and estrone)	Ovaries, placenta; small amounts in other tissues	Uterus, breast, other tissues	Stimulates the development of female sexual characteristics and breasts; bone and nervous system maintenance
Follicle-stimulating hormone (FSH)	Anterior pituitary (gonadotroph cells)	Ovaries	Gonadotropin; promotes the development of ovarian follicles; stimulates estrogen secretion
Gonadotropin-releasing hormone (GnRH)	Hypothalamus (neuroendocrine cells)	Anterior pituitary (gonadotroph cells)	Stimulates the production and release of gonadotropins (FSH and LH) from the anterior pituitary
Human chorionic gonadotropin (hCG)	Placenta	Ovaries	Stimulates the secretion of estrogen and progesterone during pregnancy
Inhibin	Ovaries	Hypothalamus, anterior pituitary (gonadotroph cells)	Inhibits GnRH production in the hypothalamus and FSH production in the anterior pituitary
Luteinizing hormone (LH)	Anterior pituitary (gonadotroph cells)	Ovaries	Gonadotropin; triggers ovulation; promotes the development of the corpus luteum
Oxytocin (OT)	Posterior pituitary	Uterus, mammary glands	Stimulates uterine contractions; stimulates the ejection of milk into the ducts of the mammary glands; involved in social bonding
Progesterone	Ovaries, placenta	Uterus, mammary glands, other tissues	Helps to maintain proper conditions for pregnancy
Prolactin (PRL) (lactogenic hormone)	Anterior pituitary (lactotroph cells)	Mammary glands (alveolar secretory cells)	Promotes milk secretion
Relaxin	Placenta	Uterus, joints	Inhibits uterine contractions during pregnancy; softens pelvic joints to facilitate childbirth
Testosterone	Adrenal glands, ovaries	Nervous tissue, bone tissue, other tissues	May affect mood, sex drive, learning, sleep, protein anabolism, and other functions

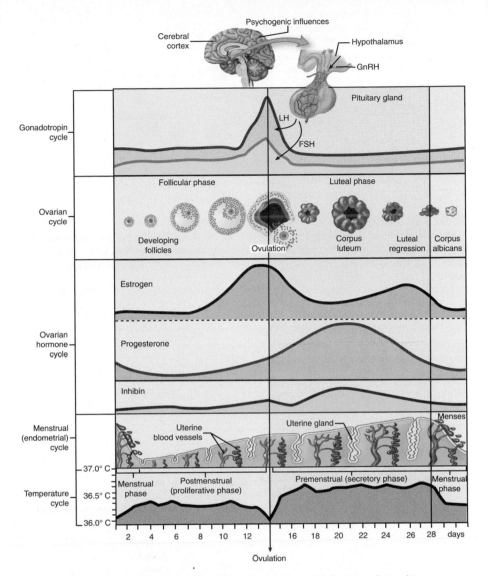

FIGURE 6-5 Female Reproductive Cycles. This diagram illustrates the interrelationships among the cerebral, hypothalamic, pituitary, ovarian, and uterine functions throughout a standard 28-day menstrual cycle. The variations in basal body temperature are also illustrated.

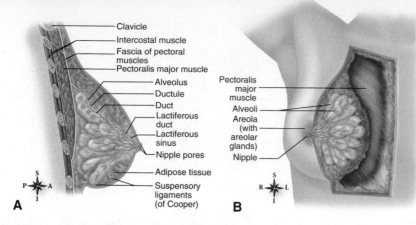

FIGURE 6-6 The Female Breast.
A, Sagittal section of a lactating breast. Notice how the glandular structures are anchored to the overlying skin and to the **pectoral muscles** by the **suspensory ligaments** (*of Cooper*). Each **lobule** of glandular tissue is drained by a **lactiferous duct** that eventually opens through the **nipple**.
B, Anterior view of a lactating breast. The overlying skin and connective tissue have been removed from the medial side to show the internal structure of the breast and the underlying skeletal muscle. In nonlactating breasts, the glandular tissue is much less prominent, with adipose tissue comprising most of each breast.

✳ TABLE 6-3   Hormones That Support Milk Production

Category	Role in Lactation	Hormones*
Mammogenic hormones	Promote tissue growth and development	↑ Estrogens ↑ Growth hormone (GH) ↑ Insulin-like growth factor (IGF-1) ↑ Insulin ↑ Cortisol ↑ Prolactin (PRL) ↑ Relaxin ↑ Epidermal growth factor (EGF)
Lactogenic hormones	Initiate milk production by secretory cells of alveolus	↑ Prolactin (PRL) ↑ Placental lactogen (hPL) ↑ Cortisol ↑ Insulin ↑ Insulin-like growth factor (IGF-1) ↑ Thyroid hormones (T$_3$, T$_4$) ↑ Growth hormone (GH) ↓ Estrogens ↓ Progesterone
Galactokinetic hormones	Promote milk ejection by stimulating myoepithelial cells that surround alveoli	↑ Oxytocin (OT) ↑ Antidiuretic hormone (ADH)/ vasopressin (AVP)
Galactopoietic hormones	Maintain milk production (after it has already started)	↑ Prolactin (PRL) ↑ Cortisol ↑ Insulin ↑ Insulin-like growth factor (IGF-1) ↑ Thyroid hormones (T$_3$, T$_4$)

*↑ = increase in hormone produces effect; ↓ = decrease in hormone produces effect.

B. Development

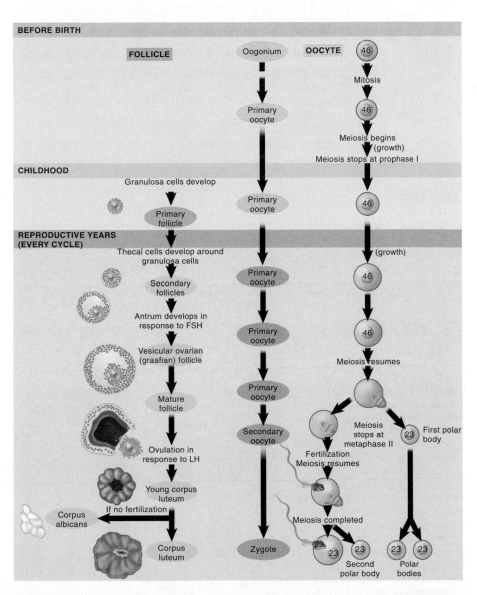

FIGURE 6-7 Oogenesis. The production of a mature **ovum** *(oocyte)* and subsequent **fertilization** are shown on the right as a series of cell divisions and on the left as a series of changes in the **ovarian follicle**.

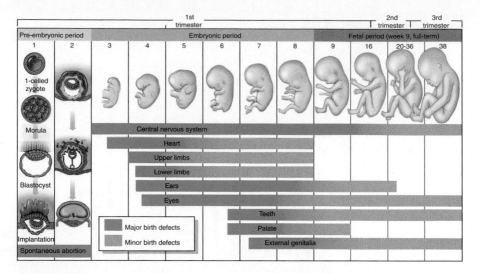

FIGURE 6-8 Critical Periods of Neonatal Development. The red areas show when teratogens are most likely to cause major birth defects, and the yellow areas show when minor defects are more likely to arise.

C. Genetics

FIGURE 6-9 Punnett Square. The Punnett square, which was named for geneticist Reginald Punnett, is a grid that is used to determine the relative probabilities of producing offspring with specific gene combinations. Phenylketonuria (PKU) is a recessive disorder that is caused by the gene *p*; *P* is the normal gene.
A, Possible results of cross between two PKU carriers. Because one in four of the offspring represented in the grid have PKU, a genetic counselor would predict that there is a 25% chance that this couple will produce a baby with PKU at each birth.
B, A cross between a PKU carrier and a normal noncarrier.
C, A cross between an individual with PKU and a PKU carrier.
D, A cross between an individual with PKU and a normal noncarrier.

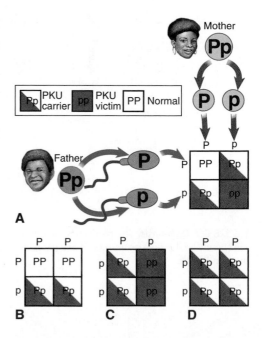

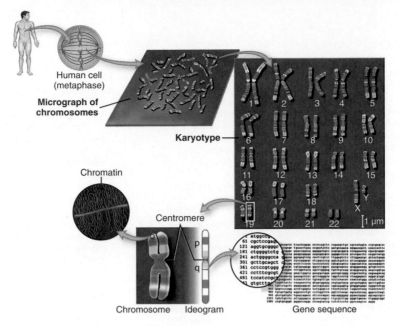

FIGURE 6-10 Human Genome. A cell that is taken from the body is stained and photographed. A photograph of **nuclear chromosomes** is then cut and pasted to arrange each of the 46 chromosomes into numbered pairs of decreasing size to form a chart called a **karyotype.** Each chromosome is a coiled mass of chromatin (mostly deoxyribonucleic acid [DNA]). In this figure, differentially stained bands in each chromosome appear as different, bright colors. Such bands are useful as reference points when identifying the locations of specific genes within a chromosome. The staining bands are also represented on an **ideogram** (a simple graph) of the chromosome as reference points to locate specific genes. The genes themselves are usually represented as the actual sequence of **nucleotide bases,** which are abbreviated as a, c, g, and t. In this figure, the sequence of one **exon** *(segment)* of a gene called *GPI* from chromosome 19 is shown. Each of these representations can be thought of as a type of genetic map.

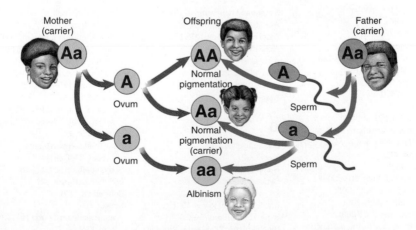

FIGURE 6-11 Inheritance of a Recessive Trait. Albinism is a recessive trait that produces abnormalities only in those individuals with two **recessive genes** *(a).* The presence of the **dominant gene** *(A)* prevents albinism.

Index

Page numbers followed by "f" indicate figures, "t" indicate tables, and "b" indicate boxes.

Common Word Parts

✳ TABLE 1 Word Parts Commonly Used as Prefixes

Word Part	Meaning	Word Part	Meaning
a-	without, not	inter-	between
a[d]-	toward	intra-	within
all[o]-	[an]other, different	iso-	same, equal
an-	without, not	macro-	large
ante-	before	mega-	large, million(th)
anti-	against, resisting	mes-	middle
auto-	self	meta-	beyond, after
bi-	two, double	micro-	small, millionth
circum-	around	milli-	thousandth
co-, con-	with, together	mono-	one (single)
contra-	against	neo-	new
de-	down from, undoing	non-	not
dia-	across, through	oligo-	few, scanty
dipl-	twofold, double	ortho-	straight, correct, normal
dys-	bad, disordered, difficult	para-	by the side of, near
ectop-	displaced	per-	through
ef-	away from	peri-	around, surrounding
em-, en-	in, into	poly-	many
endo-	within	post-	after
epi-	upon	pre-	before
eu-	good	pro-	first, promoting
ex-, exo-	out of, out from	quadr-	four
extra-	outside of	re-	back again
hapl-	single	retro-	behind
hem-, hemat-	blood	semi-	half
hemi-	half	sub-	under
hom(e)o-	same, equal	super-, supra-	over, above, excessive
hyper-	over, above	trans-	across, through
hypo-	under, below	tri-	three, triple
infra-	below, beneath		

✳ TABLE 2 Word Parts Commonly Used as Suffixes

Word Part	Meaning	Word Part	Meaning
-al, -ac	pertaining to	-malacia	softening
-algia	pain	-megaly	enlargement
-aps, -apt	fit, fasten	-metric, -metry	measurement, length
-arche	beginning, origin	-oid	like, in the shape of
-ase	signifies an enzyme	-oma	tumor
-blast	sprout, make	-opia	vision, vision condition
-centesis	a piercing	-oscopy	viewing
-cide	to kill	-ose	signifies a carbohydrate (especially sugar)
-clast	break, destroy		
-crine	release, secrete	-osis	condition, process
-ectomy	a cutting out	-ostomy	formation of an opening
-emesis	vomiting	-otomy	cut
-emia	refers to blood condition	-penia	lack
-flux	flow	-philic	loving
-gen	creates, forms	-phobic	fearing
-genesis	creation, production	-phragm	partition
-gram*	something written	-plasia	growth, formation
-graph(y)*	to write, to draw	-plasm	substance, matter
-hydrate	containing H₂O (water)	-plasty	shape, make
-ia, -sia	condition, process	-plegia	paralysis
-iasis	abnormal condition	-pnea	breath, breathing
-ic, -ac	pertaining to	-(r)rhage, -(r)rhagia	breaking out, discharge
-in	signifies a protein	-(r)rhaphy	sew, suture
-ism	signifies "condition of"	-(r)rhea	flow
-itis	signifies "inflammation of"	-some	body
-lemma	rind, peel	-tensin, -tension	pressure
-lepsy	seizure	-tonic	relating to pressure, tension
-lith	stone, rock		
-logy	study of	-tripsy	crushing
-lunar	moon, moon-like	-ule	small, little
		-uria	refers to urine condition

*A term that ends in -graph refers to an apparatus that results in a visual or recorded representation of biological phenomena, whereas a term that ends in -graphy refers to the technique or process of using the apparatus. A term that ends in -gram is the record itself. For example, in electrocardiography, an electrocardiograph is used to produce an electrocardiogram.

✳ TABLE 3 Word Parts Commonly Used as Roots

Word Part	Meaning	Word Part	Meaning
acro-	extremity	chem-	chemical
aden-	gland	chol-	bile
alveol-	small hollow, cavity	chondr-	cartilage
angi-	vessel	chrom-	color
arthr-	joint	corp-	body
asthen-	weakness	cortico-	pertaining to cortex
bar-	pressure	crani-	skull
bili-	bile	crypt-	hidden
brachi-	arm	cusp-	point
brady-	slow	cut(an)-	skin
bronch-	air passage	cyan-	blue
calc-	calcium, limestone	cyst-	bladder
capn-	smoke	cyt-	cell
carcin-	cancer	dactyl-	fingers, toes (digits)
card-	heart	dendr-	tree, branched
cephal-	head, brain	dent-	tooth
cerv-	neck	derm-	skin

Continued

✳ **TABLE 3**   Word Parts Commonly Used as Roots—cont'd

Word Part	Meaning	Word Part	Meaning
diastol-	relax, stand apart	osteo-	bone
dips-	thirst	oto-	ear
ejacul-	to throw out	ov-, oo-	egg
electr-	electrical	oxy-	oxygen
enter-	intestine	path-	disease
eryth(r)-	red	ped-	children
esthe-	sensation	phag-	eat
febr-	fever	pharm-	drug
gastr-	stomach	phleb-	vein
gest-	to bear, carry	photo-	light
gingiv-	gums	physio-	nature (function) of
glomer-	wound into a ball	pino-	drink
gloss-	tongue	plex-	twisted, woven
gluc-	glucose, sugar	pneumo-	air, breath
glutin-	glue	pneumon-	lung
glyc-	sugar (carbohydrate), glucose	pod-	foot
		poie-	make, produce
hepat-	liver	pol-	axis, having poles
hist-	tissue	presby-	old
hydro-	water	proct-	rectum
hyster-	uterus	pseud-	false
iatr-	treatment	psych-	mind
kal-	potassium	pyel-	pelvis
kary-	nucleus	pyo-	pus
kerat-	cornea	pyro-	heat, fever
kin-	to move, divide	ren-	kidney
lact-	milk, milk production	rhino-	nose
lapar-	abdomen	rigor-	stiffness
leuk-	white	sarco-	flesh, muscle
lig-	to tie, bind	scler-	hard
lip-	lipid (fat)	semen-, semin-	seed, sperm
lys-	break apart	sept-	contamination
mal-	bad	sigm-	Σ or Roman S
melan-	black	sin-	cavity, recess
men-, mens-, (menstru-)	month (monthly)	son-	sound
metr-	uterus	spiro-, -spire	breathe
muta-	change	stat-, stas-	a standing, stopping
my-, myo-	muscle	syn-	together
myc-	fungus	systol-	contract, stand together
myel-	marrow		
myx-	mucus	tachy-	fast
nat-	birth	therm-	heat
natr-	sodium	thromb-	clot
nephr-	nephron, kidney	tom-	a cut, a slice
neur-	nerve	tox-	poison
noct-, nyct-	night	troph-	grow, nourish
ocul-	eye	tympan-	drum
odont-	tooth	varic-	enlarged vessel
onco-	cancer	vas-	vessel, duct
ophthalm-	eye	vesic-	bladder, blister
orchid-	testis	vol-	volume

Common Abbreviations

Abbreviation	Term
1,25-D3	1,25-dihydroxycholecalciferol
5-HT	serotonin
α-MSH	alpha melanocyte-stimulating hormone
Å	angstrom
AAA	American Association of Anatomists
ABP	androgen-binding protein
ACF	anterior cranial fossa
Ach	acetylcholine
ACL	anterior cruciate ligament
ACTH	adrenocorticotropic hormone
ADH	antidiuretic hormone
AFM	atomic force microscopy
AFP	alpha-fetoprotein
AHF	antihemophilic factor
AHG	antihemophilic globulin
AI	adequate intake
AIIS	anterior inferior iliac spine
ANH	atrial natriuretic hormone
ANP	atrial natriuretic peptide
ANS	autonomic nervous system
APC	antigen-presenting cell
APS	American Physiological Society
ASIS	anterior superior iliac spine
AV	atrioventricular
AVP	arginine vasopressin (antidiuretic hormone)
B	bursa-equivalent tissue (as in *B cell* or *B lymphocyte*)
BBB	blood–brain barrier
BCOP	blood colloid osmotic pressure
BEAM	brain electrical activity map
BHP	blood hydrostatic pressure
BM	basement membrane
BMD	bone mineral density

Abbreviation	Term
BMI	body mass index
BMR	basal metabolic rate
BP	blood pressure
BTB	blood–testis barrier
°C	degrees Celsius or centigrade
C	calcitonin-producing (cell)
C	Calorie or kilocalorie
C	cervical
C	complement (protein)
C or Cx	coccygeal
CA	carbonic anhydrase
cal	calorie
CART	cocaine- and amphetamine-regulated transcript
cc◆	cubic centimeter
CCK	cholecystokinin
CD	collecting duct
CDK	cyclin-dependent kinase
CD-X	cluster differentiation (blood cell marker system, where *X* is the cluster number)
CN	cranial nerve*
CNS	central nervous system
CO	cardiac output
CoA	coenzyme A
COMT	catechol-O-methyl transferase
COX	cyclooxygenase
CRH	corticotropin-releasing hormone
CT	calcitonin
CT	chromosome territory
CTFR	cystic fibrosis transmembrane conductance regulator
CTL	cytotoxic T lymphocyte
DA	dopamine
DC	dendritic cell

Continued

Abbreviation	Term
DCT	distal convoluted tubule
DEJ	dermoepidermal junction (dermal–epidermal junction)
DHEA	dehydroepiandrosterone
DIP	distal interphalangeal (joint)
dl or dL	deciliter
DNA	deoxyribonucleic acid
DRG	dorsal respiratory group
dsRNA	double-stranded ribonucleic acid
E_2	estradiol
ECF	extracellular fluid
ECM	extracellular matrix
EDV	end-diastolic volume
EF	ejection fraction
EFP	effective filtration pressure
EGF	epidermal growth factor
EM	electron microscopy
ENS	enteric nervous system
EOP	endogenous opioid peptide
Epi	epinephrine
EPOC	excess postexercise oxygen consumption
EPSP	excitatory postsynaptic potential
ER	endoplasmic reticulum
ERV	expiratory reserve volume
ET	endothelin
ET-1	endothelin-1
ETC	electron transport chain
ETS	electron transport system
°F	degrees Fahrenheit
FA-1	fertilization antigen 1
FASEB	Federation of American Societies for Experimental Biology
FEV_X	forced expiratory volume (where X is the number of seconds)
FCAT	Federative (International) Committee on Anatomical Terminology (see FICAT)
FICAT	Federative International Committee on Anatomical Terminology
FM	fluorescence microscopy
FRC	functional residual capacity
FSH	follicle-stimulating hormone
FVC	forced vital capacity
G0	nondividing phase of cell life cycle
G1	first growth (or gap) phase of cell division
G2	second growth (or gap) phase of cell division
GABA	gamma-aminobutyric acid (γ-aminobutyric acid)
GAL	galanin
GAS	general adaptation syndrome
GC	glucocorticoid
GFR	glomerular filtration rate
GH	growth hormone
GHIH	growth hormone-inhibiting hormone (somatostatin)
GHRH	growth hormone-releasing hormone
GHRL	ghrelin
GI	gastrointestinal
GIP	glucose-dependent insulinotropic peptide (gastric inhibitory peptide)
GLP-1	glucagon-like peptide 1
Glu	glutamic acid, glutamate
Gly	glycine

Abbreviation	Term
GnRH	gonadotropin-releasing hormone
GPCR	G-protein–coupled receptor
HAPS	Human Anatomy and Physiology Society
$HbCO_2$	carbaminohemoglobin
hCG	human chorionic gonadotropin
HDL	high-density lipoprotein
hGH	human growth hormone
HGH	human growth hormone
HGP	Human Genome Project
H-K pump	hydrogen–potassium pump
HLA	human leukocyte antigen
HPA axis	hypothalamus–pituitary–adrenal axis
hPL	human placental lactogen
HR	heart rate
Hz	Hertz (waves per second)
IC	inspiratory capacity
ICF	intracellular fluid
IF	interferon
IFAA	International Federation of Associations of Anatomists
IFCOP	interstitial fluid colloid osmotic pressure
IFHP	interstitial fluid hydrostatic pressure
IFN	interferon
IFN-α	interferon alpha (fibroblast interferon)
IFN-β	interferon beta (leukocyte interferon)
IFN-γ	interferon gamma (immune interferon)
IGF-1	insulin-like growth factor 1
IL	interleukin
IL-X	interleukin (where X is a numeral [type])
IMP	integral membrane protein
IPSP	inhibitory postsynaptic potential
IRV	inspiratory reserve volume
IS	immunological synapse
IU◆◆	international unit
JG	juxtaglomerular
°K	degrees Kelvin
L†	lumbar
LDL	low-density lipoprotein
LES	lower esophageal sphincter
LH	luteinizing hormone
LM	light microscopy
LP factor	leukocytosis-promoting factor
μm	micrometer; micron
M	mitotic phase of cell division
M	mole or molar concentration
M	muscarinic
MAC	membrane attack complex
MALT	mucosal-associated lymphoid tissue
MAO	monoamine oxidase
MC	mineralocorticoid
MCF	middle cranial fossa
mDNA	mitochondrial deoxyribonucleic acid
Mgb	myoglobin
MHC	major histocompatibility complex
MMC	migrating motor complex
mm Hg	millimeters of mercury (unit of pressure)
MP	metacarpophalangeal (joint)
mRNA	messenger ribonucleic acid
MSH	melanocyte-stimulating hormone
mtDNA	mitochondrial deoxyribonucleic acid
mV	millivolt